Expert Psychiatric Evidence

Keith J. B. Rix MPhil LLM MD FRCPsych

RCPsych Publications

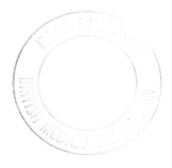

CAMBRIDGE
UNIVERSITY PRESS

University Printing House, Cambridge CB2 8BS, United Kingdom

One Liberty Plaza, 20th Floor, New York, NY 10006, USA

477 Williamstown Road, Port Melbourne, VIC 3207, Australia

314-321, 3rd Floor, Plot 3, Splendor Forum, Jasola District Centre, New Delhi - 110025, India

79 Anson Road, #06-04/06, Singapore 079906

Cambridge University Press is part of the University of Cambridge.

It furthers the University's mission by disseminating knowledge in the pursuit of education, learning and research at the highest international levels of excellence.

www.cambridge.org
Information on this title: www.cambridge.org/9781908020321

© The Royal College of Psychiatrists 2011

RCPsych Publications is an imprint of the Royal College of Psychiatrists, 17 Belgrave Square, London SW1X 8PG
http://www.rcpsych.ac.uk

First published 2011

A catalogue record for this publication is available from the British Library

ISBN 978-1-908-02032-1 Hardback

Distributed in North America by Publishers Storage and Shipping Company.

Dedicated to four generations of women in my life:

Phyllis Irene Rix,
My mother, who set me an example of hard work;

Elizabeth,
My soul-mate and ethical guide;

Virginia, Marianne and Rowena,
Who have made fatherhood so worthwhile;

And my granddaughter,
Lorna,
So full of potential

Contents

Appendices

Foreword

The Rt Hon. The Baroness Hale of Richmond,
Justice of the Supreme Court

Judges and juries need the help of experts of many kinds in order to understand matters which are not within their ordinary knowledge and experience. But they also need to know that the experts to whom they turn for help are reliable, not quacks, not hired guns, but independent professionals who understand that their principal duty is to the court and not to the person who is paying them. Nowhere is this more so than in psychiatry, which is 'not an exact science' (*R (B) v. Ashworth Hospital Authority* [2005] 2 AC 278, para 31), and unfortunately liable to be treated with even more suspicion by the non-expert than many other disciplines which regularly come before the courts.

The reliable expert is one who is not only on top of her subject, both in the books and on the ground, but also has a thorough understanding of the role and the issues which arise in the particular case in which she has been asked to advise. The reliable expert psychiatrist, therefore, is one who has read and absorbed this book. It is a mine of useful information. It is full of practical tips and do's and don'ts. It explains the difference between a witness of fact, a professional witness who has played a part in the relevant events, and an expert witness who provides an independent evaluation of the situation. It contains an extraordinarily comprehensive discussion of the many different legal contexts in which expert psychiatric evidence may become relevant. It is peppered with delightful anecdotes which show that it is the product of the real experiences of a real human being. There cannot be many psychiatrists who have appeared before an agricultural land tribunal but this one has.

In short, this book ought to increase the confidence of the court in the reliability of the expert evidence which it is hearing. But, just as important, it ought to increase the confidence of the psychiatrist who is setting out upon or developing a practice as an expert witness. We want and need psychiatrists to be prepared to do this important but challenging work. We hope that they will not be put off doing so by the recent decision of the Supreme Court, in *Jones v. Kaney* [2011] UKSC 13, that a paid expert witness can be liable in negligence to her client. There is little risk that a psychiatrist who follows the wise guidance in this book (including the need to keep continually up to date) will find herself in that unfortunate position.

Preface and acknowledgements

I prepared my first criminal report, for a defendant's solicitors, when I was an honorary senior registrar in about 1981. It was a salutary experience. The solicitors sent the report to their client. He was remanded in custody. Notwithstanding the confidentiality that attaches to communications between prisoners and their solicitors, the prison authorities read my report. They contacted my consultant to ask him if he thought that it was a good idea for the prisoner to read my opinion about him. Needless to say, in trying to uphold the ethical principle of doing justice, I had fallen foul of the principle of doing no harm.

It was the beginning of a steep learning curve. Since then I have had 30 more years of preparing expert psychiatric reports and giving evidence in various courts. I use the term 'court' for any court of law, tribunal or body concerned with the process of arbitration or dispute resolution or professional conduct committee or panel.

I have given evidence to an agricultural land tribunal. It was convened in the lounge bar of a Yorkshire Dales country hotel. The tribunal sat in a raised area, usually occupied by the band. The parties, the witnesses and experts sat at small tables but without the customary pint. We were surrounded by pictures of sheep-shearing and cattle markets, including *Sheep Shearing at Hawes*. I purchased this as a leaving present for a colleague who kept his own sheep.

I have given evidence in the panelled court rooms at the Royal Courts of Justice. There, enticingly for me, if no one else, the side walls are lined from floor to ceiling with bookshelves teeming with the law reports of the last two centuries. The most conspicuous signs of the 21st century are the laptop computers of the judges and counsel.

At the beginning I was fortunate to be trained by Dr Angus Campbell. I owe an enormous debt to many more psychiatrists, and lawyers, than I will go on to acknowledge by name. In the early 1980s, training as a psychiatric expert witness was very much on the apprenticeship model, if you were fortunate, as I was, to begin preparing reports as a trainee. If not, and as it was for me once I became a consultant, it was a case of learning on the job.

This meant learning from other experts and from lawyers, and learning from one's mistakes. I continue to make mistakes. For as long as I go on learning from them, I hope to continue as an expert witness.

My acquisition of experience has not been a smooth process.

I learned a lot and changed my practice a lot after going on a two-day course run by Bond Solon, a legal training consultancy based in London. The first day was on report writing and the second day on witness skills. So Chapters 4 ('The structure, organisation and content of the generic report') and 11 ('Going to court') particularly bear the Bond Solon stamp. The same two chapters are also particularly influenced by Babitsky *et al* (2000), *The Comprehensive Forensic Services Manual: The Essential Resources For All Experts*, albeit that it is written for an American audience, and Lord Justice Wall's *A Handbook for Expert Witnesses in Children Act Cases* (2007).

When I entered the final stage of my transition from general psychiatry to forensic psychiatry I was fortunate to join the dynamic and stimulating group of then young consultants and trainee forensic psychiatrists at the Yorkshire Regional Centre for Forensic Psychiatry (Newton Lodge). I still value its study days, to which I occasionally return.

At this time, I was responding to frequent requests from senior registrars for teaching and training. They stimulated me to publish many of my case reports and papers on medico-legal subjects. I also learned a lot from them. They confirmed the view I already had, that when you stop learning from your junior doctors it is time to stop being a consultant.

For the last few years, I have been attending courses on risk assessment run by Northern Networking Events Ltd in Edinburgh. These have influenced the way in which I carry out risk assessments and incorporate them into expert reports.

Over the last ten years the annual residential conference organised by my consulting rooms, The Grange, has provided rich fare in terms of teaching and training by other experts and by solicitors, judges, barristers and coroners. As this text took its final shape at the time of the last conference I can specifically acknowledge the influence of Mr Andrew Axon, Park Lane Plowden Chambers, Mr Bill Braithwaite QC, Exchange Chambers, Ms Bridget Dolan, 3 Serjeants' Inn, and Ms Diana Kloss MBE, St John's Buildings. I owe no lesser a debt to contributors to previous Grange conferences. If they recognise some of their pearls of wisdom, I hope that they will forgive me for not remembering their source sufficiently to acknowledge them by name. I am also indebted to those who have attended the conferences and shared knowledge, experience and ideas. In 2010 we spent a lot of time looking at how medico-legal reports can be part of the case-based discussions that are going to inform our annual appraisals and the General Medical Council's revalidation process.

This text was also nearing completion when I attended Professor Penny Cooper's inaugural lecture at the City Law School and this is reflected in what I have written about cross-examination.

The Grange itself, where psychiatrists and psychologists have consulting rooms for medico-legal work, established by Dr Peter Wood in 1998, and with its roots in the Bradford consulting rooms of the late Dr Hugo Milne, a pioneer of forensic psychiatry in Yorkshire, has been a means of achieving my continuing professional development. This is particularly through its regular educational meetings as well as the annual residential conference. Equally importantly, it has provided a support group, which is essential for psychiatrists in an area of practice where disgruntled, disappointed and sometimes vexatious litigants are only too ready to fire off complaints to the General Medical Council and are now able to sue experts.

Over the last few years I have had the opportunity to study the law, and the development of this text has also been influenced by my teachers and fellow students on the LLM in Medical Law and Ethics at De Montfort University, Leicester.

The purpose of this book is to provide assistance to trainee psychiatrists and relatively inexperienced consultants who are at, or near, the bottom of their learning curve. It is also intended to provide a resource to experts who are approaching the plateau of the learning curve. However, the law is constantly changing, as are the needs and expectations of society, so the psychiatric expert will probably never reach a plateau of expertise. I hope that parts of the book will also be of use to other medical experts and psychologists.

This book is heavily referenced to both statute and case law. They define the role of the psychiatric expert witness in a particular case. However, given the dynamic nature of the law, a book like this will never be up to date. It was meant to represent the law up to about November 2010 but I have made brief reference to the Family Procedure Rules, which came into effect on 6 April 2011, the Law Commission's report *Expert Evidence in Criminal Proceedings in England and Wales*, laid before Parliament on 21 March 2011, and the case of *Jones v Kaney* [2011] UKSC 13, which has the effect of removing expert witnesses' immunity from suit. Significant updates as to the law and other developments will be posted on my website (http://www.drkeithrix.co.uk).

I encourage readers to study carefully relevant law reports. When I was a boy, I thought that the law was 'black and white'. Of course it is not. There is no better way of trying to understand the law, in particular the interpretation of statutes and the precedents established in case law, than to study judicial thinking and reasoning, particularly those of the Appeal Court judges and the judges of the Supreme Court. Many law reports also tell a story, which I know psychiatrists find appealing, and some record, probably for posterity, the virtues, but also the failings, of expert psychiatric witnesses.

This book is intended for readership in the British Isles but the British Isles are made up of a number of legal 'jurisdictions'. There are substantial differences between the laws of these various jurisdictions. Scots law is now based on the Roman law that applied in the reign of the Emperor Justinian but in Orkney and Shetland Udal law, a remnant of Old Norse law, is still of limited application. The Viking influence also remains to this day in the Isle of Man, where the Viking term 'deemster' is used for the three permanent, full-time judges of the High Court. The inquisitorial legal systems of the Channel Islands have greater affinity with the legal systems of mainland Europe than with the adversarial systems of the rest of the British Isles.

It would have made the 'central' chapters of this book, by which I mean the chapters relating to reports for different forms of court proceedings and court cases, unnecessarily complicated, and their reading very difficult, if I had tried to weave together the laws of these various jurisdictions. It has not been an easy decision, but I have decided to build the central chapters mainly on the laws of England and Wales, but have added where appropriate 'good practice' points from other jurisdictions, and I have included a chapter in which I have set out some of the particular requirements or important features of the other jurisdictions within the British Isles (Chapter 10). Unless otherwise indicated, but not entirely so, the opening and closing 'generic' chapters should be applicable at least to a very large extent in all these jurisdictions.

It is customary in the preface to a book to deal with the issue of gender. This is particularly important for the psychiatrist who travels to what Professor Nigel Eastman terms 'Legalland'. This is where 'the reasonable man' lives, where one of the most influential figures is 'the man on the Clapham omnibus' and where, if you read only the statute law, you would be surprised that the population had not gone into extinction because all the inhabitants seem to be male. I have not followed the convention of using the male personal pronoun and asking readers to give it the meaning of male or female but have instead opted for the most part to use the plural personal pronoun.

As far as I am aware, the law does not recognise the term 'service user' and nor did it recognise the term 'client', which this term replaced, or perhaps there were some others in between which I have forgotten. 'Client', I thought, was particularly unfortunate, as it emphasises dependency, being derived from the Latin word for someone dependent on a patron, and it sits uncomfortably with the autonomy of today's patient. So, at the risk of being very old-fashioned, where appropriate I have used the term 'patient'. There are three reasons: (1) by the time this book is published, 'service user' will probably be obsolete; (2) judges continue to use the term 'patient'; and (3) the term 'patient' comes closest to the central role of the doctor, in that it derives from the Latin intransitive verb *'patior'*, which means simply 'I suffer'. It has the connotation of one who bears or endures suffering and, if doctors cannot cure, they should at least help their patients bear or endure suffering, and that includes the suffering of going to law or being on the receiving end of legal proceedings.

Also on the subject of terminology, although I have used the term 'intellectual disability' wherever possible, the meaning of some judgments would be misrepresented if I had not used the terminology of the statute or judgment where 'mental handicap' is the term used. In any event, even the *ICD-10 Classification of Mental and Behavioural Disorders* (World Health

Organization, 1992) uses the term 'mental retardation' and it is only a few years since the law ceased to use the term 'mental defective'.

I have referred to Daniel McNaughtan as the person. This is on the basis that 'McNaughtan' was the spelling of the family name. I have followed the legal convention of referring to 'the M'Naghten rules'. My specimen criminal report (Appendix 11) on Daniel McNaughtan relies heavily on West & Walk's *Daniel McNaughton: His Trial and the Aftermath* (1977). However, I have been unable to find an account of a mental state examination of Daniel McNaughtan, so I am particularly indebted to Siân Busby, the author of the novel *McNaughten* (2009), for providing me with an account of his mental state based on her study of the historical materials and elaborated with a novelist's appropriate literary licence.

Insofar as this book does not include model terms and conditions of engagement, it is incomplete. The reason for this is that mine have been drawn up and are updated by a firm of solicitors. The conditions of the licence under which I use them preclude me from publishing them. Appendix 1, which is a generic letter of response to a request for a report, does, though, cover some of the relevant points, and I am grateful to Mr James Wood of Schofield Sweeney, Solicitors, Bradford, for advice on its construction.

This book bears some similarity to one that I started to plan many years ago with Dr Rajan (Taj) Nathan. I am pleased to acknowledge my valuable discussions with him at the time. It also includes material on the reliability of admissions in police interviews which I prepared with Dr John Kent and Dr Mike Ventress and which we intended to publish as a companion to our paper on fitness to be interviewed by the police (Ventress *et al*, 2008).

I am grateful to the following publishers for permission to reproduce copyright material: the British Medical Association ('Capacity to engage in sexual activity' and 'Capacity to make a gift'); Churchill Livingstone (Professor Bluglass's case of infanticide and Box 28); the Scottish Executive (Box 11), and SEAK Inc. (Box 46). Over the course of 30 years I have made notes following discussions with solicitors and counsel, I have kept extracts from the advices of counsel and I have kept extracts from letters of instruction. I apologise if any of these are based on copyright material about which I am unaware. I will be pleased to rectify any such omissions in a second edition.

I am grateful to the following for their comments on my first draft or parts of it: Mr James Badenoch QC, 1 Crown Office Row; Mr Bill Braithwaite QC, Exchange Chambers; Dr James Briscoe; Dr Ian Bronks; Professor Patricia Casey; Mr Michael Carlin; Her Honour Judge E. A. Carr QC; His Honour Judge John Cockroft; Mr Alan Gough and Ms Helen Gough, Gough Advocates, Isle of Man; Mr David Hinchcliff, HM Coroner for West Yorkshire Eastern District; Mr Robert Holt, Mental Health Tribunal Judge; Dr Rob Kehoe; Ms Diana Kloss MBE, St Johns Buildings Chambers; His Honour Judge Simon Lawler QC; Dr Sajid Muzaffar; Mr Ben Nolan QC, Broad Chare Chambers; Dr Mike Ventress; and Dr Peter Wood.

I am grateful to my daughter, Rowena Rix, Kingsley Napley LLP, for proof-reading, to Dr Digby Jess, Exchange Chambers, for assistance with legal referencing, and to my personal assistant, Debbie Small, for all manner of general assistance. I am also indebted to my son-in-law, Chris Burgess, who built my website, from which some of the material in this book is taken.

I am also grateful to Dave Jago and his colleagues at RCPsych Publications for helping me deliver the finished product, to Ralph Footring, copy-editor, and to Shaun Kennedy in the College Library. Nevertheless, I am ultimately responsible for any mistakes, from which I intend to learn.

Keith J. B. Rix

Boxes

Statutes, statutory instruments and codes cited in the text

Statutes

England and Wales

Scotland

Statutory instruments

England and Wales

Codes of conduct and practice

England and Wales

Scotland

Cases and practice directions

As is common legal practice, in the listing below 'Re' is transposed such that, for example, *Re AB (Child Abuse: Expert Witnesses)* [1995] 1 FLR 181 appears as *AB (Child Abuse: Expert Witnesses), Re* [1995] 1 FLR 181'.

Australia

Canada

England, Wales and Northern Ireland

Hong Kong

Isle of Man

Jersey

New Zealand

Republic of Ireland

Scotland

Practice directions

Abbreviations

See also Appendix 10 (page 257), which covers the abbreviations that appear after a judge's surname to indicate judicial status.

ABH	actual bodily harm
CAFCASS	Children and Family Court Advisory and Support Service
CCRC	Criminal Cases Review Commission
CJA 2003	Criminal Justice Act 2003
CJA 2009	Coroners and Justice Act 2009
CPD	continuing professional development
CP(I)A	Criminal Procedure (Insanity) Act 1964
CP(IU)A	Criminal Procedure (Insanity and Unfitness to Plead) Act 1991
CPR	Civil Procedure Rules
CPS	Crown Prosecution Service
CP(S)A	Criminal Procedure (Scotland) Act 1995
CrPR	Criminal Procedure Rules
CV	curriculum vitae
DDA	Disability Discrimination Act 1995
DSM-IV-TR™	*Diagnostic and Statistical Manual* of the American Psychiatric Association (4th revision – text revision)
DVCVA	Domestic Violence, Crime and Victims Act 2004
ECT	electroconvulsive therapy
FME	forensic medical examiner
FPR	Family Procedure Rules
GBH	grievous bodily harm
GMC	General Medical Council
HMP	Her Majesty's Prison
ICD-10	ICD-10 Classification of Mental and Behavioural Disorders (10th revision)
IPP	imprisonment for public protection
JSB	Judicial Studies Board

LPA	lasting power of attorney
MCA	Mental Capacity Act 2005
MDO	medical defence organisation
MHA	Mental Health Act 1983 (as amended by the Mental Health Act 2007)
MHO	mental health officer
MH(CT)(S)A	Mental Health (Care and Treatment) (Scotland) Act 2003
NGRI	not guilty by reason of insanity
NHS	National Health Service
NHSLA	National Health Service Litigation Authority
NICE	National Institute for Health and Clinical Excellence
PACE	Police and Criminal Evidence Act 1984
PCC(S)A	Powers of the Criminal Courts (Sentencing) Act 2000
PDP	personal development plan
PHA	Protection from Harassment Act 1997
SCR	social circumstances report
SGC	Sentencing Guidelines Council
SJE	single joint expert

CHAPTER 1

Nature and duties of an expert witness

The dependence of the Court on the skill, knowledge and above all, the professional and intellectual integrity of the expert ... cannot be overemphasized. (Wall J in *Re AB (Child Abuse: Expert Witnesses)* [1995] 1 FLR 181)

For over 600 years at least, medical experts have assisted the courts. In 1345, a court summoned surgeons for an opinion on the freshness of a wound (*Anon* (1353) Anon Lib Ass 28, pl.5). In 1664, Dr (later Sir) Thomas Browne of Norwich gave an opinion as to whether or not certain Lowestoft women were witches, relying on the type of fits suffered by the children upon whom they had cast spells (*Witches' Case* (1665) 6 Howell's State Trials 687). In 1760, Dr John Monro, Physician Superintendent of the Bethlem Hospital, gave evidence at the trial of Earl Ferrers, who was charged with the murder of his former steward and pleaded insanity (*R v Ferrers* (1760) 19 State Trials 886).

Experts and expertise

Why do courts need experts?

Courts need experts when dealing with matters which are outside the experience of a judge or jury. If they can draw their own conclusions on the proven facts without such help, expert assistance is unnecessary. In order to receive such assistance, the courts make an exception to the general rule that opinion evidence is inadmissible and witnesses may speak only of facts they have personally perceived.

What is an expert?

An expert is someone recognised by the court as 'qualified' to give expert opinion evidence. It is for the court to decide whether or not someone is qualified to come within the exception to the rule regarding the inadmissibility of opinion evidence. Case law has established how someone might become so eligible. If the Criminal Evidence (Experts) Bill (Law Commission, 2011) becomes law, it will put on a statutory basis the meaning of being 'qualified': 'a person may be qualified to give expert evidence by virtue of study, training, experience or any other appropriate means' if the court is satisfied as to such on a balance of probabilities. To some extent it does not matter that the Bill has not been enacted or that it will apply only to criminal proceedings. When issues arise as to the admissibility of expert evidence in criminal proceedings, the contents of the Bill may be persuasive without being determinative of the issue. If it is enacted, the Act will not be binding on proceedings other than criminal proceedings but again it may influence a court's approach.

First, experts must have *relevant experience*:

if matters arise in our law which concern other sciences or faculties, we commonly apply for the aid of that science or faculty which it concerns. Which is an honourable and commendable thing in our law. (*Buckley v Rice Thomas* (1554) 1 Plowd 118)

Second, experts' opinion must come from *within their own area of special knowledge and experience*. Third, the opinion must be *based on the facts*: 'The opinion of scientific men upon proven facts may be given by men of science within their own science' (*Folkes v Chadd* (1782) 3 Doug KB, 157). Fourth, the test of expertise is *skill*:

The test of expertness ... is skill, and skill alone, in the field of which it is sought to have the witness's opinion. ...I adopt, as a working definition of 'skilled person', one who has by dint of training and practice, acquired a good knowledge of the science or art concerning which his opinion is sought. (*R v Bunnis* (1964) 50 WWR, 422)

What is an expert witness?

In short, an expert witness is an expert whose evidence is *relevant* to the case being tried by the court and whose evidence is *admitted* by the court. The critical test of *admissibility* was established in a case in which psychiatric testimony was given in a murder case:

An expert's opinion is admissible to furnish the court with the scientific information which is likely to be outside the experience and knowledge of a judge or jury. If on the proven facts a judge or jury can form their own conclusions without help, then the opinion of an expert is unnecessary. (*R v Turner* [1975] 1 All ER 70)

The court may further consider whether or not the proposed expert has the experience, expertise and training necessary, having regard to the value, complexity and importance of the case. Judges in the Chancery Division are advised that:

The key question now in relation to expert evidence is the question as to what added value such evidence will provide to the court in its determination of a given case. (Her Majesty's Courts Service, 2009)

At present, unlike in the USA, there is no requirement, or procedure, to test the *reliability* of expert evidence, although *R v Gilfoyle* [2001] 2 Cr App R 57 has indicated the approach under case law. It was held that psychiatric evidence as to the state of mind of a defendant, witness or deceased, falling short of mental illness, might be admissible in some cases when based on medical records and/or recognised criteria, but the present status of 'psychological autopsies' was not such as to permit such evidence as expert opinion before a jury.

At least for criminal cases, however, there may soon be legislation that sets out the requirements and procedures (Law Commission, 2011). If the Criminal Evidence (Experts) Bill is passed into law, judges will have to decide whether the proposed expert is qualified to give expert evidence. Impartiality, the requirement to give objective and unbiased expert evidence, and a duty to the court that overrides any obligation to the person from whom the expert receives instructions or by whom the expert is paid, will be put on a statutory basis. Expert opinion evidence will be admitted as being of sufficient reliability only if it is (1) soundly based and (2) strong enough having regard to the grounds on which it is based. Specific grounds for determining that the evidence is not sufficiently reliable will be spelled out, for example if the opinion relies on an inference or conclusion that has not been properly reached. Generic factors to which the court must have regard will be listed, such as whether or not the expert's methods followed established practice in the field, or, if not, the reason for the divergence. There will be a provision for the Lord Chancellor to set out, in a statutory instrument, other factors relevant to specific fields of expertise. The proposed schedule to the Bill sets out factors to which the court must have regard when considering the reliability of expert opinion evidence. One of these is 'Whether there is a range of expert opinion on the matter in question; and, if there is, where in the range the opinion lies and whether the expert's preference for the opinion proffered has been properly explained'. Professor Nigel Eastman, a member of a Law Commission working group looking at the Bill, has suggested that this factor, in tandem with the need for the expert to provide an opinion as to why his or her opinion is sound, summarises 'particularly well what should be the approach to medical evidence which is psychiatric in nature' (Law Commission, 2011, p. 67).

It seems likely that in criminal cases the reliability of expert evidence will be decided at a pre-trial hearing and this may mean experts having to give evidence at such a hearing if the court cannot decide from the reports themselves whether or not they meet the statutory requirements for reliability.

The *expert witness* will be distinguished from the *professional witness* and from the *witness to fact*, although an *expert witness* may give evidence of facts as the basis for his or her opinion evidence. For example, a senior house officer witnesses one patient attack another. She is a *witness to fact*. A visitor to the ward also witnesses the attack and may give similar evidence as to the facts of what happened. As to what was seen and heard, the fact that one witness is a senior house officer in psychiatry is irrelevant. The specialist registrar who documents the assailant's mental state immediately afterwards is a *professional witness* because she is using her professional knowledge and experience to ascertain relevant facts. So, the professional witness is also a witness to fact. The consultant psychiatrist engaged by the assailant's solicitors to give an opinion on whether or not the assailant has a defence of insanity is an *expert witness*. She derives her opinion, in part, from the evidence of the witnesses to fact and she may also use her expertise to give evidence of facts within her own knowledge, such as the assailant's mental state at the time she examined him. Her opinion may support the defence of insanity. Another consultant psychiatrist engaged by the prosecution may not support the defence of insanity. The material facts are the same but the opinions may differ.

If the issue is tried in court, the specialist registrar may be called to give evidence as to the assailant's mental state at the time of her examination. She does so as a *professional witness*. Once in the witness box, counsel or the judge may ask for her opinion as to insanity. If she does not think that her training and experience qualify her to give an opinion on this issue, she should say that she is giving evidence as a *professional witness*, not as an *expert witness*, and she cannot assist the court with an expert opinion on the issue. If she thinks that she is qualified to give an opinion on this issue, she should preface her response by reminding the court that she has attended as a *professional witness*, that she may not have heard all of the relevant evidence, but, if the court allows her to do so, she is now about to assist the court as an *expert witness*.

What are the duties and responsibilities of a psychiatrist acting as an expert witness?

A psychiatrist who acts as an expert witness is:
- a *citizen*
- a *doctor*
- a *psychiatrist*
- an *expert witness*.

All of these roles carry responsibilities. The responsibilities of doctors are underpinned by the four basic principles of medical ethics:
- autonomy
- beneficence
- non-maleficence
- justice.

There are also the two subsidiary principles of:
- consent
- best interests.

Sometimes two or more of these principles may clash.

Duty as citizen

A psychiatrist has a *duty as a citizen* to assist in the administration of justice:

It is a complaint made by coroners, magistrates and judges, that medical gentlemen are often reluctant in the performance of the offices, required from them as citizens qualified by professional knowledge, to aid the execution of public justice. (Percival, 1803: p. 120)

Duty as a doctor

The *duties of a doctor* are set out by the General Medical Council (GMC). *Good Medical Practice* (General Medical Council, 2006) states as core guidance:

You must be honest and trustworthy when writing reports, and when completing or signing forms, reports and other documents. (para. 63)

If you have agreed to prepare a report, complete or sign a document or provide evidence, you must do so without unreasonable delay. (para. 66)

If you are asked to give evidence or act as a witness in litigation or formal inquiries, you must be honest in all your spoken and written statements. You must make clear the limits of your knowledge or competence. (para. 67)

In *Acting as an Expert Witness* (General Medical Council, 2008) the GMC explains how this guidance applies to the medical expert witness. Also, the Academy of Medical Royal Colleges (2005) has made recommendations that derive from the GMC's core guidance.

Duty as a psychiatrist

The *duties of a psychiatrist*, who is a Member (or Fellow) of the Royal College of Psychiatrists, derive from the College's Charter as well as from the GMC. The psychiatrist who acts as an expert witness should be mindful of the objects and purposes of the College's Charter. As a Member or Fellow, in giving written expert opinion or oral testimony, she should advance the objects and purposes of the College, by furthering public education as to the science and practice of psychiatry (3(1)(a) and (b)), and she should adhere to the highest possible standards of professional competence and practice (3(2)(b)) (Royal College of Psychiatrists, 2008*a*).

The College has complemented the GMC's *Good Medical Practice* with *Good Psychiatric Practice* (Royal College of Psychiatrists, 2009), which advises that it should be read in conjunction with *Court Work* (Royal College of Psychiatrists, 2008*b*), which makes 14 recommendations with regard to 'Duties of a psychiatric expert witness' (Box 1).

Box 1 Duties of psychiatric expert witnesses

The Royal College of Psychiatrists (2008*b*) states that expert witnesses should:

- Ensure that they have had an induction in expert witness work.
- Have relevant knowledge of court procedures.
- Act with honesty, impartiality, objectivity and respect for justice, regardless of the party who instructs them.
- In criminal matters, show a willingness and ability to be instructed by either defence or prosecution.
- In Children Act cases, recognise that the interests of the child are paramount.
- Decline instructions that go beyond psychiatric expertise.
- Where advised that a report is not to be disclosed to the court, seek advice as to whether or not disclosure is in the public interest.
- Make clear to the subject of a report that:
  - the expert's role is to provide an opinion to the court
  - they may refuse to cooperate
  - the report is not confidential and may be seen by a number of different professionals
  - they may refuse to answer certain questions
  - the expert is not there to provide treatment, except in an emergency.
- Develop a pro forma addressing consent and confidentiality and devise a model consent form.
- With regard to recommendations:
  - make clear the evidence base
  - have some knowledge of the facilities available and discuss the recommendations with the relevant services
  - make evidence-based recommendations if no local facilities are available
  - if it is unlikely that they will be carried out, state why and what a second, less desirable plan might be
  - where appropriate, attribute evidence to other professionals and provide details of their qualifications and experience.
- Where there is concern about the conditions in which a subject is held, report these.
- Be prepared to provide evidence of continuing professional development (CPD) and peer group review geared to maintain competence as an expert.
- Be clinically active, belong to a CPD group (peer group), have a relevant personal development plan and be appraised at least once a year.
- Be ethical:
  - do not give evidence beyond their expertise
  - undertake CPD to maintain expertise
  - have an awareness of the possibilities for the treatment and placement of subjects
  - declare any conflicts of interest
  - rely on the evidence and specialist knowledge uninfluenced by the exigencies of the litigation and regardless of who has commissioned the report
  - be cognisant of funding arrangements and ensure value for money
  - have the integrity to resist pressure to 'adjust' the report to suit the needs of instructing lawyers or their clients
  - be clear about timescales so as to minimise delay
  - retain all notes.

Duty as an expert witness

The *duties of an expert witness* in general have been refined over the years by judges who have commented on them in particular cases. A case involving the sinking of a merchant vessel, the *Ikarian Reefer* (*National Justice Compania Naviera SA v Prudential Assurance Co Ltd 'Ikarian Reefer'* [1995] 1 Lloyd's Rep 455, CA) (Rix, 1999), remains a landmark case and guidance therein has become increasingly embodied in rules made by the courts and in protocols made, or endorsed, by the courts. The three most important sets of rules in England and Wales are the Civil Procedure Rules (SI 1998/3132) (CPR) Part 35, the Criminal Procedure Rules (SI 2010/60) (CrPR) Part 33 and the Family Procedure Rules (SI 2010/2955) (FPR) (collectively 'the Rules'). The most important protocol is the *Protocol for the Instruction of Experts to Give Evidence in Civil Claims* (Civil Justice Council, 2005) (hereinafter the *Protocol*), much of the core guidance of which is applicable to non-civil proceedings. The guidance evolves, however, as case law supersedes what is set out in the *Protocol*; indeed, guidance in the use of experts in criminal trials given by Gage LJ in *R v Bowman* [2006] EWCA Crim 417 goes further than ever previously. By the time this book is published, it is likely that there will have been further guidance issued with which experts will have to comply. The *Expert Witness Year Book*, published each year by the UK Register of Expert Witnesses, is a useful means of keeping up to date in this regard; at the time of writing the latest edition was Pamplin (2011).

The Rules make it clear that:

- the paramount or overriding duty of the expert is to assist the court on matters within his or her own expertise
- this overrides any obligation to the person from whom the expert has received instructions or is paid.

Psychiatric expert witnesses should be aware that they are accountable to the GMC as well as the courts. They owe a responsibility to those who instruct them, to the person upon whom they are reporting and to the College. The responsibilities to those instructing them and the person upon whom they report are:

- to identify weaknesses as well as strengths in their case
- to recommend any further treatment that is advisable
- to suggest any other expertise that may be required.

They have a responsibility to the College, because those whose reputation as experts in psychiatry is based on Membership or Fellowship of the College must at least uphold, preferably enhance, and certainly do nothing to damage, its reputation.

The *Protocol* sets out seven duties of experts (Box 2).

Not surprisingly, there is considerable overlap between the various sets of guidance. This book incorporates as much as possible of the guidance. Readers are referred to the original sources and should note that College recommendations in *Court Work* go further than any other rules or general guidance.

> **Box 2** Summary of the 'Duties of experts' set out in the *Protocol*
>
> The *Protocol for the Instruction of Experts to Give Evidence in Civil Claims* (Civil Justice Council, 2005) states that experts have the following duties:
>
> - A duty to exercise reasonable skill and care to those instructing them and to comply with any relevant professional code of ethics. Overriding duty to help the court on matters within their expertise.
> - Be aware of the overriding objective that courts deal with cases justly. This includes dealing with cases proportionately, expeditiously and fairly. Assist the court so to do.
> - Provide opinions which are independent, regardless of the pressures of the litigation. Useful test: the expert would express the same opinion if given the same instructions by an opposing party. Do not promote the point of view of the instructing party or be an advocate.
> - Confine opinions to matters material to the disputes between the parties and only in relation to matters within their expertise. Advise without delay if questions or issues are outside their expertise.
> - Take into account all material facts, set out those facts and any literature relied upon, indicate if opinion is provisional or qualified or if further information is needed before giving final and unqualified opinion.
> - Inform those instructing them without delay of any change of opinion on any material matter and the reason.
> - Be aware that failure to comply with Rules or court orders or any excessive delay for which they are responsible may result in a financial penalty to those instructing them and may lead to their evidence being debarred.

Rewards and penalties for the expert witness

Fulfilling the duties of a psychiatric expert witness will enhance the confidence which the courts have in admitting and relying on psychiatric evidence and enhance the professional standing and public understanding of psychiatry. Failure in discharging these duties will undermine the professional standing of psychiatry, risk injustice in cases where the courts need psychiatric expertise and set back the public understanding of psychiatry.

It is common for experts to be asked to change their opinion. If you are asked to change your opinion for no other reason than to improve the case being put forward by those instructing you, you should refuse, as this is unethical and unprofessional. Your first duty is to the court and not to those instructing you. If you do change your opinion to please your paymaster, and get away with it, remember that the solicitor and barrister will not forget. Your next contact with the same barrister may be in a case where she is instructed by the other side. Do not be surprised if she gives you a hard time and do not be surprised if she does not recommend you for other cases. If you acquire a reputation among barristers as a 'hired gun' you may have some short-term gains but when the barristers are sitting as recorders or have been elevated to the bench you should not be surprised if your opinions carry little weight with them. If, but only with good reason, you refuse to budge, this will enhance your reputation as an expert and judges who have known you when they were barristers will be more likely to respect your opinions.

Do not be afraid to provide an opinion which those instructing you wish that they had not obtained. Your report may go in the confidential waste or the shredder and never see the light of day in court, but when the solicitor or barrister wants an opinion upon which she knows that she can rely, she will come back to you.

If you are asked to change your opinion on the basis of new information or because you have misunderstood the legal test or have misinterpreted the facts, this is a different matter. As John Maynard Keynes said, 'When the facts change, my opinion changes'. However, your opinion has to remain your opinion and not that of those instructing you. If you change your opinion, the basis for doing so should be crystal clear. If it is not and if the earlier version of your report has already been disclosed, or is disclosed inadvertently, or otherwise falls into the hands of the other side, any change of opinion, especially if it suggests partiality to those instructing you, will be put under the microscope and, if the reason for the change is not crystal clear and justified, you will be accused of being biased, partisan or even a 'hired gun'.

It is worth bearing in mind that expert reports are often filed by barristers under the name of the expert, so that an expert's reports can be compared. The expert whose opinion has been 'black' when instructed by the claimant's solicitors and 'white' when instructed by the defendant's solicitors in similar cases, or where the facts and issues are similar, should expect a hard ride under cross-examination in the witness box.

I once witnessed the cross-examination of a psychiatrist who had prepared his first report in the mistaken belief that he was being instructed by solicitors acting for the defendant. His second report was very different, as by this time he had realised that he was instructed by the claimant's solicitors. By the time the case came to trial, it was too late to avoid what counsel for the defendant described afterwards as 'the iron fist in the velvet glove'. Lest it be thought that this book is a vehicle for poking fun at some psychiatric experts, let me admit at this stage being forever haunted by an early cross-examination of my own, as an expert witness instructed by the prosecution, at the end of which Mr Norman Jones QC turned to the psychiatrist instructed by solicitors for the defendant and whispered 'game, set and match'. It just so happened that on this occasion there were half a dozen of our fellow consultants in court and many more of our trainees. Perhaps 'haunted' is the wrong word but when my cross-examiner became the Recorder of Leeds, it was salutary, every time I gave evidence before him, to reflect on our meeting many years previously, when I was lower down on my learning curve.

There are other potential penalties if the expert witness falls short.

In extreme cases, the expert's name may be erased from the Medical Register. This happened to a professor of microbiology who indicated an intention to mislead the Legal Services Commission in order to obtain financial advantage and expressed a willingness to provide a false estimate of the number of hours likely to be worked in the preparation of an expert report in order to obtain an enhanced fee from the Commission.

There may be a financial penalty of a 'wasted costs order' where, by their evidence, psychiatrists have caused significant expense to be incurred through flagrant disregard of their duties to the court. In the case of *Phillips and Others v Symes and Others* [2004] EWHC 2330 (Ch), an application was made for the psychiatrist who had given evidence to be joined to the proceedings as a respondent for the purposes of costs only. The basis of the application was that the psychiatrist 'was in serious breach of his duties to the Court by acting recklessly, irresponsibly and wholly outside the bounds of how any reasonable psychiatrist preparing an opinion for the Court could properly have acted having regard to his duties'. In this case the psychiatrist had given evidence that Mr Symes, a bankrupt, not only lacked capacity to participate in the Chancery proceedings but had lacked capacity since a stroke in 1980, thus rendering null and void every transaction in which he had participated since then. However, the court had found that he did not lack capacity and there was criticism of the psychiatrist for five reasons. First, he had formed his initial opinion on a wholly inadequate basis. Second, he had not considered the manner in which Mr Symes had actually been able to conduct his business and legal affairs since his stroke. Third, he refused to reconsider his opinion in the light of further material sent to him and, indeed, refused to look at the material until directed by the judge to do so at the trial (after doing so, he was forced to admit that Mr Symes was capable of managing his affairs and that his original opinion could not be sustained). Fourth, in verifying his two reports as his evidence in chief, the psychiatrist failed to act in conformity with his expert's declaration (1) to mention all matters which he regarded as relevant to his opinions, (2) to draw attention to matters of which he was aware that might adversely affect his opinion and (3) to comply with his duty to correct or qualify his report when necessary. Fifth, by ignoring and disregarding any evidence or material which was inconsistent with his position, and actively trying to find material to support it, he assumed a role as an advocate for Mr Symes.

Smith J did not reach a decision as to whether or not the psychiatrist was guilty of a breach of his duty but he held that he did have a case to answer and he found that a wasted costs order could be made against an expert in the event that his evidence was 'given recklessly in flagrant disregard for his duties'. A wasted costs order has the effect of making the person against whom it is made pay costs wasted by their misconduct, default or serious negligence.

A penalty need not be financial. It may be in the form of a judicial criticism of the psychiatrist, for example as irresponsible for expressing views at the end of long-running personal injury litigation which are not easy to reconcile with his recent examination of the plaintiff for family proceedings and in the course of which he indicated that there had been a dramatic improvement in the plaintiff's health (*Vernon v Bosley (No. 2)* [1999] QB 18, CA). Judicial criticism can in fact have far-reaching consequences. In his lecture at the 2006 Grange annual conference, a lawyer specialising in mental health tribunal cases quoted criticism of the independent psychiatric expert in a reported case before a mental health tribunal (*R (on the application of PS)* [2003] EWHC 2335 (Admin)). The judge devoted four paragraphs to his criticism, under the heading 'Misgivings about Dr [Z]'s evidence' and ended with references to his 'evasive and overdefensive approach in answering questions when cross-examined' and 'his continuing willingness to base an unqualified and dogmatic opinion on limited evidence'. After the lecture, the speaker had to be almost physically separated from the expert, whom he had not named, but who happened to be in the audience and who took exception to the speaker's reference to him.

In *Rhodes v West Surrey & North East Hampshire Health Authority* [1998] 6 Lloyd's Rep Med 246, an obstetrician was found not to have told the truth on two matters – his experience as a surgeon and as an expert witness. Margaret Puxon QC MD FRCOG, commenting on the case, asked whether the GMC had an interest in these matters. It does.

It has now been suggested that a judge may have powers under the CrPR to require an expert instructed by the defence to disclose any past adverse criticism by a judge and, although this may not be a ground for refusing the admission of the expert's evidence, it might lead to second thoughts about the advisability of calling the expert (*R v Henderson and Others* [2010] EWCA Crim 1269).

A psychiatrist was reported to the GMC for organising covert surveillance of a police officer he had examined in a police pension case.

Professor Sir Roy Meadow strayed outside his field of paediatrics into statistics, making an honest error without any intention to mislead (*Meadow v General Medical Council* [2006] 1 WLR 1452, CA). Although he was successful in appealing against the GMC's finding of serious professional misconduct (by a majority decision, the Master of the Rolls dissenting), Auld LJ found him guilty of some professional misconduct because he fell below the standards expected of him by his profession and Thorpe LJ found his evidence flawed.

One of the experts, albeit not a doctor, in the eighteenth-century Wells Harbour case of *Folkes v Chadd* (Rix, 2006a) was threatened with an action for perjury because he got his tides going in the wrong direction.

Further reading

Pamplin, C. (ed.) (for the UK Register of Expert Witnesses) (2011) *Expert Witness Year Book*. JS Publications.
Royal College of Psychiatrists (2008b) *Court Work*. RCPsych.

CHAPTER 2

Training, contractual, administrative and other practical matters

Experts should be spared piles of documents which [are] of little relevance. The cost of expert involvement [is] unnecessarily inflated by over-burdening them with insignificant papers. (*Re S (Care Proceedings: Assessment of Risk)* (2008) *The Times*, 7 April, CA)

This chapter refers to some standardised or semi-standardised letters and documents that your secretary should have stored as templates (Box 3). Some of the materials presented here and in the appendices are composites, so it is important to delete what is not appropriate in a particular case, for example a case not covered by CPR, and adapt them as necessary. These and other useful materials are available on my website (http://www.drkeithrix. co.uk). This material is freely available for use and adaptation by experts. If you do improve on them, share the improvements with colleagues.

Getting started – advice for trainees and their consultants

Trainees sometimes ask how they can get started preparing and giving expert psychiatric evidence (Rix, 2011). Some opportunities should exist for pre-Membership trainees if they are attached to consultants who prepare medico-legal reports. Specialist registrars in forensic psychiatry are likely to be involved in the preparation of expert reports as a matter of routine. Specialist registrars in other subspecialties may be able to arrange special-interest sessions with a consultation forensic psychiatrist, or other suitable consultant, for the purpose of learning how to write expert psychiatric reports and deliver expert psychiatric testimony.

A prerequisite is some knowledge and understanding of law and legal procedures. *The Expert Witness: A Practical Guide* (Bond *et al*, 2007) has useful chapters on 'The English legal system', 'The criminal courts' and 'The civil courts'. *The Criminal Justice System: An Introduction* (Gibson & Cavadino, 2008) is also useful, as it has a glossary of words, phrases, acronyms and

> **Box 3** Standardised and semi-standardised letters and documents to
> be stored as templates
>
> - Positive letter of response to an enquiry/letter referring to, or including, terms and conditions of appointment (see Appendix 1)
> - Terms and conditions of appointment
> - File front sheet (see Appendix 2)
> - Time sheet (see Appendix 3)
> - Appointment letter (see Appendix 4)
> - Information for people attending for an appointment (see Appendix 5)
> - Letter to prison for authorisation to use laptop computer (see Appendix 6)
> - Consent form (see Appendix 7)
> - Covering letter for report (see Appendix 8)

abbreviations. *Experts in the Civil Courts* (Blom-Cooper, 2006) is a more detailed and very comprehensive introduction to the role of the expert in civil proceedings. Lord Justice Wall's *A Handbook for Expert Witnesses in Children Act Cases* (Wall, 2007) is not only the book for experts in family proceedings but many of the chapters are applicable to experts in general. Baroness Hale's *Mental Health Law* (2010) should be on every psychiatrist's bookshelf already.

Before preparing a report, trainees should read a number of their consultants' reports. The next stage is for the consultant to provide the trainee with a report from which the 'Opinion' and 'Summary of conclusions' have been omitted. The trainee should then prepare their own 'Opinion' and 'Summary of conclusions' for discussion with the consultant. This can also be done on a group basis, particularly in a forensic psychiatry setting, where there are a number of trainees learning to prepare reports.

A trainee's first report should probably be a 'ghost report'. The trainee interviews and examines someone who has been referred to the consultant for a report. The consultant will need to obtain at least the consent of the subject of the report for the trainee to be so involved and probably also the permission of the instructing solicitor. In the same way that a pre-Membership trainee 'clerks' a new patient in the consultant's out-patient clinic and then presents the case to the consultant, so the trainee will present the history and examination findings to the consultant and there will be the opportunity for the consultant to check the history, take any additional history necessary and confirm the mental state findings. The trainee should then prepare a report in the consultant's name and include a sentence giving their own name and status along the lines: 'I have been assisted in the preparation of this report by Dr William Batty, Specialist Registrar...'. It will be necessary to include the trainee's curriculum vitae (CV) as an appendix. Consultants do need to 'own' the opinion and will need to make sure that the final form and content are of the same standard as reports they prepare in their own right.

Specialist registrars should be able to progress to preparing reports in their own right; however, their preparation must be supervised by the consultant. It will be necessary for those instructing the consultant to give permission for a specialist registrar to prepare the report unless the instructions provide for delegation, as sometimes happens with instructions to consultants in forensic services.

When first instructed in your own right, do not hesitate to ask a sufficiently experienced consultant to read the report in draft and provide advice.

Getting it wrong and the negligent expert

Trainees sometimes ask what happens if they 'get it wrong'. If properly trained and supervised, this should not happen. Experts who realise that they have got something wrong need to revise their opinion without delay and advise those instructing them and/or the court (see p. 50).

Your opinion may not be accepted by the court but that does not mean that you 'got it wrong'. If, in the witness box, you realise that you have got something wrong, admit it and apologise. It may be embarrassing but your reputation will be damaged more by attempts to cover up, blame someone else or deny that you have got it wrong.

The case of *Jones v Kaney* [2011] UKSC 13 is of relevance here. This is the decision of the Supreme Court to allow the aggrieved Mr Jones to bring a negligence action against the expert witness, a clinical psychologist, Ms Kaney, who reported on him for his solicitors in a road traffic accident case. It is important to look at the facts of the case. In relation to Mr Jones' road traffic accident, Ms Kaney prepared two reports. In the first she diagnosed post-traumatic stress disorder and in the second she expressed the opinion that Mr Jones was still suffering from depression and some symptoms of post-traumatic stress disorder. A consultant psychiatrist, instructed as an expert by the defendant's solicitor, expressed the view that Mr Jones was exaggerating his physical symptoms. A meeting of the experts was ordered by the court, at the end of which the expert instructed by the defendant (the psychiatrist) prepared a joint statement recording agreement that: the claimant's psychological reaction to the accident was no more than adjustment reaction; it did not reach the level of a depressive disorder or post-traumatic stress disorder; the claimant had been deceptive and deceitful in his reporting; and his behaviour was suggestive of 'conscious mechanisms', which raised doubts as to the genuineness of what he had reported. The claimant's solicitors taxed Ms Kaney about the discrepancies between the joint statement and her earlier assessments and what the trial judge described as this 'unhappy picture' emerged:

1   She had not seen the reports of the opposing expert at the time of the telephone conference.

2   The joint statement, as drafted by the opposing expert, did not reflect what she had agreed in the telephone conversation, but she had felt herself to be under pressure to agree to it.

3   Her true view was that the claimant had been evasive rather than deceptive.

4   It was her view that the claimant did suffer post-traumatic stress disorder, which was now resolved.

5   She was happy for the claimant's then solicitors to amend the joint statement.

Ms Kaney should not have 'attended' the experts' meeting without seeing the opposing expert's reports. If the draft joint statement did not reflect what she had agreed, she should have amended it and the experts should have carried on amending it until they could both sign it, having regard to the statement of truth that was either at the end of the statement or would have been regarded by the court as applying to it. She should not have allowed herself to be pressurised into signing it if it did not reflect her opinion accurately and fully. It was her responsibility to amend the statement and not that of her instructing solicitors. If she had changed her opinion on an issue, she should have set out in full the reasons for this in the joint statement or in an accompanying letter to those who had instructed her. Whether or not Ms Kaney's acts or omissions were such that she failed the *Bolam* test for negligence (see Box 32, p. 122) was not decided by the Supreme Court but Ms Kaney had already admitted negligence.

Address and correspondence

It is not advisable to you use your home address in correspondence and reports or to give your home address when asked in court for your address. You may put the safety of your family and neighbours at risk as well as your own. My former next-door neighbour, whose semi-detached house mine adjoined, when she is addressing medico-legal audiences shows a picture of her hedge that was burnt down by one of my arsonists who had recognised me in a local shopping centre and followed me home. We remain on good terms but when she moved she was quite alarmed to meet my successor in my National Health Service (NHS) post and discover that another psychiatrist was living only doors away from her new home. But all is well that ends well. When she became the lead postgraduate dean for psychiatry in England and Wales, she knew something about the importance of psychiatry in general and forensic psychiatry in particular.

If you do not have a professional address that you can use for correspondence, get a PO box address or consider joining a document exchange. The advantage of having a document exchange box is that it improves communications with solicitors and barristers, most of whom belong to one of the document exchanges, and if industrial unrest, for example, brings many communications to a halt you should still be able to continue to deliver hard copies of your reports and receive documents from your instructing solicitors.

Responding to the letter of enquiry

To accept or decline

Upon receipt of a letter of enquiry as to whether or not you can provide an expert opinion in a particular case, ask yourself a number of questions (Box 4). If they can all be answered in the affirmative, you may decide to accept instructions and proceed to prepare an expert report.

The positive letter of response or engagement letter

Send your positive letter of response to an enquiry or engagement letter and your terms and conditions of appointment. Box 5 sets out what should be

---

Box 4 Questions to be answered in the affirmative before accepting instructions to prepare an expert psychiatric report

- Am I in good standing with the College?
- Have I been appraised in the last year?
- Am I up to date with continuing professional development?
- Does my personal development plan address the issue of my competence as an expert witness?
- Have I had an introduction to expert witness work?
- Have I received training in the role of an expert witness in the last five years?
- Am I available to attend the trial (if the trial date has been fixed)?
- Can I deliver the report by the required deadline?
- Can I declare that I have no actual or potential conflict of interest or personal interest?
- Do I understand exactly what questions I am being asked or what the issues are?
- Do I have relevant knowledge or direct experience of, and expertise in, this area of psychiatry?
- Does the question or issue fall within my own expertise?
- Am I able to give an honest, trustworthy, objective and impartial opinion without it being prejudiced by any views I may have as to the age, colour, culture, disability, ethnicity, national origin, gender, lifestyle, marital or parental status, race, religion or beliefs, gender, gender orientation or social or economic status of the subject of the report?
- Can I provide sufficiently detailed information as to my proposed fees for those instructing me to decide if they are proportionate to the matters in issue?
- Do I understand the specific framework of law and procedure within which this case is taking place?
- Am I familiar with the general duties of an expert?
- Do I understand my duty to the court?

included in the letter and Appendix 1 is a sample letter. It has been drawn up to comply with paragraph 4.2 of the Practice Direction *Experts in Family Proceedings Relating to Children* (1 April 2008) but it can be used as it is or modified for other cases.

The *Protocol* advises that terms of appointment should be agreed and it sets out what they should normally include (Box 6). Although this guidance is for civil cases, it is guidance of general applicability.

Fees

At present, most experts usually charge by the hour for preparation and report writing, and by the half-day or day for conferences with counsel and attendance at court, but fixed fees may be introduced for some expert witness work. You should be in a position to provide an estimate based

---

Box 5 Matters to be covered in positive letter of response to an enquiry

- Confirm that there is no conflict of interest, or draw attention to any that, it has been agreed, does not disqualify you
- State that the work is within your expertise
- State that you can comply with the timetable
- If the trial has been fixed, indicate dates and times to avoid if possible. If it has not been fixed, indicate how to obtain an up-to-date commitments list
- If evidence is to be by telephone conference or video-link, indicate how much notice will be needed to make arrangements
- If, for example in a family case, you do not want to be named, or otherwise identified, in any public judgment, say so

---

Box 6 Terms of appointment to be agreed at the outset in a civil case

- The capacity in which the expert is to be appointed (e.g. party-appointed expert, single joint expert or expert advisor)
- The services required of the expert (e.g. provision of expert's report, answering questions in writing, attendance at meetings and attendance at court)
- Time for delivery of the report
- The basis of the expert's charges (either daily or hourly rates and an estimate of the time likely to be required, or a total fee for the services)
- Travelling expenses and disbursements
- Cancellation charges
- Any fees for attending court
- Time for making the payment
- Whether fees are to be paid by a third party
- If a party is publicly funded, whether or not the expert's charges will be subject to assessment by a costs officer

---

on the amount of reading and preparation, the time spent in consultation with the subject of the report and any informant(s) and the time spent preparing the report. Especially where payment is from public funds, there may be a narrow range of hourly rates and only in exceptional cases will it be possible to negotiate higher rates. Where private funds are involved it may be easier to negotiate a more favourable hourly rate. In any case, the hourly rate will depend on a number of factors: the experience and reputation of the expert, the scarcity of the relevant expertise, the nature and complexity of the case and the source of funding. Overall, the need to do more than break even, in terms of covering overheads, has to be balanced against the obligation to assist in the administration of justice and ensure that expertise is available to people of limited financial means who do not qualify for public funding. The ethical expert will do some work completely on a *pro bono* basis and some at rates below or around the hourly rate necessary to cover overheads.

Terms and conditions

The United Kingdom Register of Expert Witnesses has produced a handy 'little book', *Expert Witness Fees* (Pamplin, 2007) and expert witness bodies such as the Academy of Experts and the Expert Witness Institute produce model 'terms and conditions'. These can be adapted to cover all of the matters in Box 6 but nonetheless it is advisable and some would say necessary for each practitioner to obtain legal advice in the drafting of their own terms and conditions. It is surprising how some model terms and conditions miss some vital points. Mine are written by a lawyer who has taken action for and against experts numerous times and hence they include clauses to deal with the practical issues that arise. He also regularly instructs experts and deals with issues on such matters as questions to experts and joint statements. Thus, what he has devised are terms and conditions that would equally help him as an instructing party. He says that his particular favourite, at the moment, is the term that deals with the expert making an application to court at the expense of the instructing party. This is particularly useful when an expert is being pulled in different directions on, say, a joint statement, and the true effect of the term is to allow an expert to take the ultimate measure to ensure that she remains impartial. From a lawyer's perspective, he suggests that the threat of putting an issue before the judge may well be enough to ensure fair play.

Curriculum vitae

You may be asked to provide your CV. Occasionally it may be necessary to provide a full-length CV but have a one-page CV, or preferably a selection of them, tailored to the type of work required (for example personal injury, criminal, family), or even use a highly specialised one where, for example, you are responding to a letter of enquiry about a type of case about which you have published research or written. If the solicitors have not previously instructed you, it can make all the difference between being instructed and being passed over. Make sure that your CV is accurate and contains no exaggerations, untruths or material omissions, otherwise this may become the beginning, and even the end, of your cross-examination. 'A poorly drafted CV can provide substantial ammunition to an attorney set on discrediting an expert' (Babitsky *et al*, 2000, p. 77). If you have exaggerated your CV, it will be argued that you have exaggerated your opinion.

Balance of claimant and defendant work

You may be asked at the outset about the balance of claimant, defendant and single joint expert (SJE) instructions in civil cases and the balance of prosecution and defence instructions in criminal cases. Prepare a 'breakdown of new instructions' every year and send this out when requested (or make it available on your website). In order to avoid an imbalance of claimant or defendant instructions in personal injury cases – which might suggest that you have a bias towards one or other – once you are established, and start to receive defendant instructions, run two waiting lists, as Dr Donald Johnson taught me, so that the number of claimant and defendant reports is approximately equal. This balance will probably not be possible in criminal cases as there are fewer prosecution and court instructions; this is because they tend to be reactive to defence reports and many defence reports are not disclosed or, if disclosed, may not trigger a prosecution or court report if they are accepted as independent and impartial.

Qualified acceptance of instructions

If some questions set out in Box 4 are answered in the negative, it may be that, with further information, they can all be answered in the affirmative. If the trial date is not convenient, it may be possible for the trial to be moved or for you to give your evidence by video-link. It may be possible for the deadline for delivery of the report to be extended. An actual or potential conflict of interest or personal interest may not affect your suitability as an expert. It may be possible to clarify sufficiently the questions being asked or the issues to be addressed. The instructing party may be able to provide sufficient information as to the specific framework of law and procedure involved in the case, perhaps including the legal test or tests to be applied. In such instances, either modify the 'positive letter of response to enquiry' or, especially if there is a lot to find out, clarify or negotiate, send an individualised letter. An experienced medico-legal secretary or personal assistant may be able to do this for you but remember that first impressions count and often solicitors will have sent the same letter of enquiry to a number of experts.

Getting ready for starter's orders

If the instructing party accepts your terms and conditions, it is time to do the preparatory work.

First, reconsider the questions or issues to be addressed. They may relate to a particular legal test that has a statutory or common law basis. If so, ask those instructing to explain it because 'it is a good thing for the expert to have given to him the legal test' (*Routestone Ltd v Minories Finance Ltd* [1997] BCC 180). This is particularly important if your report is for a jurisdiction other than your own and where the law may be different to that in England and Wales. Experts in Scotland are required to 'ensure that they are up-to-date with the current legal criteria before they give an opinion as to insanity or diminished responsibility, although it is the responsibility of the commissioning agent to ensure that the medical practitioner is provided with the relevant information' (Scottish Executive, 2005, ch. 3, para. 13).

Second, make sure that all relevant documents have been supplied. What is relevant will depend on the nature of the case. Almost always, it will be necessary to see the subject's general practice records or some other medical records. Without them, the history will be uncorroborated 'hearsay' (see p. 45) and thereby vulnerable to attack. Make sure that the 'Lloyd George' cards have been supplied for the period that pre-dates or overlaps with the computerisation of general practice records. Check that all correspondence has been provided; the practice may have hard copies of older correspondence that has not been scanned into the practice computer. Use the general practitioner records to identify which mental health, community psychiatric nursing or counselling records should be obtained. If they exist, decide whether they are needed before the consultation or can be obtained later.

If there is anything about which you are uncertain, speak to those instructing you. Good communication is essential. It can prevent problems occurring later that delay the litigation, add to the cost of the proceedings, add to the stress of the case for you, those instructing you or their client, or otherwise prejudice the good working relationship which will become more and more important as the case progresses and if it goes to trial.

Records

Your records should be stored safely, securely and according to a system that enables them to be easily retrieved and in compliance with the Data Protection Act 1998 (see Pamplin, 2010). Bear in mind that, at least until the case is concluded, you may need to store lever-arch files, ring-binders and combinations of these. Your main file should indicate what separate files, such as lever-arch files, ring-binders and even 'bankers' boxes' exist and where they are stored. Archive storage may be necessary in addition to storage for active cases. If you are informed that your report, an addendum or a letter has been disclosed, mark your file copy 'Disclosed'.

You may find it helpful to have an index/contents page for each file, on which you can record the progress of the case, including all incoming and outgoing communications, and keep track of what has been disclosed in the course of the proceedings (see Appendix 2).

Deadlines and timetables

Ensure that your report is delivered on time. Remember that a defence solicitor may want to take instructions on your report from the client and have to arrange to see the client in prison to do so. Solicitors acting for the defendant in a civil case may want to take instructions from their insurance clients. The report may be needed for the 'trial bundle', which a judge may study a day or more before the trial starts. If problems arise and you cannot meet the deadline, inform those instructing you as soon as possible, explain why and explain how much longer you need. There is a reasonable expectation that an expert should be able to produce the report within four weeks of conducting an examination or receipt of the papers. There is a tight deadline for serving on the court a joint statement prepared following an experts' meeting (see pp. 137, 162). Answers to questions put to an expert usually have to be provided within a specified time. Undue delay can lead to a complaint to the GMC.

What is often difficult to judge, but very important, is how easy it will be to comply with the later stages of the court's timetable. Most civil cases will not go to trial, but if they do, and the expert evidence is central and contentious rather than peripheral and largely agreed, a great deal of time may be necessary for reading further documents, re-reading documents, organising files and attending experts' meetings and conferences with counsel.

Information technology

The practice in the Commercial Court and High Court of providing the court with electronic copies of reports is now spreading to all courts with the increased use of modern technology. Be prepared for this but have safeguards in place so that reports cannot be amended by anyone else and make provision for encryption or password access as appropriate. I worked late one night on a report recommending a hospital order and fell asleep upon completion of it. The following day my registrar telephoned me to say that the magistrates had made the order but she asked if I had seen the signature page of my report. Underneath the signature block were the words: 'Goodnight Dad. Gone to bed'!

Commitments list

If you have not already been notified of when you may be required to give evidence in court, you may be notified after your report is received. Maintain and keep up to date a list of your forthcoming commitments and make this list available when requested. I make mine available on my website with a password that has to be obtained from my personal assistant. Free access to your commitment list may mean free access to your home by burglars when you are away.

The commitments list should include your holiday dates but perhaps not destinations. Otherwise an enterprising solicitor will identify a hotel with videoconferencing facilities and you will need to take a few lever-arch files in your holiday luggage and travel in the middle of the night to attend a conference with counsel or court by video-link.

The list should include the names of cases, the court and the instructing solicitors. This facilitates communication between solicitors if there is a potential clash. A few solicitors are embarrassed about issuing a witness summons and still consider it a discourtesy to issue one to a professional person. Most solicitors, though, like many experts, realise that it is the best way of securing the attendance of the expert and establishing priority or precedence if more than one is issued for the same period or if only one firm has done so at all. It is a contempt of court and you are liable to punishment if you do not attend in response to a witness summons. However, experts can challenge a witness summons. They can expect the solicitors and the courts to help to manage clashes where two or more summonses have been issued for the same date. Grounds for challenge include where the summons is for more time than the expert is likely to spend giving evidence. Some solicitors issue summonses, or ask experts to reserve dates, for the whole period of a trial, which is hardly ever appropriate.

Holidays

In *Matthews v Tarmac Bricks and Tiles Ltd* [2000] 54 BMLR 139, the case was fixed for a particular date but one of the doctors was on holiday abroad and the other was going to be in court in another town. Woolf MR noted that no request had been made to the doctor who was going on holiday to consider whether his holiday could be changed and he said:

It was very important that in cases where doctors were involved as much notice as possible was given for the date of the hearing. However, it was essential that it was appreciated that, whereas the courts would take account of the important commitments of medical men, they could not always meet those commitments in a way which would be satisfactory from the doctor's point of view. ...Doctors who held themselves out as practicing [*sic*] in the medico-legal field had to be prepared to arrange their affairs to meet the commitments of the courts where that was practical.

So, it looks like open season on doctors' holidays, but not so on judges' holidays: a circuit judge received some bad press when he would not start a rape trial because it was not going to end before his holiday, which was scheduled to begin with the opening of Wimbledon. HHJ Robert Taylor wrote in *The Times* (7 July 1999):

A holiday is for recreation, being deprived of which is not going to make people better judges. As an American Supreme Court Justice once said: 'I can do a year's work in 10 or 11 months – but not in 12!'

So, one rule for the doctors and another rule for the judges?

Staff care

An expert is only as good as his personal assistant or secretary. Ensure that he or she is adequately remunerated, has a comfortable office, all modern facilities and as generous terms and conditions as you expect for yourself. If income from medico-legal work is boosting your pension, you should have equally generous private pension provision for your staff.

Getting paid

Have a system for making sure that you get paid according to your agreed terms and conditions. If your instructing solicitors need credit, they should get it from a bank and not from you. As more and more firms of solicitors, and not just the small firms, go into administration owing individual experts hundreds or even thousands of pounds, it may be worth adopting the practice in the Republic of Ireland where experts do not send their report to the solicitor until they have received payment for it. Some experts use this practice when instructed by medical reporting organisations (agencies which obtain expert medical reports for solicitors), some of which, also, have also gone into administration owing experts a lot of money. Some experts send the report initially unsigned and in draft form and provide a signed, final version only upon receipt of payment.

Marketing

The key to marketing your services as an expert witness is to prepare reports and give testimony of such high quality that solicitors and barristers recommend you to other solicitors. It is useful to have an entry in at least one of the expert witness directories used by solicitors. In the age of the internet, your own website can be very useful. Mine is copyright but psychiatrists and other medical experts are welcome to use it as a model and copy contents subject to their own website including the following acknowledgment: 'Based on/adapted from the website designed by Chris Burgess for Dr Keith Rix (http://www.drkeithrix.co.uk)'.

Appraisal

For your annual appraisal, you should include feedback letters from solicitors, comments from judges and, if there are any, copies of law reports that refer to your evidence. In most cases these should be complimentary, but you must also disclose any adverse comment, however trivial or unjustified it seems. In particular, you must provide details and documentation relating to actual complaints made about you in your role as an expert.

Probity and compliance

Make sure that, as appropriate, your practice complies with data protection law and employment law, including employer liability law. Maintain and archive for the requisite period sufficiently detailed financial records for compliance with taxation laws and preparation of annual accounts by an accountant. It may be necessary to register for value added tax.

Keep a careful record of the time spent on the case (see Appendix 3). Like solicitors, I bill by six-minute units (that is, ten units per hour). In a long, complex or expensive case include the time spent on, for example, the various parts of a report. The more detail you provide on your invoice, the less likely it is that the fee will be queried or challenged. If, as may happen, the courts require more detailed estimates before agreeing to the instruction of the expert, collation of information from invoices in similar cases may assist.

A well-known psychiatrist was asked, at the opening of his cross-examination in a murder trial, how long he had spent with the prisoner. After he had replied, the QC reached down and lifted up a huge and heavy tome, with much huffing and puffing, and through the pages of which he slowly leafed, building up a sense of suspense, until he came to the date of the psychiatrist's visit to the prison. This was the prison's 'gate book', which recorded the time of the psychiatrist's arrival at, and the time of his departure from, the prison. Say no more!

Further reading

Bond, C., Solon, M., Harper, P., et al (2007) *The Expert Witness: A Practical Guide* (3rd edn). Shaw & Sons.

Pamplin, C. (2007) *Expert Witness Fees.* (United Kingdom Register of Expert Witnesses Little Book Series.) JS Publications.

Pamplin, C. (2010) Data protection and the expert. *Expert Witness Institute Newsletter,* autumn, 13–15.

Pamplin, C. (ed.) (for the UK Register of Expert Witnesses) (2011) *Expert Witness Year Book.* JS Publications.

CHAPTER 3

The medico-legal consultation

I must say that, as a litigant, I should dread a lawsuit beyond almost anything else, short of sickness or death. (Judge Learned Hand, quoted by Shapiro, 1993, p. 304)

In legal cases where medical issues arise, the medico-legal consultation lies at the heart of the process of assisting the court in the resolution of disputes and the administration of justice. It provides the psychiatrist with the opportunity to use her training, skill and experience to explore the subject's psychological complaints in the context of the family history, personal history, personality and medical history and to assess current mental state. Where the report is to be prepared without a personal consultation with the subject, the psychiatrist is reliant on the records made by others as to the subject's history and mental state.

The medico-legal consultation is an important and potentially stressful experience for subjects. It is very likely that the litigation itself is a major stress in their life. It may have dominated their life not just for weeks or months but sometimes for years. Their liberty, reputation, career or financial security may be at stake. They may have been waiting for the appointment for some time. They may have had to travel a long distance and suffered other inconvenience to get to the appointment. If you are seeing a prisoner in custody, however carefully your arrangements have been made, they may not be expecting you or they may have been wrongly informed as to who you are and the purpose of the visit. If you are instructed by 'the other side', they may be expecting a hostile consultation because they have been told to expect this, often by friends rather than their solicitor, or because they have seen another expert instructed by 'the other side' who has been abrupt or unsympathetic. It may be the first time that they have seen a psychiatrist. They may have various inappropriate expectations arising out of the popular misunderstanding of such practices as psychoanalysis, so-called 'sectioning' and electroconvulsive therapy (ECT). They may be afraid of the psychiatric label or angry that their solicitors have suggested that a psychiatric opinion is needed.

In short, the medico-legal consultation comprises history-taking and examination, supplemented where appropriate by tests or investigations and, if possible, information from an informant. It calls for the highest standards of psychiatric history-taking and mental state examination and it should be conducted with an awareness and understanding of the potential effects of the proceedings on the subject.

Arrangements for the consultation

Fix a date for the consultation and send out an 'appointment letter' (Appendix 4). The subject needs due notice, although sometimes it is necessary, usually for the subject's benefit, to arrange appointments at short notice. Take into account how far away the subject lives and, if appropriate, the complexity of the journey on different forms of public transport. Anyone travelling long distances by public transport will have difficulty attending appointments early in the day. In my experience parents in family proceedings are particularly likely to find travel difficult.

The appointment letter should include or enclose:
- the nature and purpose of the consultation
- the length of the consultation
- who has requested the consultation
- where, when and at what time the consultation will take place
- a request for details of any special requirements (such as a downstairs consulting room, an interpreter)
- any requirements as to proof of identity
- contact details sufficient to enable the appointment to be changed, a warning to be given of late arrival or for directions sought en route
- how to complain.

Include with the appointment letter travel directions, details of car parking arrangements and, if appropriate, information as to how and where refreshments may be obtained.

Appendix 5 sets out the information that I provide on my website to subjects of reports.

The essential ingredients

The essential ingredients of the medico-legal consultation are *courtesy, respect, sympathetic objectivity* and *patience*.

Courtesy

It is surprising how often subjects report that experts they have seen 'for the other side' have treated them unpleasantly, abruptly or condescendingly.

Respect

However distasteful or objectionable the behaviour the subject admits to or is alleged to have carried out, whatever your own views about the merits of the litigation, or however appalled you feel about a parent's behaviour towards a child, the subject is a fellow human. It is not for you to judge them and they are entitled to your respect.

Sympathetic objectivity

A sympathetic approach helps to build rapport and helps you to elicit a reliable history. The subject wants to know that someone is prepared to listen to them, to believe them and to try to understand what it feels like for them. But, sympathy has to be combined with objectivity. It is not necessary to believe everything that the subject says. It is a forensic investigation and the doctor's or psychiatrist's usual therapeutic objectives must almost always take second place to the requirement of the courts for evidence that assists in achieving the overriding principles of achieving justice and fairness.

Patience

Some people find it difficult enough describing their problems and history to any specialist. It may be even more difficult when it is a psychiatrist and the more so if it is the first time that they have seen one. Time and patience are needed for a history and examination that enable justice to be done. A hurried and inaccurate history is not in the subject's interests, it is not in the interests of justice and it is not in the interests of the expert, who may have this failing exposed in the witness box. The subject needs time, patience and often encouragement to tell their story.

The venue

Safety

Consider the venue carefully, having regard to safety issues. There has to be a reasonable balance between adhering to the safety measures that apply in a hospital emergency consultation room and providing an environment in which the subject feels as comfortable as possible. If you are using a consulting room, have an agreed method of summoning assistance. If you are seeing the person outside usual clinic hours, consider whether or not it is safe to do so or what special precautions need to be taken.

If you are seeing the subject in a prison or hospital, ask the staff whether or not you should see them on their own. It may be necessary for you to have a member of staff with you. If the hospital staff have personal safety alarms, ask if you can be provided with one. In prison, familiarise yourself with the arrangements for summoning help. On one occasion I had to use the senior medical officer's room and, in response to hearing the prison alarm, the prisoner and I rushed to the door with a view to offering assistance. There we collided with a posse of prison officers coming into the room. The senior medical officer had an alarm button underneath his desk and as I made the most of his office chair, which was on castors, I had accidentally pressed the button with my knee. A senior registrar in neurology, doing a prison clinic for his consultant, finished his first consultation and pressed the button on the wall to summon the next patient, with similar consequences.

Safety issues are particularly important if the subject is to be seen at their own home. If you do not know the area, discuss this with those instructing you and ask them if they would see the subject in their home. Consider taking someone with you. Make sure that a family member or friend knows the time and location of your consultation. Solicitors are often only too happy for you to see their client at their offices, regardless of which side has instructed you.

If you are going to see the subject in your own home, reconsider whether or not you should be doing this work. A retired consultant psychiatrist in Leeds was killed in his home by a former patient. His name was on a gate-post at the end of his drive. The patient had been looking first for another of his former consultants but he had moved.

The consulting room

So far as it is within your control, make the consulting room welcoming. Carpet, curtains and fresh flowers help. Sit on a chair identical to that of the subject or at least sit at the same level. If your consulting room is also an office, try to organise it so that, whatever else happens in the room at other times, the subject feels that they are your priority for the time you spend with them, that you were expecting them and you had prepared for their arrival. A box of paper tissues is essential and if the subject cannot bring in a hot beverage there should at least be water available.

Use of NHS or private facilities

The use of NHS or private facilities may need to be negotiated with managers or employers.

Be prepared

Chaperones and interpreters

Consider, and if necessary make, arrangements for an interpreter or chaperone. It is inadvisable to use family or friends of the subject as interpreters. Chaperoning may be necessary for physical examination, where there is a history of abuse, including abuse by professionals, where particular gender issues arise or in order to respect cultural conventions.

Security clearance and related requirements

If the subject is in prison custody, allow time for security clearance and compliance with requirements such as those relating to the use of a laptop computer. Pay attention to what you are not allowed to take into a prison. If you have to return several times to the visitors' centre to leave yet more items in your locker, do not be surprised if it is 'dinnertime' or 'teatime' shortly after, or even before, you get to the prisoner. Consider using a standard letter to the prison service requesting permission to use laptop (Appendix 6).

Timetabling

Ensure that sufficient time is available and consider whether or not more than one consultation may be needed. Have a means of contacting the subject in the event that the consultation is going to be delayed or postponed. Allow sufficient time to read the documents and records prior to the consultation, either a day or so ahead or just before the time the consultation is scheduled to start. How prepared you are will affect the subject's perception of you. The appointment should take place when you are unlikely to be interrupted or have to deal with something else but, if an interruption is expected, explain this to the subject at the beginning of the consultation. Try to make sure that the appointment starts on time. A delayed start may make the subject more anxious, give the impression that they are not important or cause them to rush as they think that they are not going to have enough time.

The consultation

Your professional demeanour

Before you go to fetch the subject from the reception or waiting area, or before someone brings them to your room, remind yourself that their solicitor may well ask the subject how you treated them. Cultivate an appropriate professional demeanour. Introduce yourself and find out how the subject wishes to be addressed.

Should anyone else be present?

In most cases, it is best to see the subject on their own. In some cases, indicated above, a chaperone may be advisable and in some cases the subject may be too nervous to be seen on their own. In one case, however, the Court of Appeal refused an application by a nervous subject to have a friend present (*Whitehead v Avon County Council* (1995) 29 BMLR 152 CA). What matters is that the subject should be sufficiently at ease to develop a rapport and give a reliable history. On the other hand, a subject may be inhibited from giving a full and frank history if a partner or friend is present. Experts who have allowed a family member to be present have sometimes been criticised in court on the basis that the history the expert reports may have come not from the subject but from the accompanying person, or may have been influenced by their presence or their non-verbal communication. Sometimes it is advisable to see the subject and accompanying person for the introductory part of the consultation and then, if the subject is willing, for the accompanying person to leave. There are exceptions. For example, in the assessment of severely brain-injured claimants, it is commonly regarded as essential to have either a family member or another familiar person present. Likewise, in the assessment of capacity, it may be necessary to establish what the claimant can achieve with the assistance of a family member, a friend or a professional who works with them.

If there is a third party present, seating should be arranged so that you can control communication.

Introducing yourself, and explaining and obtaining consent

Explain who you are, who has asked for the report, the nature of the consultation, the purpose of the consultation and the limits of confidentiality.

In order to disclose information about the subject to a third party you need express consent. This is respect for the subject's autonomy. Express consent does not have to be in writing but it helps if it is, especially if the subject later complains, for example, that something was not explained or that they did not know the purpose of the consultation. Create or adapt a 'written consent' form and have this ready for the beginning of the consultation (Appendix 7). A consent form can create a useful framework for explaining the nature and purpose of the consultation and obtaining express consent.

Experts in Scotland are advised to seek the subject's consent: (1) to carry out the interview; (2) to prepare the report; (3) to contact any other person for further information; and (4) to access relevant documents or records.

It should be made clear that the subject does not have to answer all or even any of the questions, although if they choose not to answer certain questions this may limit the usefulness of the report (but perhaps not significantly). The subject may disclose sensitive information, in which case it can be agreed to identify this as such in the report, but the subject needs to know that the solicitors and court may not be able to restrict circulation of this information. The subject needs to know that any information that is given 'off the record' will have to be divulged if the psychiatrist is ordered to do so by the court or, in any event, to prevent death or serious harm. If it is information that is relevant to your opinion, make this clear and state that you will not be able to deal with a particular issue unless the subject agrees to the information disclosure. In a family case, however, nothing is 'off the record': any information that is relevant must be disclosed.

Occasionally a subject may not be able to consent and they may lack the capacity to do so. In a criminal case, this may be someone who is unfit to plead and stand trial. In a civil case, it may be a brain-injured claimant who lacks the capacity to litigate in their own right. In such a case, it may be in the subject's best interests to prepare a report without their consent. This should be justified in the report. Guidance as to working out 'best interests' is provided in the Mental Capacity Act 2005 (MCA) and its accompanying Code of Practice. It may be that you have to consult with others, such as carers or relatives, before deciding whether to proceed in an incapacitated individual's best interests.

History-taking and examination

It is probably sensible not to discuss the alleged offence or the cause of the action (that is, an accident or allegedly negligent treatment) at the beginning. In a criminal case, it is a good idea to take the whole history prior to the alleged offence and then ask, if appropriate, about the alleged offence. In a personal injury case, it is a good idea to take a family history, personal history and medical history prior to the accident or allegedly negligent treatment and then ask about the incident or circumstances giving rise to the personal injury action. In a criminal case, the subject's history between the alleged offence and the consultation must be distinguished from the history prior to the alleged offence.

In a personal injury case, the subject's history subsequent to the accident or allegedly negligent treatment will be of critical significance, but it will need to be considered against the background of the subject's history up to the potentially injurious event or events and compared with what the person's personal and medical history might have been if the accident or allegedly negligent treatment had not occurred.

Sometimes subjects attempt to dismiss any enquiry as to their life prior to the alleged offence or the accident. It may be helpful to explain that the expert needs to understand them as a person: in a civil action, their unique reaction to a traumatic event may be more, or only, understandable in the light of their history prior to the accident; and in a criminal case, their life up to the alleged offence may assist in understanding why they acted as they did. Also, in many civil cases, it is helpful to explain that in order to give an opinion as to the effects of the accident on how the subject copes with life, relationships, employment and social functioning, it is necessary to understand what their life was like before the accident. Additionally, such a detailed history is essential for choosing between treatment options, determining the likely response to treatment and giving an overall prognosis.

What the psychiatrist is best placed to do is to obtain a detailed and accurate history of psychological or psychiatric symptoms. This often includes a painstakingly detailed account of an event, or series of events, such as a criminal offence or a road traffic accident, and its effects. It is this part of the psychiatrist's report which is likely to be analysed in depth by the lawyers and compared with the account given to the other side's psychiatrist, perhaps accounts given to other experts, the contents of the medical records or police interviews, and the subject's proof of evidence or witness statement. It takes time to obtain such an account.

A mental state examination is mandatory. This may need to include extended cognitive testing. It starts when you collect the subject from the waiting room and it finishes when you return them to the waiting room. For some neurologists, the examination ends when they have observed the claimant, from behind the curtains of their upstairs consulting room, making their way down their long drive to the road.

Certain investigations may be indicated. It may be appropriate to use particular rating scales and questionnaires, although their interpretation and validity in the medico-legal context may be questioned, as they are unlikely to have been validated in that context, where they are even more prone to bias than in ordinary clinical practice. They should not be confused with screening instruments, favoured much more by psychologists than psychiatrists, which can be used to alert the expert to the need to look in detail at particular areas. However, a thorough psychiatric assessment should reveal the presence of any significant psychiatric disorder. It is therefore arguable that the use of screening instruments should be unnecessary and indeed in some cases their use may be counterproductive if they suggest psychopathology about which the expert is subsequently going to enquire.

A history from an informant

It is often helpful and sometimes advisable to obtain a history from an informant. It is often useful to hear about the impact of the subject's condition from the person who may know them best, albeit they are not likely to be a disinterested party. It provides a check on the accuracy of what the subject says. This is not just about being alert to exaggeration. Especially in the case of a person with a brain injury, dementia, an intellectual disability, memory problems, lack of insight, confabulation, slow information processing, and so on, it can be easy to underestimate or misunderstand the degree of handicap or disability unless a history is additionally obtained from an informant.

Records

The consultation should be recorded on paper or electronically and be structured, clear, legible and comprehensive so that it can be studied by another expert, who should be readily able to see why and how certain opinions have been reached. If it is disclosed, however good your handwriting, expect counsel or the judge to make a joke about doctors' handwriting. Record the times of the start and finish of the consultation.

Further enquiries

You should not hesitate to recommend a further consultation, ask for other records or obtain more evidence if, without this, you will have to express only a provisional or qualified opinion. Occasionally it may be necessary to recommend the instruction of another expert.

CHAPTER 4

The structure, organisation and content of the generic report

[A] well constructed expert's report containing opinion evidence sets out the expert's opinion and the reasons for it. If the reasons stand up, the opinion does. If not, not. (Jacob J in *Pearce v Ove Arup Partnership Ltd* (2002) 25(2) IPD 25011)

The purpose of the report is to communicate your opinion so as to assist the court in reaching conclusions on matters in issue and to enable it to do so justly. Aim it at the intelligent professional with no medical knowledge. Make it easy to understand and easy to follow. Spare a thought for the bored, tired judge, one who is past his 'sell-by date' or any judge presiding over the afternoon 'graveyard' slot. Especially when it is going to be the basis of evidence before a jury, it has to tell a story that the jury can understand, and hold their interest. As the jury rarely sees the report itself, you will have the opportunity to précis the report in language suitable for the jury when you give your evidence.

Consider using a model form. The models produced by the Academy of Experts and the Expert Witness Institute have been approved by judges and, although many reports will not be read by judges, it is in cases that go to trial that the 'judge-friendly' format may be critical. Whether or not the report is used in court, readers are going to be assisted if the report is easy to navigate and is easily compared with other reports because they are similar in format.

For valid reasons, perhaps depending on the nature of the case or the nature of the instructions, or to meet the requirements of a particular jurisdiction, it may be appropriate to depart from the model format. This may be necessary, for example, in reports for sentencing in criminal cases (p. 104).

See Appendix 11 for a specimen criminal report, on the case of Daniel McNaughtan, laid out according to the Academy of Experts and Expert Witness Institute model form.

Length of the report

Not many psychiatrists remember the days when it was said that a report should be no more than two pages of foolscap. Today's reports are much longer but this may change. Increased control by judges over expenditure on expert reports may lead to experts' fees being reduced if their reports are considered to be too long. Judges prefer shorter reports. As one said, quoting a Spanish saying, 'Something good, if it is short, is twice as good'. Judges say that they have little time to read and digest reports. They look for findings and conclusions. Some suggest that the facts, or assumed facts, which justify the conclusions, but which counsel need for examination and cross-examination, can be confined to appendices.

Basic requirements of the report

The points of presentation, content and style that are preferred (if not mandated) by the courts are set out in Box 7. If it is not the first report, it should state: 'Second report of...'. Remember that the report will probably become part of a trial bundle, perhaps in a lever-arch file, and when looking for a document, or a page in a document, most people flick through the bottoms of pages.

Structure of the report

Box 8 shows a suggested structure.

Front page

The *front page* contains key information.
 The top section shows:
- the name of the court top left (e.g. 'In the Central Criminal Court')
- the case number top right
- the title of the action (name of the case) below and central (e.g. *R v Daniel McNaughtan*).

The second section identifies the author of the report (e.g. 'Report of Dr E. T. Monro, Consultant Psychiatrist'). This section may be omitted and incorporated in the fourth section but it must stand out somewhere on the front page. I once saw a report which was signed illegibly and nowhere in the report was the name of its author.
 The third section should include:
- 'On the instructions of' – name and address of those instructing the expert
- 'Who act on behalf of' – person or party, such as 'The defendant'
- 'Their reference'
- 'Specialist field' – e.g. 'Child and adolescent psychiatry'
- 'Subject matter' – e.g. 'Psychiatric examination of the Defendant'
- 'Date of report' (often missing!)
- 'Report reference'

Box 7 Presentation and style of the report

- Typed
- First person
- Short sentences and paragraphs
- Headings and subheadings
- Fact distinguished and separated from opinion
- Clear, concise, succinct, objective, reliable and of high quality
- Straightforward and not biased, intentionally misleading or false
- Not promoting the view of the instructing party or advocacy
- Not omitting material or information that does not support the opinion expressed or conclusions reached
- The product of an independent investigator, regardless of the pressures of the litigation
- Showing the weaknesses as well as the strengths of the case
- Properly and fully researched
- A 'stand-alone' document
- Good quality paper
- Margins wide enough for written comments – at least 5 cm
- Font size 11
- Arial typeface
- Line spacing 1.5 (saves paper) or 2
- Numbered paragraphs
- Paper hole-punched for use in a standard lever-arch file or ring-binder
- Presented in a slide binder (because it allows the report to be removed for copying – avoid comb-binders, staples and paperclips)
- Plastic covers
- Front cover clear so that the title page can be read without opening the folder
- Report printed on one side of the page only
- Use of 'headers' and 'footers'

The header zone (on all pages except the front page) should set out at the right:

Report of: Dr E. T. Monro
Specialism: Psychiatry
On the instructions of: Monteith and Company
Prepared for: The Central Criminal Court

The footer zone should feature:

- the title of the action
- the name of the subject of the report (who may not always be a party to the action)
- your name, in the format 'Report of Dr E. T. Monro'
- the date of the report
- page number in the bottom right corner (on all pages including appendices but except the front page).

Box 8 The structure of the report

Front page
Contents page
1   Introduction
   1.1   The writer
   1.2   Synopsis
   1.3   Instructions
  (1.4   Summary of conclusions/Executive summary)*
   1.5   Disclosure of interests
2   The background to the case and issues
   2.1   The relevant parties
   2.2   The assumed facts and substance of all material instructions
   2.3   The issues to be addressed
   2.4   The assumptions adopted
3   Investigation of the facts and assumed facts
   3.1   Methodology
   3.2   Interview and examination/Basis of report
   3.3   Investigations
   3.4   Documents and materials
   3.5   Medical terms and explanations
4   The facts and assumed facts
5   Opinion
6   Summary of conclusions
7   Declaration
8   Statement of truth
Signature block
Appendix 1: qualifications and experience of the writer
Appendix 2: Documents and materials studied
(Appendix 3: Publications and authorities)*
Appendix 4: Glossary of medical and other terms

Sometimes omitted

- 'Date of examination'
- 'Place of examination'
- 'Consent' – 'Written', 'Verbal' or 'Not applicable'.
  The fourth section should include:
- name of expert
- status/appointment
- academic and professional qualifications;
- GMC number

- contact details, including:
  - full professional/correspondence address
  - telephone number(s)
  - fax number
  - email address
  - perhaps also name of secretary/personal assistant (including their email address and telephone number if different).

Contents page

The list of contents helps readers to navigate their way round the report. How detailed it is will depend on the report's length and complexity. Only in very short reports is it unnecessary.

Introduction

The first section is 'The writer'. Briefly introduce yourself just enough to orientate the reader, as your full details are in Appendix 1 of the report:

I am John Monro, a licensed and registered medical practitioner approved under section 12 of the Mental Health Act 1983 (as amended by the Mental Health Act 2007) and registered with the General Medical Council as a specialist in general psychiatry according to the provisions of Schedule 2 of the European Specialist Medical Qualifications Order 1995. Full details of my qualifications and experience entitling me to give expert opinion evidence are in Appendix 1.

The second section is 'Synopsis'. Set out concisely the general nature of the case: 'Daniel McNaughtan ("the Defendant") is charged with the murder of Edward Drummond, private secretary to the Prime Minister, and there is an issue as to the Defendant's mental state'.

The third section is 'Instructions'. It overlaps with 'The assumed facts and substance of all material instructions' (see p. 40) and makes it clear at whose request the report has been prepared. It can be very brief: 'I have been instructed by the Defendant's solicitors to examine him and prepare a psychiatric report for use at his trial'.

The fourth section (unless there is an executive summary or summary of conclusions – see p. 50) is 'Disclosure of interests'. Either state any actual or potential conflict of interest or personal interest, such as connections with any of the parties or witnesses, which might be considered as influencing your opinions, or state that there are none. Make it clear that you do not consider that any interest disclosed affects your suitability as an expert witness on any issue on which you have given opinion evidence. Confirm that you will advise those instructing you if, between the date of the report and the final hearing, there is any change in circumstances which affects these statements. It is particularly important to make it clear if you have treated the subject of the report in the past or are currently treating the subject. In *Vernon v Bosley* [1997] 1 All ER 577, CA, Thorpe LJ observed that 'In the field of psychiatry it may be more difficult for those who have treated the plaintiff (claimant) to approach the case with true objectivity. That was certainly the case here'. However, some solicitors and counsel prefer to have the treating clinician provide the expert report. Braithwaite & Waldron (2010) do not agree that there is any principle that the treating doctor cannot prepare a report for the purpose of litigation and point out that 'the treating doctor is likely to know far more about the patient than an outsider who has seen the patient for a few minutes or an hour or two' (p. 128). In the Republic of Ireland it is normal practice for the treating doctor to prepare the report for litigation.

The background to the case and issues

The first section is 'The relevant parties' and is often limited to the name of the defendant in a criminal case or the names of the claimant and defendant(s) in a civil case. In most cases it probably adds nothing and can be omitted. It is of use in a complex case, such as a case of allegedly negligent psychiatric care, where it is a list of the staff, patient, family members, and so on who feature in your narrative account, like a *dramatis personae*, for example 'Dr Alexander Morison – on-call senior house officer'. Sometimes in a criminal case it is helpful to list the key witnesses who feature in your narrative account, such as 'Mary Ferrers, estranged wife of the Defendant'.

Second is 'The assumed facts and substance of all material instructions'. This is a background narrative of the facts provided by the instructing party. Include any information given orally, for example by telephone. Usually, it is based on the letter of instruction. Although some experts attach a copy of the letter of instruction, it is legally privileged and its inclusion needs the approval of the instructing party. Usually it is not disclosed, but if there is reason to believe that the statement of the substance of the instructions is inaccurate or incomplete, or you have misled the court as to the substance of your material instructions, the court can order disclosure and allow cross-examination on the matter.

Third is 'The issues to be addressed'. This is a list that corresponds closely, if not entirely, to the letter of instruction. It reminds you not to waste time and money and incur criticism for dealing with matters other than those material to the issues before the court, however interesting or important they appear to you. If you think that another matter or matters should be addressed, write to those instructing you. In order to avoid question or criticism about matters on which you have not expressed an opinion, consider a footnote along the lines: 'Unless I have indicated otherwise, these are the only matters I have been asked to address. The absence of an opinion on a particular issue does not mean that I have no opinion on the issue. It means only that I have not been asked to address the issue.'

In many cases, it is useful for this section of the report to include a statement of the relevant law as understood by the psychiatrist. This is not the psychiatrist proclaiming expertise about the law. It is an indication that the psychiatrist knows the relevant legal tests. Of course, sometimes you may get it wrong but this then provides the opportunity for the instructing solicitor to give you the correct legal test and for the opinion to be adjusted accordingly.

If any issue falls outside your expertise, make it clear, although your instructing party should already have been informed.

'The assumptions adopted' is the fourth section. In a psychiatric report, this may be the assumptions that what the subject has said is true and that the contents of the medical records are accurate unless otherwise indicated. If you have made such assumptions or any other assumptions as to facts or made any deductions from factual assumptions, make this clear. Occasionally you are asked to adopt an assumption. Set this out fully. If it is unreasonable or unlikely, make this clear.

Be careful because in cross-examination 'probably the most useful grounds that [counsel] can focus on are the validity and merits of any assumptions applied by the expert' (Smethurst, 2006).

Investigation (of facts and assumed facts)

The purpose of this part of the report is to explain how the expert opinion has been reached. Some readers may not know, or may misunderstand, how a psychiatrist works.

The first section is 'Methodology'. This may become particularly important if the Law Commission's proposals on the determination of evidentiary reliability are implemented (Law Commission, 2011) (see p. 3). It may, however, in the meantime, be wise, if not necessary, to indicate that clinical practice, including psychiatric practice, depends partly on knowledge for which there is a sound scientific evidence base and partly on experience-based knowledge which has stood the test of time but lacks a robust foundation in the rigorous research that now forms the basis of 'evidence-based medicine'. Indicate that, in relying on both categories of knowledge, you have done so in accordance with what would be regarded as a responsible body of psychiatric practice.

Thus, in this section, explain how the diagnosis has been reached, explain how, for example in a personal injury case, the opinion on causation has been reached, explain how the particular prognosis has been reached and explain why you recommend particular treatment or have commented, as you might do, on the treatment already given.

Particularly in relation to treatment in family cases it is now common practice to ask that recommendations for treatment comply with guidelines produced by the National Institute for Health and Clinical Excellence (NICE). This is not always going to be possible. Thus, it may be necessary to point out that you have relied on approaches that have wide acceptance by psychiatrists and, where possible, given weight to treatments for which there is the strongest evidence base with regard to effectiveness and safety. However, as in medicine in general, there are many treatments that are accepted as effective but for which there have not been trials that satisfy the most stringent criteria of evidence-based medicine or which have not been endorsed by NICE.

Already in family cases, you have to describe your own professional risk assessment process and the process of differential diagnosis. Other courts may soon expect this. The key is transparency. Where the report involves risk assessment, indicate its limitations (Royal College of Psychiatrists, 2008c).

Under 'Interview and examination', set out the details of the consultation. Say whether anyone else was present, and if so, what part, if any, they took *during* the consultation. State that, unless otherwise indicated, the history is that obtained from the subject of the report *at the consultation*. It is hearsay, which will either be admitted (without being proved) or may have to be proved (see p. 45).

Refer to any particular circumstances of the consultation, such as the place, time and any constraints, for example inadequate time to complete the assessment owing to prison routine, or the potentially inhibiting effect of someone else being present, such as a police or prison officer or a partner or care worker.

If a trainee has assisted you, name them and cross-refer to an extra appendix that gives details of their qualifications, training and experience.

Make it clear at this point (reflecting the wording in the 'Statement of truth') that, unless otherwise indicated, the only facts within your own knowledge are your findings on examination of the subject.

If an informant has been interviewed, identify them and explain this. In family cases it is assumed that the opinion will be based on collateral information as well as the interview with the subject, and in reports for sentencing in criminal cases it is expected that a history and information will be obtained from members of the defendant's family.

Occasionally reports are prepared without consulting with the subject, because:

- the subject is dead
- the court has ordered it
- the subject has consented to this.

If so, modify this section and head it 'Basis of report', and make it clear that the report is based on a study of records only, why this is so, and indicate any limitations this may create. Justify the decision to proceed on such a basis. Indicate a willingness to reconsider your opinion following a consultation.

If someone, such as a psychologist, has carried out testing, they should be identified under 'Investigations', with a cross-reference to an appendix which sets out their qualifications, relevant experience and accreditation. State whether or not you supervised the testing. Experiences of asking psychologists to allow you to supervise their testing will make an interesting paper for *The Psychiatrist* or, more controversially, for *Clinical Psychology Forum*!

Under 'Documents and materials' refer to Appendix 2 of the report, in which documentary and other evidence is listed, such as audiotapes, DVDs and photographic exhibits. Some counsel and solicitors hold that all documents and materials should be listed. Other counsel and solicitors hold that if you list everything, the other side is entitled to see all of the material and so you should not refer to documents that your instructing solicitors do not intend to disclose for the time being, such as draft witness statements in a civil case, a draft proof of evidence in a criminal case or a report on liability and causation in a medical negligence case (see p. 126) because, if they are listed, the other side will be entitled to see them. The actual test is whether or not the other side needs to read the document in order to understand your opinion or if you have used that document as a significant part of the process of forming your opinion. In an application for disclosure of a document or report, it is likely that the other side will succeed if you have seen it and relied on it but not if you have seen it, read it and definitely not relied on it. An application for disclosure may also succeed in the unlikely event that there is some reason to believe that there is something inaccurate or misleading about your statement of the instructions you have received.

If documents are missing, illegible or incomplete, point this out. Be prepared for a judge to criticise you for not having made more effort to obtain documents or even to get the illegible handwriting of general practitioners transcribed.

Identify materials that have not been produced with the report; these may be, for example, original medical or other professional records, or an instruction from a party. Be prepared to reveal everything.

If important documents have not been supplied or obtained, say so and explain why they have not been obtained. Make a list of these and indicate why they are important. Make it clear why and how information from such documents may make a material difference to your opinion.

All documents and materials need to be retained at least until the case has gone to trial and some need to be retained in the event of an appeal. Box 9 presents a guide to retention in criminal cases. Except in criminal cases, where records must be retained for more than six years, a sensible guide is to retain documents for six years because this is the period during which, other than exceptionally, the GMC will investigate a complaint against a medical practitioner and it is the limitation period for a case of alleged professional negligence. The clock starts when the case is discontinued or concluded.

If you rely on published or unpublished research or other authoritative material, state that under 'Research' or 'Authorities' and cross-refer to Appendix 3 of the report, a list of the published and unpublished works. Supply copies or extracts, with sufficient pages from before and after the extract for it to be seen in context. If you have not included descriptions from ICD-10 or DSM-IV- TR™ in the glossary, they can go in Appendix 3.

Box 9 Retention requirements for records in criminal cases

- Cases involving homicide, riot, Official Secrets Acts, treason and other offences against the state, terrorist offences, schedule 1 offenders, kidnapping and all cases in which a sentence of life imprisonment has been imposed: 20 years
- Other criminal cases tried on indictment: 10 years
- All cases tried summarily: 1 year
- All other criminal cases: 1 year

These times are from the date on which the court or tribunal finally disposed of the case.

A reference to 'Medical terms and explanations' can either be included in this part of the report or it can go at the end of the Introduction. Explain that any medical or technical terms will be highlighted, for example **emboldened**, and included in a glossary that appears as Appendix 4 of the report. Some experts also give a definition or explanation as a footnote whenever a medical term is first used. The glossary may include symptoms, signs, diagnoses, drug names, forms of treatment, Mental Health Act provisions and definitions of grades such as 'specialist registrar' and 'staff grade psychiatrist'.

The facts and assumed facts

So far you should not have expressed any opinion. Similarly, in this section there should be no opinion – not even a snippet. If you need to comment, do so in parentheses and follow the comment with your initials.

This section sets out facts and assumed facts. Your opinion is only as strong as the facts upon which it is based.

Usually the only facts about which you can testify are your findings on mental state or physical examination. All the rest of the information with which you are provided, such as what the subject of the report or any informant tells you and what the witnesses say, are assumed facts, which may or may not be agreed between the parties or proved in evidence. Remember that the judge or the jury decides the facts and:

Where an expert relies on the existence or non-existence of some fact which is basic to the question on which he is asked to express his opinion that fact must be proved by admissible evidence. (*R v Abadom* [1983] 1 All ER 364)

The corollary of this is that:

If the doctor's evidence is based entirely on hearsay and is not supported by direct evidence, the judge will be justified in telling the jury that the defendant's case ... is based on a flimsy or non-existent foundation. (*R v Bradshaw* (1985) 82 Cr App R 79)

Hearsay, or 'second-hand' evidence, is evidence by one person of the evidence of another and statements in documents that are offered to prove the truth of what is written. The general rule is against the admission of hearsay evidence. The main reason why it is inadmissible is that the original statement was not given under oath and its reliability cannot be tested by examination, cross-examination and re-examination of the person who made it (verbally or in a document). However, there are statutory and common law exceptions to the exclusion of hearsay evidence and these are known as 'admissible hearsay assertions'. Thus, in civil cases most hearsay statements are admissible and medical records are admissible as evidence of the facts stated in them. In criminal cases, under s.114 of the Criminal Justice Act 2003 (CJA 2003), hearsay is admissible if there is a statutory provision for it to be admitted, if there is a common law exception to its inadmissibility, if all the parties agree or if its admission is in the interests of justice. Where psychiatrists give evidence as to the condition of a person, they can report the symptoms they have elicited and rely on these symptoms to explain the diagnosis they have reached, but if the existence of these symptoms is in issue, they must be proved by admissible evidence. Likewise, although medical records are admissible in evidence, they are evidence only that the patient reported a particular symptom or a doctor observed a particular sign. If there is an issue as to whether or not the patient had that symptom or indeed whether or not the doctor did observe a particular sign, the symptom or sign will have to be proved by admissible evidence.

You can assume a fact, for example that prior to an alleged offence the defendant had been sleeping for only about three hours a night, but the jury will decide whether or not to accept this as true. You can assume it to be true that a claimant in a personal injury case has completely lost interest in football but later covert surveillance may challenge this assumption. So these are 'assumed facts'.

Usually the only 'facts' to which you can testify are your findings on examination, for example that the subject sat in a downcast posture, made little eye contact, did not laugh or smile, was intermittently tearful, was slow to respond to questions and gave minimal responses. The tribunal of fact is likely, but not bound, to accept this as a depressive mental state, but this will depend on your expert interpretation of the facts. Separate headings are needed to distinguish the history (assumed facts) and the mental state/psychiatric examination (facts).

Where you rely on assumed facts outside your knowledge, identify the source, preferably with the appropriate page number if there is one.

In this section you are likely to set out assumed facts which are not otherwise within the knowledge of the court, specifically the contents of medical records and, at least to some extent, the history you have obtained from the subject. Some experts, barristers and judges, however, prefer these to be in an appendix.

There should be an account of the subject's background history. Views differ as to how detailed this should be. One school of thought is that this should be a full and detailed account of family history, personal history and personality, like that documented by psychiatrists at the beginning of an episode of psychiatric care. This school believes that this is necessary in order to bring the subject of the report alive and to show that all potentially relevant aspects of the history have been considered. Another school of thought is that this section should be very brief and limited to that information which is necessary in order to demonstrate, and allow reference to, the evidence base for the opinions reached. Thus, no more confidential information is revealed than is necessary and the report is much shorter.

There should be a separate account of the subject's medical history.

Usually, relevant information from the medical records should be set out under 'Medical history as taken from medical records' and not combined with 'Medical history as given by the defendant/claimant'. If much depends on the comparison of the subject's account with the documented history or if it would otherwise be difficult to convey the relevant chronology, they can be integrated, but only so long as the two sources of information can be distinguished.

Usually, information from medical records is set out chronologically, with information from general practitioner and specialist records integrated. Wherever possible, identify sources of information by page number. With a computerised word-processing package, there is no excuse for setting out the information from the medical records in the same haphazard way in which documents have been filed and entries made on the general practice or hospital computer. It is sometimes argued that, in the absence of paginated records, finding the source documents is easier if the notes are reviewed in the order in which they have been supplied, but the overriding consideration should be to set out the material so as to assist the reader in understanding the case.

A section here should summarise the findings of any investigations you have carried out or caused to be carried out; the details should go in an appendix.

In this part of the report, where you rely on the opinions of other experts, such as a neurologist, make this clear so that their opinion is one of your assumed facts.

The guiding principle is that different types of fact must be identified and distinguished. This is usually achieved through the use of headings and, in particular, by separating what the subject has told you from what others have said or is in other documentary sources. It can be confusing if the reader cannot distinguish between what, for example, the defendant told you about their state of mind at the material time, what they told the police when interviewed and what they told another expert at a different time. If these are different accounts, the court may have to decide how much weight to attach to each one. However, if, for example in a case of alleged negligence, where a detailed chronology needs to integrate what staff recorded at the time and what they subsequently say they did at the time, a different type can be used, such as ordinary type for what is in the contemporaneous records and italic type for information taken from their witness statements or the evidence they gave at the inquest.

This section should usually end with an account of the mental state examination or psychiatric examination.

This section is the launch-pad for the 'Opinion'. The reader will need to see how each and every opinion can be properly deduced from the facts in this section, supplemented, if appropriate, by facts in the material instructions.

Be sure to have included all material facts. Do not deliberately leave out relevant information, for example material that is inconsistent with, or does not support, your opinion. You must not mislead by omission.

What the court expects from you is an objective, independent, well-researched, thorough opinion, which takes account of all relevant information and which represents your genuine professional view on the issues submitted to you. (Wall, 2007, p. 29)

Opinion

The framework for this section is 'Issues to be addressed'. Each issue, or question, becomes a heading. This way you make sure that you address the questions asked. Under each, state your conclusion and show how this properly derives from the facts, but try to avoid their repetition. You want the reader to accept your conclusion, so the important word will be 'because'; the conclusion or opinion has to be reasoned:

What really matters in most cases is the reasons given for the opinion. (*Routestone Ltd v Minories Finance Ltd* [1997] BCC 180)

The opinion has to be objectively sound and genuinely held.

Try setting out the opinion on the issue or the answer to the question as a short, stand-alone sentence (as I was taught to do by Dr Stephen Hart when I last attended risk assessment training by Northern Networking). Follow this by one or more sentences of argument and reasoning. Try to have just one such paragraph for each question or issue. When you produce your 'Summary of conclusions' (see below), this will then comprise the opening sentence from each paragraph in the 'Opinion'.

Highlight the strengths of your arguments but also set out any material facts or matters that might undermine, or detract from, your opinion and any points that should fairly be made against it. Explain why they do not affect your opinion. Identify any unusual, contradictory or inconsistent features of the case. Take into consideration any relevant factors arising from ethnic, cultural, social, religious or linguistic contexts at the time the opinion is expressed.

It must be a balanced opinion. The use of a balance sheet listing factors that support or undermine the opinion can assist greatly.

Avoid being dogmatic or using extreme forms of expression. Avoid wording that might be regarded as pejorative or pre-judgmental.

Where there is a range of reasonable opinion, summarise that range and give reasons for your own opinion. Imagine the subject being presented at a case conference and imagine the most extreme views of your reasonable colleagues. Also, consider the views of your unreasonable colleagues, as occasionally they may be instructed as experts. In particular, if you have seen the other expert's report, comment briefly on that opinion and explain why, if it be so, you do not accept it. If you have not seen that report, try to anticipate what might be said in it. This is not about getting into an adversarial frame of mind; it is about providing the court with as much information as possible to allow the court to choose between competing opinions.

Where there is a conflict of factual evidence, set out alternative opinions based on the different factual scenarios. Do not express a preference for a particular scenario unless it depends on the application of psychiatric expertise. For example, there may be an inconsistency between the subject's reported symptoms and evidence from other sources which would not be obvious other than to a psychiatrist.

Be careful not to answer questions that have not been asked, although sometimes you may be invited to offer an opinion on any other matters you consider relevant. If properly instructed, you will have been asked to deal only with matters that are in issue in the case. If you waste time and money on matters that are not in issue, you may not be paid, or at least not in full.

One significant exception is where the set of questions does not call for an actual diagnosis. In such an instance, it is reasonable to set out this first and as the basis from which some of the other opinions will be derived. Or it may be that a separate condition has intervened, which those instructing you may not know about or understand, that potentially changes the course of the case.

Another significant exception is where the subject is not having treatment they ought to have. Whether asked to do so or not, make a recommendation for treatment that accords with the best practice of psychiatry, ask that this recommendation is passed to the subject's ordinary medical attendant and ask to be informed that this has been done (see Appendix 8). If the instructing party, for whatever reason, does not pass on the recommendation, seek legal advice as to whether or not you should communicate the recommendation directly. Beneficence may override your duty of confidentiality to those instructing you. Beware of writing to the subject's general practitioner. If you do so, and if time permits, discuss this with your instructing solicitor; be careful not to include any privileged information in your communication with the general practitioner and send a copy of any letter to your instructing solicitor.

If advancing a proposition, make clear whether it is a hypothesis, especially if it is controversial, or an opinion deduced in accordance with peer-reviewed and peer-tested technique, research and experience accepted as a consensus in the professional psychiatric community.

Do not to usurp the role of the judge, jury or coroner. Experts have been warned that:

they should restrict themselves to questions of fact, diagnosis and opinion, refraining from argument or the expression of views which appear to usurp the function of the court. (*Re LM (Reporting Restrictions: Coroner's Inquest)* (2007) EWHC 1902 (Fam)

The coroner will decide if it was suicide. The judge will decide if the defendant hospital trust was negligent. The jury will decide the defendant's guilt. This does not mean that you cannot give an opinion on the ultimate issue. Indeed, in a civil case the judge will want your opinion on whether or not the trust's psychiatrist exercised the ordinary skill of an ordinary competent psychiatrist. Under s.3(1) of the Civil Evidence Act 1972:

where a person is called as a witness in any civil proceedings his opinion on any relevant matter on which he is qualified to give expert evidence shall be admissible in evidence.

So there is no need, as the judge stated in *Routestone Ltd v Minories Finance Ltd* [1997] BCC 180, to 'simply creep up to the opinion without giving it'. Indeed, in a criminal case the judge will want you to tell the jury whether or not the defendant was insane according to the 'M'Naghten Rules' (*M'Naghten's Case* (1843) 10 Cl & F 200).

Make it clear if this is not a final opinion. If it is provisional or qualified this must be clear. Perhaps critical records remain to be obtained. Perhaps account needs to be taken of the opinion of another expert who has not yet reported. If appropriate, suggest the instruction of another expert who will bring expertise not possessed by those already involved. Rarely, be prepared to recommend a second opinion on a key issue.

Before you have concluded your opinion, ask yourself if you have satisfied the test of independence:

The area of expertise in any case may be likened to a broad street with the plaintiff walking on one pavement and the defendant on the opposite one. Somehow the expert must be ever mindful of the need to walk straight down the middle of the road and resist the temptation to join the party from whom his instructions come on the pavement. (Thorpe LJ in *Vernon v Bosley* [1997] 1 All ER 577, CA)

Summary of conclusions

Finally, set out a summary of the conclusions. I was taught that the summary should go at the beginning so that if judges could not be bothered to read the whole report, at least they would read the conclusions. But there are occasions when the judge will not need to read more than the conclusions in order to keep the case moving, such as when a case is for 'mention only', which means that the judge is dealing mainly with procedural aspects.

In a civil case, the summary has to be at the end of the report. Occasionally, in a complex case, it may assist to add an executive summary in the Introduction. It orientates the reader. If there is no requirement for the summary to be at the end, many experts prefer it at the beginning. Where it has to be at the end, there is no reason why it should not also be at the beginning, but, if so, point this out.

Declaration

Reports in criminal, civil and family proceedings require a declaration that the expert understands and has complied with their duty to the court. The minimum content of these is set out in the appropriate chapters.

Statement of truth

Reports in criminal, civil and family proceedings also require a statement of truth. These are also set out in the appropriate chapters.

Signature block

After the body of the report comes the signature block. The date of the report can be added.

After-thoughts

If you change your opinion on any material matter subsequently, you should, without delay, notify those instructing you and advise the reason. In a criminal case, if the report has been disclosed, inform all parties and the court. An undertaking to do so can be included in your Declaration. If the instructing party fails to disclose the change of an opinion already disclosed, inform the court but seek legal advice as well.

Appendices

Appendix 1 of the report sets out, preferably in no more than a page, your qualifications, relevant experience and, if any, accreditation, in three sections:
- academic and professional qualifications in full
- your clinical training and experience in psychiatry, ending with your present appointment(s) and any current positions of responsibility in, or related to, the profession
- details of research and publications.

Tailor this appendix to the case so that it is clear why it is appropriate for you to give expert evidence. Remember that if the case goes to trial it may be the basis on which your expertise is compared with that of the other side's expert. It may be used for the barristers to play the game 'My expert's better qualified than your expert', but, if your qualifications and experience do not seem to be as impressive as those of the other side's expert, remember that this is not necessarily going to be determinative.

Even in a case where your opinion is unopposed but forms the basis of oral testimony, this appendix will be the basis on which counsel for the side that has instructed you will seek to persuade the judge or jury to accept your evidence.

Appendix 2 lists the documents and other materials provided.

Appendix 3 lists published and unpublished authorities on which you rely.

Appendix 4 is a glossary of medical and other terminology.

Add other appendices as appropriate.

Further reading

Bond, C., Solon, M., Harper, P., *et al* (2007) *The Expert Witness: A Practical Guide* (3rd edn). Shaw & Sons.

CHAPTER 5

Reports for criminal proceedings

Medical science and the law have moved a long way since 1982. We hope that the safeguards now in place will prevent others becoming victims of similar miscarriages of justice. The courts must ensure that lessons learnt are translated into more effective protections. Vigilance must be the watchword of the criminal justice system if public confidence is to be maintained. (Henry LJ in *R v Roberts* (1998), quoted in Gudjonsson (2003, p. 493))

In a criminal case, the defence, the prosecution or the court itself may instruct you. Usually the request is to examine a defendant. Occasionally it is to examine, or report on, the complainant or another witness or to prepare a report on a convicted prisoner in relation to parole or release on licence.

Issues in criminal proceedings

Box 10 lists the issues you are most likely to have to address in reports for criminal proceedings but it is not an exhaustive list.

Documents and materials to be considered

It is usual to have access to the indictment (in a Crown Court case) or charge sheet (in a summary case, that is, a magistrates' court case, dealt with 'summarily'), the outline of allegations (in a Crown Court case), prosecution witness statements, the record of the police interview, the custody record and a list of previous cautions and convictions. Sometimes it may be appropriate to view CCTV tapes of the defendant in the custody suite. Sometimes it is necessary to listen to, or watch, recordings of the interview. Sometimes an extended version of the list of previous convictions may be available, one that gives some detail of the offences committed. Sometimes witness statements on which the prosecution does not seek to rely, called 'unused material', contain information relevant to psychiatric

---

Box 10 Issues in psychiatric reports for criminal proceedings

- Pre-trial and preliminary issues
  - Bail
  - Discontinuance
  - *Nolle prosequi*
  - Abuse of process
  - Fitness to be interviewed/reliability
  - Out-of-court silence
  - Fitness to plead and stand trial and vulnerable defendants
- Trial issues
  - Diminished responsibility
  - Insanity
  - Automatism
  - Intent
  - Loss of control
  - Duress and coercion
  - Miscellaneous
- Sentencing
  - Sentence for public protection
- Appeals
- Parole

---

issues. For example, there may be references to a defendant reporting particular symptoms, exhibiting certain signs or having certain personality characteristics. Unused material is not routinely made available to experts and it may be worth enquiring as to its availability and potential relevance. Defendants remanded in custody will have a prison inmate medical record and this should be seen. It is essential to request to see the general practitioner records but they cannot always be obtained (for example because the subject is not registered with a practice). If the defendant has been convicted, there may be a pre-sentence or social circumstances report (SCR) prepared by the probation officer in the case.

Consent issues

Under s.3(6) of the Bail Act 1976, the court may make it a condition of bail that the defendant cooperates with the preparation of a medical report. However, even in such cases, the defendant's express consent should be sought in the usual way.

If the defendant is pleading not guilty, be careful asking about the alleged offence. In the course of obtaining consent, explain that defendants are entitled not to answer questions about, or give an account of, the alleged

---

Box 11 Matters to be addressed in a report in a criminal case in Scotland

The Scottish Executive (2005, ch. 6, para. 102) recommends that the following points are addressed in a criminal report:

Preliminary information

- At whose request the assessment was undertaken, circumstances of assessment (place, time, any constraints on assessment, such as inadequate time to complete assessment owing to prison routine)
- Sources of information used (interview with the person, interviews with others, documents examined)
- The person's capacity to take part or refuse to take part and the person's understanding of the limits of confidentiality
- If any important sources of information could not be used, there should be a statement as to why this was the case

Background history

- Family history
- Personal history
- Medical history
- Psychiatric history
- Recent social circumstances
- Personality
- Forensic history

Circumstances of offence or alleged offence

Progress since offence or alleged offence

Current mental state

Box continues opposite

---

offence. Their account to you may be compared with the account given to the police and compared with their statement to the solicitors. If you are seeing a defendant for the prosecution, they are particularly likely to exercise their right to silence, but this may lead to difficulties, for example in relation to the assessment of fitness to plead and stand trial (see p. 77).

Consent to prepare a psychiatric report in a criminal case should include, if the defendant agrees, consent to the report being made available to the National Probation Service and/or the prison health service (see Appendix 7). The same consent form can be used to record consent to the expert

Box 11 *continued*

Opinion should cover some or all of the following matters:

- Fitness to plead
- Presence of mental disorder currently and whether the criteria for the relevant order are met
- Presence of mental disorder at the time of the offence
  - The relationship between any mental disorder and the offence (this is still relevant even if the person has been convicted, as it may affect choice of disposal)
  - Whether the person was insane at the time of the offence
  - In murder cases, whether there are grounds for diminished responsibility
- Assessment of risk in the presence of mental disorder
  - The risk of harm to self or others
  - The risk that the person might pose of reoffending
  - The relationship between this risk and any mental disorder present
  - Whether the person needs to be managed in a secure setting, and if so whether this should be at a state (high secure) hospital
- What assessment or treatment does the person require?
  - Does the person need further assessment?
  - Where should this take place?
  - Does the person need a period of in-patient assessment and what level of security would be required?
  - Why is assessment required, and what issues remain to be clarified?
- Does the person require treatment for a mental disorder or condition?
  - What treatment is needed and where should this be given?
- State any matters that are currently uncertain and the reasons why they remain uncertain

obtaining medical and other relevant records, such as probation, social services or educational records.

Report requirements

The report has to comply with the CrPR. Failure to comply may lead to judicial criticism (*R v Redbridge Magistrates' Court* [2009] EWHC 836 (Admin)). Additional requirements are in *R v Bowman*, including a statement as to the range and extent of the expertise and any limitations on it. Reports for sentencing should comply with *Good Practice Guidance: Commissioning, Administering and Producing Psychiatric Reports for Sentencing* (Her Majesty's Courts Service, 2010).

In Scotland, the Scottish Executive has set out in even more detail the matters it would expect to be addressed in a psychiatric report (Box 11) and its recommendations are equally applicable outside Scotland.

The declaration

The declaration should include at least the following standard statements:

I understand that my duty is to help the court to achieve the overriding objective by giving assistance by way of objective, unbiased opinion on matters within my expertise, both in preparing reports and in giving oral evidence. I understand that this duty overrides any obligation to the party by whom I am engaged or the person who has paid or is liable to pay me. I confirm that I have complied with and will continue to comply with that duty.

I have read Part 33 of the Criminal Procedure Rules and Schedule 5 to the Criminal Procedure Rules 2010, SI 60, and I have complied with their requirements.

The statement of truth

The report should include the following statement of truth:

I confirm that the contents of this report are true to the best of my knowledge and belief and that I make this report knowing that, if it is tendered in evidence, I would be liable to prosecution if I have wilfully stated anything in it which I know to be false or do not believe to be true.

Additional requirements when instructed by the police or Crown Prosecution Service

When instructed by the police or the Crown Prosecution Service (CPS) you have to comply with *Disclosure: Experts' Evidence and Unused Material – Guidance Booklet for Experts* and include a 'Declaration of understanding' (of disclosure obligations) and a 'Self-certificate' (Rix, 2008) (see Appendix 9).

Pre-trial and preliminary issues

Assessments in police custody and for bail

Once charged with an offence a person must either be released on police bail or held in police custody in order for a magistrates' court to decide whether they should be released on bail or further remanded in custody. The Bail Act 1976 created a right to bail and specified exceptions to that right. Unless one or more of the exceptions applies, the accused must be granted bail. If bail is not granted, the accused is remanded to a local prison, usually for not more than eight days at a time, before conviction or acquittal, but longer remands in custody, of up to 28 days, are possible in certain circumstances.

Psychiatric reports may be requested in relation to applications for, or the granting of, bail. They may be ordered as a condition of bail. A

Box 12 Issues to be addressed in a report on a person in police custody

The Scottish Executive (2005, ch. 2, para. 7) recommends that the following points are addressed in a custody report:

- Does the person *appear* to be suffering from mental disorder?
- Does the person currently pose a risk to self or other people?
- Does the person require assessment or treatment in hospital?
- If so, how urgently is this required?
- Is the person fit to be interviewed; if so, do they require an appropriate adult?
- Is the person fit to plead were they to appear in court?
- May the person require community care mental health services?

---

further point of relevance is that residence at a psychiatric hospital may be made a condition of bail. The proliferation of magistrates' courts mental health assessment and diversion schemes has created a situation in which psychiatric assessments by doctors, nurses and sometimes social workers are available to accused persons very early in the criminal process and sometimes at their first court appearance. In some schemes such assessments are carried out at the request of the magistrates and in some schemes reports are prepared before the first court appearance on accused persons identified by bail information officers, police or solicitors as being likely to require such assessment.

The main issues to be addressed in reports at this stage are helpfully set out for psychiatrists in Scotland (Box 12) but this guidance can usefully be applied in any jurisdiction.

Magistrates must now consider the issue of bail every time an accused person appears before the court but, in addition, the person's solicitor can make a specific application for bail to be granted to a person who has been remanded in custody. If the application is rejected, the solicitor cannot reapply to the magistrates for bail unless there has been a change in the detained person's circumstances, but an application can be made to a judge 'in chambers'.

In order to understand the relevance of psychiatric opinion in relation to bail applications, it is necessary to consider some of the exceptions to a person's right to bail (Box 13).

At the accused person's first appearance before the magistrates, it is particularly important to make an accurate diagnosis of the person's condition. Court schemes were established because, in some parts of the country, particularly in London, magistrates were being faced with considerable numbers of persons who had a mental disorder and, in the absence of any alternative provisions, having to remand them in custody to ensure that they received medical attention specifically for their own

---

Box 13 Some exceptions to a person's right to bail

- Having been arrested for absconding or breaching bail conditions
- For the person's own protection
- There being substantial grounds for believing that the accused would fail to surrender to custody
- There being substantial grounds to believe that the accused person would commit an offence
- There being substantial grounds for believing that the accused person would interfere with witnesses or otherwise obstruct the course of justice

---

protection. The success of such schemes in reducing the number and length of custodial remands may in part be attributable to assessments identifying conditions for which a remand in custody is not necessary and to which alternatives can be suggested. Thus, psychiatric assessment must lead to an accurate diagnosis and detailed description of the person's condition so that the magistrates are sufficiently confident, in appropriate cases, to grant bail rather than remand in custody.

The magistrates and judges are also going to be concerned about the prognosis for any mental condition identified. This has implications for their decision-making.

If the person will be at greater risk of self-harm or suicide if at liberty than if remanded in custody, this will influence the decision as to whether or not to refuse bail on the grounds that a remand in custody is necessary for the person's own protection.

Where an alleged offence involves a particular person or class of person and it appears to have arisen as consequence of some specific psychiatric condition, for example a depressive disorder or one involving delusions, the psychiatrist may be able to advise whether or not the accused person is likely to commit further offences, in particular involving the original complainant (or others similarly connected with the delusions), or interfere with witnesses, particularly the complainant. This aspect of the assessment of prognosis may be relevant if the magistrates or judge would otherwise refuse bail on the grounds that the accused person might commit further offences or interfere with witnesses.

Depending on the nature or severity of the psychiatric disorder identified, there may be a case for offering psychiatric admission, and in the case of a person who can give valid consent to be admitted to hospital informally and comply with bail conditions, the court may be willing to grant bail on the basis that hospital treatment will make it significantly less likely that the person will commit further offences or interfere with witnesses.

In any case, if a person is assessed at court, there is a responsibility not only to make an assessment which provides sufficient information for the magistrates to decide whether to grant bail or remand in custody, but also a responsibility to give full regard to the person's mental health needs and consider how those needs ought to be met, regardless of whether the person is released on bail or remanded in custody. It may be that no psychiatric intervention is needed. If there is a need for non-urgent out-patient or community treatment, arrangements can be made to facilitate this in the event of the person being granted bail, but in case the person is remanded in custody, the report needs to identify the need for treatment as a matter to be addressed by the prison health service. Where there is a more urgent need for treatment, but not necessarily as an in-patient, it is particularly important that appropriate arrangements are made in the event of the person being granted bail, and if the person is remanded in custody, the prison health service needs to be advised, so that it can arrange the treatment with the appropriate degree of urgency. Since, in many cases, the psychiatrist who makes the assessment does not know if the person will be granted bail or remanded in custody, it is important that one copy of the report is designated as being for the attention of either the person's general practitioner or the prison medical officer. Exceptionally it may be best to send a copy of the report by facsimile to the particular prison healthcare centre (it can be difficult to get email addresses that will guarantee it gets to the right person). Similar considerations apply to notifying the prison health service in cases where there is an urgent need for hospital admission and either a bed is not available or the magistrates are not willing to allow the person to go to a bed of the level of security considered appropriate by the psychiatrist.

If bail is granted, it is the person's right that it should be without any conditions being attached, although there are exceptions to this right (Box 13). Conditions may be attached under certain circumstances and in particular to facilitate the preparation of reports.

If it is a condition of bail that a person is admitted to a psychiatric hospital, it is important to pay regard to the wording of the bail conditions. A requirement that the person should simply reside in a particular hospital entitles the patient to go out all day and arrive back late at night! This may not enable the most appropriate observation or treatment of the person. Through local policies and agreements it should be possible ensure that the condition usually incorporates the requirements to obey the directions of the doctor or nurse in charge and comply with hospital rules. Thus, a patient who insists on leaving when refused permission to do so may be in breach of their bail conditions. Such a condition begs the question 'what are the hospital rules?' However, it is a simple matter to draw up a list of rules, including, for example, compliance with hospital policies concerning personal searches and the use of alcohol and recreational drugs, and to obtain the person's written agreement to these rules before offering the bed. The wording of the 'contract' and the person's written consent to it are important because these should overcome any ethical objections, on the grounds of patient confidentiality, to notifying the police that the person is about to be discharged for failure to comply with the hospital rules. If the police cannot be informed that the person is being discharged, they will not be able to consider arresting the person for breach of bail conditions and there will be a risk of the person committing further offences on bail or interfering with witnesses. Although local arrangements should ensure that the police cooperate when a patient is being discharged under such circumstances, it is preferable, if there is no urgency, to identify a date, preferably at least three working days away, on which the patient will be discharged and notify the court and the patient's solicitor so that a date can be set for a hearing to consider the breach of bail.

A person admitted to hospital as a condition of bail cannot be detained or forced to have treatment unless detained appropriately under the Mental Health Act 1983, as amended by the Mental Health Act 2007 (MHA). If such a person is detained under Part II of the MHA their solicitor should be informed as soon as possible so that discussion can take place concerning the person's fitness to attend court. A person granted bail with a condition of residence in a psychiatric hospital and then detained under the MHA has the same rights as any other patient detained under the MHA.

In the case of a person who might not be expected to comply with bail conditions, the magistrates and the Crown Court have the power to remand a person to hospital for assessment under s.35 of the MHA. It is not an alternative to a remand on bail with a condition of residence in a psychiatric hospital but an alternative to a remand to prison. Thus, it is essentially a provision for obtaining a psychiatric report which could not be obtained if the person was remanded on bail, perhaps because they could not be relied upon to comply with conditions of hospital residence, or to observe the hospital's rules or the directions of the doctor or nurse in charge.

A remand for assessment cannot be ordered unless a registered medical practitioner approved under s.12 of the MHA recommends it and gives evidence in writing or orally that there is reason to suspect that the person is suffering from mental disorder within the meaning of s.1 of the MHA. There does not have to be a firm diagnosis but there has to be reason to suspect mental disorder.

This provision applies only (1) where the offence charged is an imprisonable offence or (2) the person is suspected of having a mental disorder and has been arrested for a breach of an occupation order or a non-molestation order under the provisions of ss.47 and 48 of the Family Law Act 1996.

The powers under s.35 in a magistrates' court are limited to cases in which either the court is satisfied that the person did the act or made the omission charged or the person has consented to the exercise of the powers.

A person remanded under s.35 can be prevented from leaving the hospital and in theory they could be admitted to an unlocked ward. However, as it is a criterion that 'it would be impracticable for a report on his mental condition to be made if he were remanded on bail' (s.35(3)(b)), someone who can be relied upon to comply with the requirement to stay in hospital could probably be remanded to hospital on bail. Thus, remands under this section are more likely to be to secure hospital facilities, since the physical security may be necessary to ensure that the person does not leave hospital.

As well as needing an appropriate medical recommendation, for a s.35 assessment the court requires confirmation that arrangements have been made for admission on the day the order is to be made, or within seven days of the making of the order. This confirmation can be given by the registered medical practitioner who would be responsible for making the report or by someone representing the managers of the hospital. If the person cannot be admitted immediately the order is made, the court may direct conveyance to, and detention in, a place of safety, which is usually a prison.

In the first instance, a remand for assessment cannot be for more than 28 days, though further remands of up to 28 days can be ordered but for no more than 12 weeks in total. Written or oral evidence from the registered medical practitioner responsible for the report is necessary in order for there to be a further remand, but the person does not have to return to court as long as they are represented legally in court and their legal representative has the opportunity of being heard.

A person who absconds from the hospital to which they have been remanded, or while being conveyed to or from it, can be arrested without a warrant and must be taken as soon as practicable to the court that remanded them. It is not legal for the police to return the person to the hospital.

If the assessment is completed well within the period for which the person has been remanded, the adjourned court hearing can be brought forward and, if necessary, an alternative form of remand, in custody or on bail, can be substituted.

The Code of Practice of the MHA advises that a report prepared as a result of a remand under s.35 should include: a statement as to whether the patient is suffering from a mental disorder and if so its relevance to the alleged offence; relevant social factors; and recommendations on care and treatment, including where and when it should take place and who should be responsible.

Discontinuance of proceedings

Once a person has been summonsed, arrested on warrant or charged by the police, the CPS takes over the prosecution but first has to make sure that it is right to proceed with the prosecution. After satisfying themselves that the evidence can justify proceedings ('the evidential stage'), crown prosecutors have to decide whether or not it is in the public interest to proceed with a prosecution ('the public interest stage'). *The Code for Crown Prosecutors* (Crown Prosecution Service, 2010) identifies some common public interest factors against prosecution. They include one that relates to the mental condition of the accused person (Box 14). Crown prosecutors, in considering the alternatives to prosecution, have to consider, where appropriate, 'the availability of suitable rehabilitative, reparative, or

---

Box 14 A public interest factor against prosecution relating to the mental condition of the accused

The defendant is elderly, or is, or was at the time of the offence, suffering from significant mental or physical ill health, unless the offence is serious or there is a real possibility that it may be repeated. The CPS, where necessary, applies Home Office guidelines about how to deal with mentally disordered offenders. Crown prosecutors must balance the desirability of diverting a defendant who is suffering from significant mental or physical ill health with the need to safeguard the general public.

Code for Crown Prosecutors (Crown Prosecution Service, 2010, para. 5.10(g))

---

restorative justice processes'. Compliance with suitable conditions aimed at rehabilitation or reparation can be part of a 'conditional caution'.

Psychiatric reports prepared where discontinuance of proceedings is a potential issue are usually requested by the defendant's solicitors, but especially in particularly grave or high-profile cases the CPS may commission its own report. Box 15 lists the matters to be considered in a report where discontinuance is the issue.

Bear in mind that many people, especially those with no previous convictions, will be unhappy about being charged with a criminal offence and anxious about going to court. This is not the same as 'significant mental ... ill-health'. Likewise, threats to commit suicide if the prosecution goes ahead have to be evaluated with the utmost caution lest the CPS is manipulated into discontinuing proceedings where there is no real risk of suicide.

If the crown prosecutors are satisfied, they may 'discontinue' the proceedings under s.23 of the Prosecution of Offences Act 1985, by withdrawal of the case or simply offering no evidence.

Box 15 Matters to be considered in a report where discontinuance of proceedings is the issue

- Previous offences which may indicate an ongoing or recurrent mental disorder
- The likelihood of mental disorder leading to further offending
- Alternatives to prosecution
  - voluntary treatment as an in-patient, out-patient or in the community
  - rehabilitation under a conditional caution
- The accused's insight into the need for treatment
- The accused's likely compliance with a conditional caution or voluntary treatment
- The likely effect on the accused's mental state of the continuation of the prosecution

---

Nolle prosequi

The Attorney General has a power to stop or 'stay' a criminal prosecution by the entry of a *nolle prosequi*. It is a power limited to the Attorney General and it is a power with which the courts may not interfere. It is directed to be entered following application either by the prosecution or by the accused person by way of a letter. Although it brings the criminal process to an end, it does not amount to a discharge or an acquittal.

A *nolle prosequi* is now usually directed to be entered in cases where the accused person cannot be produced in court to plead or stand trial owing to physical or mental incapacity which is expected to be permanent. Psychiatrists asked to prepare reports in possible support of such applications should therefore pay particular regard to the severity of the accused person's medical condition and to the prognosis, insofar as it must be a permanent condition. Relatively severe forms of intellectual disability and some forms of dementia might be grounds for directing entry of a *nolle prosequi*.

Abuse of process

Courts also have the power to stay proceedings. Judges are enjoined to pause long before staying proceedings and magistrates are advised to be most sparing in their exercise of the power to stay criminal proceedings. There are various grounds for staying proceedings and one of these is the power to protect the legal process from the abuse into which it might fall without such powers. Thus, the law recognises 'abuse of process' as a limited discretionary power to prevent a prosecution proceeding. It has been defined in *Hui Chi-Ming v R* [1992] 1 AC 34, PC, as 'something so unfair and wrong that the court should not allow a prosecutor to proceed with what is in all other respects a regular proceeding'.

The power to protect against an abuse of process may be exercised where the fairness of the trial would be compromised because the proceedings are going to be 'oppressive and vexatious' for the accused person. They might be so in the case of a person who is too ill to be tried or too ill for the trial to continue.

Although it is clear that a stay of proceedings may be sought in the case of someone whose illness, but for its lack of permanency, might be the basis for an application for a *nolle prosequi*, there is not such a clear distinction between what nature or degree of mental disorder should lead to an application for a stay of proceedings and what should lead to an enquiry as to fitness to plead and stand trial. In practice what happens is that the psychiatrist who prepares a report in relation to an application for a stay of proceedings has to consider the mental state of the accused person in relation to participation in a trial and inevitably has to consider some matters that touch on fitness to plead and stand trial. The difference is that the psychiatrist is usually directed not to give an opinion on fitness to plead and stand trial but on whether or not, having regard to the mental condition of the accused, the proceedings would be so oppressive that it would be an abuse of the legal process for the accused to stand trial. It is sometimes the case that, if the application for a stay of proceedings is unsuccessful, the defence then raises the issue of the defendant's fitness to plead and stand trial, just as the defence may proceed to apply for a stay of proceedings after a failed application for a *nolle prosequi*.

A stay of proceedings is only a stay and this means that the court may order accused persons to be re-examined at a later date or dates to ascertain whether they have recovered sufficiently to stand trial. It is not unknown for accused persons to fabricate or exaggerate mental disorder in order to postpone, indefinitely, they hope, a criminal trial. The investigation of such cases requires the most careful examination of all the medical records of their treatment after the stay has been granted since, as time goes by, it may become increasingly difficult for the accused to avoid saying or doing something that 'gives the game away'. Just as criminals who think they got away with the perfect crime may eventually make just one small but fatal mistake that incriminates them, so the malingering accused person may eventually let something slip in conversation, or be observed or reported doing something which shows that their mental disorder is being fabricated or exaggerated in order to avoid standing trial.

Fitness to be interviewed and reliability of police interviews

In order to avoid obtaining interview evidence that is subsequently excluded on the grounds that it would have a substantial adverse effect on fairness – under s.78 of the Police and Criminal Evidence Act 1984 (PACE) – the police apply a number of safeguards that are set out in Code C of the PACE Codes of Practice. Recognising that although 'people who are mentally disordered or otherwise mentally vulnerable are often capable of providing reliable evidence, they may, without knowing it or wanting to do so, be particularly prone in certain circumstances to provide information that may be unreliable, misleading or self-incriminating' (Code C, Annex E, Guidance Note E2). Code C includes particular provisions relating to those termed people with 'mental disorder', as defined in s.1 of the MHA, and people with 'mental vulnerability', which means anyone who, 'because of their mental state or capacity, may not understand the significance of what is said, of questions or of their replies' (Code C, Guidance Note G). If there is any doubt that mental disorder, in this context, includes personality disorder, case law makes this clear:

The expert evidence of a psychiatrist or psychologist may properly be admitted if it is to the effect that a defendant is suffering from a condition not properly described as mental illness, but from a personality disorder so severe as properly to be categorised as mental disorder. (*R v Ward (Judith)* (1993) 96 Cr App R 1)

But this is not enough:

the abnormal disorder [sic] must not only be of a type which might render a confession or evidence unreliable; there must also be a very significant deviation from the norm shown. (*R v O'Brien* [2000] All ER (D) 62)

Determining whether or not a detainee is 'fit to be interviewed' is usually, at least in the first instance, the responsibility of the forensic medical examiner (FME).

However well safeguards are implemented for police interviews, there will continue to be cases in which expert evidence by psychiatrists and psychologists, as to reliability, will be necessary in order to avoid people who are mentally disordered or mentally vulnerable being convicted of crimes they have not committed. This may be before trial or in connection with an appeal against conviction.

Assessing the reliability of admissions or confessions made to the police by people who may have a mental disorder or other mental vulnerability builds upon an understanding of the assessment of fitness to be interviewed (Ventress *et al*, 2008) and includes: consideration of a range of records and documents, of which the complete transcripts of the police interviews and sometimes the FME's contemporaneous records are of critical importance; consideration of the role of the appropriate adult; a full mental state examination; and, often, specialised investigations such as intelligence testing and measurement of characteristics such as vulnerability and compliance.

In the context of a police interview, reliability is essentially about the capacity of the detainee for truthfulness and for accuracy that is not impaired by mental disorder or mental vulnerability or, where such dangers exist, that steps are taken to negate their potential effect on the interview (Ventress *et al*, 2008). It therefore has two main elements: internal – relating to the detainee; and external – relating to circumstances or things that are said or done that might affect detainees and what they say. Assessment therefore focuses not only on the mental state of detainees but on what effect the circumstances of their detention and the things said or done by the police may have had on them.

Box 16 sets out a framework for the forensic investigation of such cases. One objective is to reconstruct the suspect's mental and physical state while in police custody (Gudjonsson, 2003, p. 313) and then to determine the reliability or otherwise of the contents of the interview or of any confession made.

Central to the assessment are the actual interviews and the circumstances in which they took place. There has to be an analysis of the interviews that demonstrates how the detainee's mental disorder or mental vulnerability appears to have given rise to unreliability. It may be advisable to work in tandem with a forensic psychologist.

It is not enough to give an opinion that the detainee has, or had at the time of the interview(s), a mental disorder or mental vulnerability. There has to be evidence in the interviews themselves, or evidence of things said

---

Box 16 A framework for the investigation of a case where psycho-logical or psychiatric factors may be relevant to the admissibility or reliability of police interview material

- Detailed psychiatric history from the defendant
- Review of general practice, psychiatric, prison medical and social service records
- Review of witness statements and other evidence
- Review of the custody record, noting particularly
  - disclosure by detainee on reception, or suspicion by police, of a history of mental disorder or anything suggesting mental vulnerability
  - drugs in the possession of detainee
  - findings of the FME
  - the detailed written notes of any psychiatric examination
  - observations of behaviour by custody officers
- Examination of rest, sleep patterns, refreshments
- Examination of timings of interviews in relation to arrest and time of day
- Untoward events, such as collapse, hospital admissions, recall of FME
- Listen to taped police interviews/watch video-taped police interviews
- Read the transcripts of police interview
- Understand and examine the role of the appropriate adult in this case
- Understand and examine the nature of the police interview and questioning
- Detailed examination of the detainee, noting mental state, functional intellectual ability, presence of mental disorder or mental distress or other vulnerabilities
- Arranging appropriate specialised psychological investigation, such as intellectual functioning, suggestibility and compliance testing, personality testing

---

or done outside the interview, that can be demonstrated to call into question the reliability of what was said. Thus, in *O'Brien* it was held that 'the real criterion must simply be whether the abnormal disorder [*sic*] might render the confession or evidence unreliable'.

Where someone with a mental disorder or mental vulnerability has not been afforded the assistance of an appropriate adult, or where the appropriate adult has not intervened at all, or appears to have failed to intervene when they should, it will be necessary to give an opinion as to how the interview would have been different had there been interventions, or further interventions, by the appropriate adult.

It is best to work with a complete transcript of the interviews, which is something the solicitors can usually arrange to have prepared from the police tapes. The police invariably produce edited transcripts and these may omit sections that are of importance to the psychiatrist. For example, very often the beginning of the interview and the cautioning of the detainee are excluded. The difficulties the police have in explaining the caution and sometimes the complete failure of the detainee to understand it may be important clues to the nature of the interviewee's difficulties and an important ground for arguing that the interview evidence should be excluded. Box 17 lists aspects of the interview that may have a bearing on reliability.

Whether or not a suspect was suffering from a mental disorder at the time of the interview(s) is an objective test. In *R v Everett* [1988] Crim LR 826, where the medical evidence was that the detainee had an IQ of 61, the Court of Appeal held that it did not matter what the police officers thought, if anything, about the detainee's mental condition. The test was the detainee's actual condition as subsequently diagnosed by the doctor.

It may be necessary to try to re-examine the basis for a judgment, by the doctors involved at the time of the interview, that the suspect was fit to be interviewed or did not need an appropriate adult. Gudjonsson (2003, p. 269) quotes a case where the trial judge held that the two doctors had failed to approach 'the question of fitness on the basis of considering whether or not any answers given by Mr S ... to any questions asked of him by the police officers were necessarily reliable' but had instead only 'considered that the ordeal and stress and strain of being interviewed, particularly on

---

Box 17 Some pointers to unreliable police interviews

- Failure to understand the police caution
- Failure by the solicitor or appropriate adult to seek a break to consult with a detainee who has become distressed
- Failure by the solicitor or appropriate adult to seek a break if interview is lengthy or interrogation sustained and there is evidence of the detainee becoming confused, incoherent or rambling
- Failure by the police to respond appropriately to interventions by the solicitor or appropriate adult, for example to take a break, use shorter words, explain terminology (such as 'bail', 'custody')
- Evidence of acquiescence when leading questions are put, especially when put with some force
- 'Yes' responses to questions which the detainee probably did not understand
- Evidence of the defendant being led
- The police minimising the gravity of the offences (*R v Delaney* (1988) 88 Cr App R 338)
- The police suggesting that treatment, not punishment, is the likely outcome (*R v Delaney*)
- The police shouting, using bad language, being rude or being discourteous (*R v Emmerson* (1991) 92 Cr App R 284)
- A desire by the detainee to obtain release from detention as quickly as possible (*R v Delaney*; *R v Crampton* (1991) 92 Cr App R 369; *R v Aspinall* [1999] 2 Cr App R 115)
- Misunderstanding of, or failure to understand, questions or what is being put to the detainee
- Changing answers in response to negative feedback (interrogative suggestibility)
- Confessing to crimes that could not possibly have been committed (false confessions)

such a serious charge as this, was something that in their judgment the suspect could sustain without suffering any consequential harm to either his physical or mental health'.

Under s.76 of PACE the court must exclude the confession if it finds that it was obtained by 'oppression' or under circumstances likely to render it 'unreliable'. What amounts to oppression by interviewing police officers can depend on the detainee:

What may be oppressive as regards a child, an invalid or an old man or somebody inexperienced in the ways of the world may turn out not to be oppressive when one finds that the accused is of tough character and an experienced man of the world. (R v Priestley (1965) 51 Cr App R 1)

What police interviewing techniques may be oppressive or render the suspect's evidence unreliable is a specialised area (Gudjonsson, 2003, pp. 75–114). Not all of the 'oppressive' tactics identified by Gudjonsson are unacceptable and, even when they are used, their identification is not in itself sufficient to prove the evidence elicited to be unreliable. Furthermore, not all impropriety necessarily involves oppression. The critical question is whether or not reliability is compromised.

In R v Paris (1993) 97 Crim App R 99, where the detainee was on the borderline of 'mental handicap', the Court of Appeal identified as oppressive an interview in which he was 'bullied and hectored' and said that the evidence derived from it should have been excluded. It also pointed out that the interview would have been oppressive even for a detainee of normal intelligence. However, in L [1994] Crim LR 839, similar tactics seem to have been regarded as acceptable as long as they did not affect the reliability of the confession.

What is oppressive will depend to some extent on the detainee. Thus, in R v Emmerson (1991) 92 Crim App R 284, the court did not accept that the police's rude and discourteous questioning, accompanied by some shouting and bad language, was oppressive but it might be so in someone who could easily be overwhelmed by such behaviour. In the case of R v Miller [1986] 1 WLR 1191, it was held that it might be oppressive to put questions to someone known to be mentally ill so as 'skilfully and deliberately' to induce a 'delusionary' state. While an 'experienced professional criminal' might expect a vigorous interrogation (R v Gowan [1982] Crim LR 821), it was held that there had been oppression in the case of R v Hudson (1980) 72 Cr App R 163, where a middle-aged man of previous good character had been subjected to a lengthy and in some respects unlawful interrogation.

It is not just 'oppressive' interviewing which needs to be identified. In R v Waters [1989] Crim LR 62 it was sufficient to have identified merely 'improper' questioning, which had resulted in ambiguous and potentially unreliable answers.

It will often be advisable to have a formal assessment of IQ by a psychologist. This is because clinical impressions by prison medical officers and psychiatrists about intelligence are often wrong (Gudjonsson, 2003, pp. 322, 469). Furthermore, it is important to note the effect of the judgment of the court in *R v Kenny* [1994] Crim LR 284, which was that it is not appropriate to take IQ test results from one case and apply them slavishly to another case, because every case has its individual features.

In addition, psychological test results, even in the absence of a mental disorder, may be evidence of mental vulnerability, rendering evidence unreliable. It used to be the law that a mental abnormality had to fall into a recognised category of mental disorder for expert evidence to be properly admissible (*Ward*) but in *O'Brien* the court questioned this and indicated that the operative consideration was simply whether the abnormality might render the confession unreliable. However, the court added that the abnormality had to be such as to amount to a 'very significant deviation from the norm'. It also needs to be established that there was evidence of these vulnerabilities prior to police interview. Such evidence can be found sometimes in medical records, prosecution witness statements, defence witness statements, social services and other records.

Abnormal suggestibility and abnormal compliance are vulnerabilities of particular importance when determining the reliability of admissions to the police. Suggestibility may be particularly important in people who have an intellectual disorder or disability, who have a greater tendency to go along with a story that is put to them and the more so if they are put under pressure. The case of *R v King* [2002] 2 Cr App R 391 is illustrative. King was convicted of murder in 1986. His defence had been that the confession he made to the police had been obtained under pressure and was as a result of his accepting suggestions put to him by the interviewing officers. At his trial there were three medical reports. One described him as being of dull average intelligence, a second placed him in the lower end of the average range of intellectual abilities and the third stated that his full-scale IQ was 89. At his appeal in 1999 a psychologist gave evidence that, although he was then found to have a full-scale IQ of 78, his scores for suggestibility and compliance were in the abnormal range. The court held that he was 'more vulnerable than was understood at the time, and abnormally ready to accept what was put to him'.

When you prepare the report, be familiar with all of the other evidence in the case and be prepared to place your findings within the context of the totality of the case (Gudjonsson, 2003, p. 328). But do not to fall into the trap of assuming that, because there is evidence that a confession is true, there is no issue of reliability. In the case of *R v Cox* [1991] Crim LR 276, where the defendant had an IQ of 58, at the *voir dire* (a trial within a trial at which the judge decides an issue in the absence of the jury), Cox admitted one of the offences with which he was charged. The trial judge admitted this confession but was held to have been wrong to do so. Likewise, in the case of *R v Crampton* (1991) 92 Cr App R 369, concerning a drug addict, it was held that, if acts were done or words were spoken which were likely to induce unreliable confessions, then an admission was inadmissible, whether or not it was true.

Finally, your assessment may not end with the completion of the report. If the defendant gives evidence on a *voir dire*, you should be in court to observe the defendant. In the case of *R v Weeks* [1995] Crim LR 52 it was held that the demeanour of the defendant when giving evidence on the *voir dire* could assist the prosecution in showing that he was not affected by the threats allegedly made at the interview.

The presence of an appropriate adult is meant to provide safeguards for the detainee but the mere presence of the appropriate adult may not be sufficient. Para 11.17 of Code C of the PACE makes it clear that the appropriate adult is not expected to act simply as an observer. Careful consideration of the transcripts of the interviews may reveal a failure on the part of the appropriate adult to advise the person being interviewed, improper or unfair interviewing about which the appropriate adult is silent, or a failure to facilitate communication with the detainee so that misunderstandings are apparent. You should also ask for an audiotape of the interview, as pauses, tension, shouting or distress may be evident. The précis of a transcript may omit material that is of psychological or psychiatric significance.

In a case that was dismissed by magistrates after they had heard the evidence of a psychologist that the defendant was someone who needed an appropriate adult (*DPP v Cornish* (1997) *The Times* 27 January), an appeal by the prosecution led the court to set out the approach which ought to be adopted in such cases, including receiving prosecution evidence about the interviews. It was stated that the court needed to know:

who was there at the time of the interview and how the interview went, so that the court could form some impression of the effect of the absence of the appropriate adult upon the conduct of the interview and other matters of that kind.

The psychiatrist or psychologist needs to study the interview records and decide what the effect was of the absence of the appropriate adult, or what the effect was of an appropriate adult being present but failing to advise the person, failing to intervene in response to improper or unfair questioning or failing to facilitate communication.

Box 18 Possible reasons for seeking to disqualify the appropriate adult

- Detainee has no empathy with the appropriate adult
- Detainee expressly objected to the appropriate adult
- Appropriate adult is incapable of fulfilling the functions as a result of being intellectually or mentally disordered
- Appropriate adult has some involvement in the offence, for example as a victim or witness
- Appropriate adult is involved in the investigation
- Appropriate adult has already received admissions from the detainee

Even if an appropriate adult was present, there may be questions as to the appropriateness of the appropriate adult and whether or not the appropriate adult afforded the safeguards expected. Box 18 lists some of the grounds upon which appropriate adults have been found to be inappropriate.

The case giving rise to the requirement that the detainee should have some empathy with the appropriate adult is that of *DPP v Blake* [1989] 1 WLR 432, 89 Cr App R 179. The appropriate adult was the juvenile's estranged father, whom she did not wish to see. Mann LJ said that the appropriate adult 'cannot … be a person with whom the juvenile has no empathy'. It has now been argued that '*any person* to whom the suspect expressly objects is *per se* inappropriate' (Mirfield, 1997, p. 289, original emphasis).

Although case law supports the exclusion of a person with intellecual disability or mental disorder from counting as an appropriate adult, as happened in *R v Morse* [1991] Crim LR 195, where the father of the juvenile detainee, acting as appropriate adult, had an IQ of between 60 and 70, was virtually illiterate and was probably incapable of appreciating the gravity of his son's situation, the proper issue is whether or not the appropriate adult is capable of fulfilling the functions of that role. Thus, in *Ward*, where the mother of the detainee, acting as appropriate adult, was almost certainly psychotic at the time of the interview and had an IQ of 76, the trial judge accepted the evidence of a forensic psychiatrist that she was capable of fulfilling her functions and ruled that she did count as an appropriate adult. Her psychosis concerned her neighbours and so, arguably, it did not affect her perception of what was happening to her child. The Court of Appeal did not overturn the trial judge on either his description of the appropriate adult as having 'some intellectual deficit as a result of her chronic psychosis' or on his judgment of her overall capability of functioning as an appropriate adult. In the trial judge's view, the interview had been conducted fairly and

---

Box 19 Potential failings of the appropriate adult

- Appropriate adult failed to understand role
- Appropriate adult failed to ascertain that detainee understood legal rights
  - right to silence (i.e. the caution)
  - right to free, independent legal advice
  - right to consult the Codes of Practice
  - right to have another person informed of detention
- Appropriate adult failed to advise the detainee, for example, to obtain legal representation or to tell the truth
- Appropriate adult adopted a purely passive role
- Appropriate adult overlooked detainee's failure to understand questions
- Appropriate adult overlooked detainee's incoherent answers
- Appropriate adult took on role of interrogator or sided with police
- Appropriate adult failed to stop interview when detainee became too distressed

properly, it had not been over-long and it had not involved the detainee being put under any pressure.

An appropriate adult is not rendered inappropriate just because he or she is a 'somewhat critical observer and participant', as in *R v Jefferson* [1994] 1 All ER 270, where a father acted as appropriate adult for his 15-year-old son and 'intervened robustly from time to time, sometimes joining in the questioning of his son and challenging his exculpatory account of certain incidents'.

Failings of the appropriate adult which may render an interview inadmissible or lead to a challenge to reliability are set out in Box 19.

In the case of people with an intellectual disability, s.77 of PACE is very occasionally relevant. It applies when the case against the accused depends wholly or substantially on a confession by the accused and it was not made in the presence of an independent person, such as a solicitor or appropriate adult. It provides for the jury to be given a special warning about the need for caution before convicting the accused in reliance on the confession. In practice such confessions are likely to be excluded under s.76 or s.78 of PACE. The role of the psychiatrist is to provide evidence as to whether or not the person is 'in a state of arrested or incomplete development of mind which includes significant impairment of intelligence and social functioning' (s.77(3)). Careful analysis of the case to reveal its individual features is more important than a slavish application of IQ results (*R v Kenny* [1994] Crim LR 284).

Out-of-court silence

Detainees who do not answer questions put to them by the police will be at risk of the court allowing an adverse inference to be drawn from this silence (ss.34, 36 and 37 of the Criminal Justice and Public Order Act 1994). However, the courts have made special allowances for people who have a mental disorder or who are otherwise mentally vulnerable. In *R v Argent* [1997] 2 Cr App R 27, the court established a subjective test to be applied to a detainee who did not answer the questions put by the police. It includes taking into account such matters as the time of day and the detainee's age, experience, mental capacity, state of health, sobriety, tiredness, knowledge and personality. *R v Howell* [2005] 1 Cr App R 1 confirmed that 'the suspect's ill-health, in particular mental disability' was relevant.

In such a case, a psychiatrist may be instructed in order to confirm, if it be so, that, at the time of the interview, one or more of these conditions applied. In such a case, and where the solicitor has advised the detainee not to answer questions, a request should be made for access to what should be the full and comprehensive record of all the factors that the solicitor has taken into consideration. The solicitor will be aware that, if relied upon by the psychiatrist, this information will no longer be legally privileged. See Rix (1998) for a case in which the defendant's personality disorder was accepted as a condition relevant to drawing an inference from his out-of-court silence.

Fitness to plead and stand trial and the vulnerable defendant

At the York Spring Assizes in 1831, Esther Dyson was indicted for the wilful murder of her bastard child by cutting off its head (*R v Dyson* (1831) 7 Car & P 303). She had always been 'deaf and dumb'. A sign-language interpreter said that it was impossible to make her understand that she could object to such members of the jury as she pleased and that, although she had been instructed in the 'dumb alphabet', she could not put words together. The jury was told that, if they were satisfied that she had not, from the defect of her faculties, intelligence enough to understand the nature of the proceedings, they ought to find her not sane. Her incapacity to understand the mode of her trial or to conduct her defence was proved. She was ordered to be kept in strict custody until His Majesty's pleasure was known.

When Pritchard, who was also 'deaf and dumb', was indicted for the capital offence of bestiality a few years later, the trial judge referred to the procedure followed in *Dyson* (*R v Pritchard* (1836) 7 C & P 303). However, the adoption by Parker LCJ, in *R v Podola* [1960] 1 QB 325, of the direction to the jury in *Pritchard* (Box 20), has made *Pritchard* the leading case. There is now a Law Commission consultation taking place to determine whether the law should be changed so that the focus is on whether the defendant can play a meaningful and effective part in the trial and make relevant decisions about the defence (Law Commission, 2010). It is also proposed that there should be applied a defined psychiatric test to assess whether or not the defendant has decision-making capacity.

The present procedure for determining whether an accused is 'under a disability' is governed by the Criminal Procedure (Insanity) Act 1964 (CP(I) A) as amended by the Criminal Procedure (Insanity and Unfitness to Plead) Act 1991 (CP(IU)A) and the Domestic Violence, Crime and Victims Act 2004 (DVCVA). If the issue is raised by the defence, it bears the burden to establish that the accused is under a disability on a balance of probability; if raised by the prosecution or the judge, it has to be proved beyond reasonable doubt. In practice, the issue is almost always raised by the defence.

Box 20 The *Pritchard* test

In *R v Pritchard* (1836) 7 C & P 303 the jury were given the following direction:

Is the accused 'of sufficient intellect to comprehend the course of proceedings on the trial, so as to make a proper defence – to know that he might challenge [any jurors] to whom he may object – and to comprehend the details of the evidence, which in a case of this nature must constitute a minute investigation ... if you think that there is no certain mode of communicating the details of the trial to the prisoner, so that he can clearly understand them, and be able properly to make his defence to the charge; you ought to find that he is not of sane mind.

The CP(I)A does not apply to summary proceedings, where the usual course, if there is evidence of unfitness to plead and stand trial, is to determine the issue of whether the defendant did the act or made the omission charged as charged, and if so satisfied, to make a hospital order under s.37(3) of the MHA or indeed make no order at all. In such a case, if the court does not have sufficient medical evidence to decide on an order under s.37(3), s.11(1)(a) of the Powers of the Criminal Courts (Sentencing) Act 2000 (PCC(S)A) gives the court the power to remand the defendant in custody for up to three weeks, or on bail for up to four weeks, for a medical report, and if remanding on bail, to impose a condition under s.11 that the defendant cooperates. The focus of such a report will be narrow and will in essence have to address the criteria for a hospital order under s.37 of the MHA but including a risk assessment that informs the recommendation and which sets out the proposed treatment, particularly if there is to be no recommendation of a hospital order and it is proposed to care for the defendant in the community.

Under the DVCVA, the issue is now decided by a judge alone. According to s.4(6) of the CP(I)A, the court may not determine the issue except on the evidence (written or oral) of two or more registered medical practitioners, at least one of whom must be approved under s.12 of the MHA, but this does not apply to summary proceedings (see above). Where the medical evidence is unanimous, the medical evidence may be read, but the judge is entitled to reject it, in which case, as where it is contested, oral testimony will be necessary.

The test for fitness to plead and stand trial was helpfully operationalised by HHJ Jones QC, in *R v Whitefield* (see Rix, 1996a) and a similar operationalisation by HHJ Roberts QC was approved by the Court of Appeal in *R v M (John)* [2003] EWCA Crim 3452 CA (Box 21). However, there are some common misunderstandings about fitness to plead and stand trial (see Box 22).

In *R v M (John)* the Court of Appeal endorsed the trial judge's explanations of parts of the test. The following should be read in conjunction with Box 21.

Instructing solicitors and counsel involves being able (1) to understand the lawyer's questions, (2) to apply one's mind to answering them, and (3) to convey intelligibly to the lawyers the answers which one wishes to give.

Following the course of the proceedings means that defendants must be able (1) to understand what is said by the witness and counsel in their speeches to the jury and (2) to communicate intelligibly to their lawyers any comment they may wish to make on anything that is said by the witnesses or counsel (for example, they may consider that a witness is saying something that is not true).

Giving evidence if he wishes in his own defence means that defendants must be able: (1) to understand the questions they are asked, (2) to apply their mind to answering them, and (3) convey intelligibly to the jury the answers which they wish to give.

Box 21 The *Pritchard* test as operationalised in *R v M (John)*

The *Pritchard* test was operationalised as follows in *R v M (John)* [2003] EWCA Crim 3452 CA; here, expansions *in italic* are based on HHJ Jones QC in *R v Whitefield* (1995, unreported):

Are any of the following beyond the defendant's capabilities?

- Understanding the *nature and effect of the* charges
- Deciding whether to plead guilty or not
- Exercising his right to challenge jurors
- Instructing solicitors and counsel *so as to prepare and make a proper defence in this case. This includes understanding the details of the evidence which can reasonably be expected to be given in his case and to advise his solicitor and counsel in relation to that evidence. This applies to his ability to instruct his legal advisers before and/or during his trial*
- Following the course of the proceedings
- Giving evidence in his own defence

Box 22 What does not necessarily amount to unfitness to plead and stand trial

- A complete loss of memory for the events at the material time (*R v Podola* [1960] 1 QB 325)
- Being unable to remember some of the matters giving rise to the charges (*R v M (John)* [2003] EWCA Crim 3452 CA)
- Not being capable of acting in one's best interests (*R v Robertson* [1968] 3 All ER 557, CA)
- Being deluded as to the material facts (*Robertson*)
- Having delusions that might lead to a wrong or unwise challenge of a juror (*Robertson*)
- Having delusions about the punishment liable to be inflicted (*R v Moyle* [2008] EWCA Crim 3059)
- Having a delusional belief that the jury were possessed (*Moyle*)
- Having delusions that might at any moment interfere with a proper action (*Robertson*)
- A grossly abnormal mental state and being unable to view actions in any sort of sensible manner (*Hinz v Berry* [1970] 2 QB 40)
- Giving instructions that are implausible, unbelievable or unreliable or not being able to recognise them as such (*M (John)*)
- Being unable to make valid or helpful comments on the evidence and counsels' speeches (*M (John)*)
- Failing to see what is or is not a good point in his defence (*M (John)*)
- Being unable to remember at the end of a court session all the points that may have occurred to the defendant about what has been said (*M (John)*)
- Being unable, in his own defence, to give answers that are plausible, believable or reliable or not being able to recognise them as such (*M (John)*)

Allowance needs to be made for the adjustments that can reasonably be made to the trial to assist a defendant and ensure effective participation. Practice Direction *(Criminal Proceedings): Further Directions* [2007] 1 WLR 1790 sets out 'vulnerable defendant' provisions that apply to defendants who suffer from a mental disorder under the MHA or who have any other impairment of intelligence or social functioning. The steps that should be taken are to be judged having regard to such matters as the age, maturity and development (intellectual, social and emotional) of the defendant and all other circumstances of the case.

Defendants may benefit from visiting the courtroom out of court hours and before the trial to familiarise themselves with it. Consideration should be given to suggesting that the judge, counsel and court officers dispense with wigs and robes and sit on the same level as the defendant. It may be appropriate for defendants to sit, if they wish, and security considerations permitting, in the well of the court, with members of family or others in a like relationship and with a suitable supporting adult who can explain the proceedings as they unfold. It may be advisable for the number of members of public in court to be limited. Frequent and regular breaks can be introduced for those with impairments of attention or concentration and to allow the defendant's solicitor, or a supporting adult, to explain evidence, in language the defendant can understand, and take instructions. When the defendant gives evidence, counsel and the judge can be advised to put questions that are short, clear and simple, or even very simple. There may be an argument for the defendant giving evidence by a live television link. Another special provision for a vulnerable defendant is the use of a facilitator or intermediary.

The use of a 'facilitator' was approved by the Court of Appeal in *R v SH* [2003] EWCA Crim 1028. This was the case of an adult with an intellectual disability. The role of the facilitator was to assist the defendant communicate with the judge and counsel by putting questions into language the defendant could understand. In the same case, approval was also given to two measures to assist a defendant who had a poor memory and this was hampering his ability to give evidence. The first was to read out the defendant's defence statement, to help the jury understand his evidence. The second was to allow the defendant to refer to his proof of evidence or, if he could not read, allow leading questions from such a document to be put to him.

Although this 'facilitator' role is similar to that of an 'intermediary' who is allowed to facilitate communication with a witness, there had been no such statutory provision for defendants until the passing of the Coroners and Justice Act 2009 (CJA 2009), s.104 of which adds a new s.33BA to the Youth Justice and Criminal Evidence Act 1999 permitting the use of an intermediary in the case of accused persons under the age of 18 years whose ability to participate effectively is compromised by their level of intellectual ability or social functioning and in the case of accused persons over the age of 18 years who suffer from a mental disorder within the meaning of the MHA or otherwise have an impairment of intelligence and social functioning and for that reason are unable to participate effectively in giving oral evidence. The function of the intermediary is to communicate questions put to the accused person, communicate their answers to any person putting the questions and to explain such questions or answers so far as is necessary to ensure that they are understood by the accused or the person in question.

These allowances are particularly likely to apply to the young and those who have an intellectual disability. However, they need to be considered in any case where the psychiatrist is of the opinion that the defendant is not fit to plead and stand trial because otherwise the court or another expert may suggest that, with certain provisions, the defendant will be able to plead and stand trial.

Assessment is best approached, following a minimum of introduction, by asking defendants to explain their attendance at your consulting room. Their response may indicate that they understand the adversarial criminal proceedings and the nature of the offence(s) with which they are charged. Questions as to plea may reveal whether or not they understand the available pleas and their effects. If pleading not guilty, defendants can be asked to explain why they are pleading not guilty, although, if the assessment is at the request of the prosecution, they may have been advised not to discuss their defence. Then it will be more difficult to decide whether or not they can give instructions. If there are co-defendants, the accused's relationship with them should be explored, as any vulnerability might be such as to require consideration of special provisions, such as not sitting with the other defendants or even a separate trial. To test defendants' ability to give instructions and their understanding of the evidence, it is necessary to put some of the evidence and ask them to comment or explain. It is important to realise that they have to understand the detail of the evidence. The issue is case specific ('a case of this nature' – *Pritchard*; 'in his case' – *Whitefield*). There is a world of difference between understanding the evidence in a complex fraud case and understanding the evidence in a shoplifting case. All of this questioning will also shed light on the ability of the accused to give evidence. The test of challenging a juror is satisfied if defendants are capable of understanding that they should tell their lawyers if they know or recognise a juror and can tell them so. The case should not be considered in isolation: how the defendant conducts the affairs of everyday life will shed light on the defendant's possession of the abilities needed to understand evidence, give instructions and give evidence. Witness statements, reports and medical records should be searched for evidence of the accused's ability, or otherwise, to function in everyday life. As fitness to plead and stand trial may change over time, re-examination on the day of the trial may be advisable and this is usually done on a joint basis with the other expert(s).

Cases involving people with intellectual disability are often the most straightforward. Borderline cases can be problematic, however. Although it will often be advisable to have the evidence of a psychologist, the test is a legal test and not a matter of IQ or performance on some particular psychological test. Furthermore, psychologists cannot be approved under s.12 of the MHA unless they are also registered medical practitioners. Cases involving dementia ought to be straightforward but, as with Ernest Saunders in the Guinness case, when the case is over it may be decided that the diagnosis was mistaken (see Howard *et al*, 1992). The most difficult cases involve depressive disorders. These often involve hitherto, or still, law-abiding professional or business people who are understandably unhappy when charged with an offence such as fraud and fear not just financial and professional ruin but years of imprisonment, to which they will be unaccustomed. It is necessary to remember that many defendants are unhappy at being prosecuted and are fearful of the outcome but are not under a disability. Memory and concentration impairments severe enough to interfere with understanding evidence, giving instructions or giving evidence are easy to assert and for some not difficult to represent. Careful forensic assessment is needed to judge their genuineness. The recollection of a recent event can call into question alleged memory impairment. An admission to spending six hours a day going over statements and documentary exhibits with a solicitor can call into question impairment of concentration. Careful study of medical records and witness statements may reveal evidence inconsistent with the symptoms alleged.

Wood & Guly (1991) provide helpful accounts of the approach to the assessment of fitness to plead and stand trial in the cases of three people charged with murder and manslaughter.

If the accused is found to be under a disability and, on a trial of the facts, is found by a jury to have done the act or made the omission, the court may make: a hospital admission order, with or without restrictions on discharge; a supervision order; or an order for absolute discharge. If the jury is not satisfied, they must acquit. Additionally, s.5A of the CP(I)A permits the making of orders under ss. 35, 36 and 38 of the MHA prior to final disposal of the case where there has been a finding of disability (or insanity).

Be prepared for the court seeking assistance as to the disposal in the event that the jury does not acquit. If it is a case in which the court ought to consider imposing restrictions on discharge, make this clear in the report, as some judges take the opportunity to hear oral evidence on this issue, with the opportunity for cross-examination, during the enquiry into unfitness. It is then unnecessary to recall the psychiatrist to give evidence if the jury's verdict is that the accused did the act(s) alleged.

It can be a ground for appeal against conviction that the appellant was not fit to plead and stand trial. *R v Moyle* [2008] EWCA Crim 3059 is a case in which the Court of Appeal had evidence from three psychiatrists to the effect that the appellant had been unfit to plead at the time of his trial but the court was unable to accede to this submission. The reasons given by the court helpfully point to matters that should be carefully considered in such cases at the time of the trial and where the issue arises on appeal (Box 23).

In addition to provisions for defendants who are unfit to plead and stand trial, there is also a provision under s.35 of the Criminal Justice and Public Order Act 1994 for the court to refrain from giving the 'adverse inference' direction to the jury in respect of the defendant's silence at trial if 'it appears

---

Box 23 Reasons for not finding an appellant to have been unfit to plead and stand trial

The following reasons were given by Pill LJ in *R v Moyle* [2008] EWCA Crim 3059:

- The appellant was represented at trial by leading and junior counsel and a solicitor. Notwithstanding the evidence available from the psychiatrist, they found no reason to query, or investigate further, the appellant's fitness to plead. The trial was conducted by a judge experienced in criminal cases, who allowed it to proceed. Given the appellant's instructions, the plea and the issues raised were entirely appropriate.
- The appellant gave evidence at his trial and did so in a way which does not create doubts about his ability to understand questions put to him and to give the answers he saw fit to give. The trial involved a consideration of the events at the material time and the appellant's part in them. There is no indication that he failed to understand the evidence given or to respond to it with his own account, albeit an account which the jury disbelieved.
- There is no reason to doubt that the appellant understood that the proceedings were serious proceedings, that he was being tried for a serious offence and that the aim of the trial was to determine whether he was guilty of wrongdoing.
- The appellant's evidence did demonstrate a tactical awareness difficult to reconcile with unfitness to plead as understood in the authorities. For example, he gave evidence about the timing of his punching the victim which was inconsistent with an account given to the police. He gave a reason for having told the police what in evidence he claimed to be an untruth.
- The medical witnesses acknowledged the possibility of guile by the appellant in his approach to the case. Their main concern was that the appellant's delusions were such as to impede his communication with his legal advisors and his understanding of proceedings.
- The appellant's embarrassment at his predicament and his inability to accept that his conduct was the cause of death were reactions not uncommon in those charged with serious crime and certainly not supportive of unfitness to plead.
- Clearly, beliefs, one hopes always delusional, that the court is biased cannot extinguish a person's right to be tried or the public's right to have that person tried. A false belief about the punishment liable to be inflicted does not impair the defendant's ability to be tried.
- Even if, at times during the trial, the appellant was not acting in his own best interests, in the evidence and instructions he gave, that does not, in itself, create or contribute to a finding of unfitness to plead.
- The appellant's condition has not changed substantially since his trial. His present legal advisors have sought specific instructions from him and appear to have had no difficulty in obtaining them.

to the court that the physical or mental condition of the accused makes it undesirable for him to give evidence'.

The courts differ in the way they approach the relationship between this provision and the provisions for fitness to plead and stand trial. Grubin (1996) described what appears to have been one of the first cases in which this provision was applied. This was a case in which there did not appear to be any issue with regard to the defendant's fitness to plead and stand trial, he was not suffering from any form of mental disorder within the meaning of the MHA and no psychiatric diagnosis could be made of mental illness or personality disorder, but it was suggested that:

his personality was such that under the stress of cross-examination he was likely to become anxious, frustrated and confused, and that this could cause him to behave in an inappropriate manner, with the risk of prejudicing the jury against him.... He had already demonstrated a wide repertoire of behaviours ... [any of which], while not being an indication of his guilt or innocence, could distract from the content of his evidence and lead the jury to make inappropriate inferences. (Grubin, 1996, p. 650)

There was also an argument that although he did not suffer from a form of mental disorder, he might appear to do so to a lay individual, as he had appeared to his solicitor and barrister, and this was what the terminology 'mental condition' was intended to reflect. The court stressed that the overriding concern had to be the risk that the jury could misinterpret his behaviour and obtain an inappropriate picture of the defendant and his defence. The defendant did not give evidence on his own behalf and he was acquitted.

It has been suggested by Gray *et al* (2001) that there are a number of psychiatric and psychological disorders that may amount to a 'condition' within the meaning of s.35(1):

severe mental health problems, learning disabilities, dementia or head injury that may lead to the evidence that they give at trial being misinterpreted by a jury and consequently leading to a potentially biased view being formed of both the defendant and the defence. (Gray *et al*, 2001, p. 55)

Whereas in the case reported by Grubin (1996) the issue addressed by s.35(1) was treated as being separate from the issue of fitness to plead and stand trial, Gray *et al* (2001) reported a case in which defence counsel argued that it should be included as a new and additional criterion in the evaluation of fitness to plead and stand trial and in which case both psychiatrists who had been instructed concurred in their opinion that if the court 'considers that ability to give evidence in your own defence is vital for someone to be fit to plead and stand trial, on the basis of his inability to give evidence on his own behalf, [we] consider Mr M unfit to plead and stand his trial'. The defendant was then found unfit to plead and stand trial. On a trial of the facts he was found to have done the act alleged and he was made subject to a guardianship order. Insofar as the evidence of the psychiatrists was that he was unable to give evidence on his own behalf, it could be argued that, in any event, he should have been found unfit to plead and stand trial on the basis that he was incapable of giving evidence on his own behalf according to the Dyson/Pritchard rules as usually applied, in which case the s.35(1) provision was unnecessary. Gray *et al* (2001) state that since their reported case they have been aware of a small number of other cases in which 'the ability to give evidence in one's own defence had been included in the criteria of fitness to plead and stand trial'. However, the ability of defendants to give evidence on their own behalf is still determined by the original 'Pritchard test' (Box 20).

Insofar as, in the case reported by Grubin (1996), the defendant was fit to plead and stand trial, and this included being *capable* of giving evidence on his own behalf, and s.35(1) refers to the *desirability* of the defendant giving evidence on his own behalf, it would appear that it is the distinction between 'capacity' and 'desirability' which is the key to understanding the s.35(1) provision. The cases described by Grubin (1996) and by Gray *et al* (2001) are of defendants who were going to appear or behave in such a way as to prejudice the jury against them. As already indicated (Box 22), not being capable of acting in one's best interests (*R v Robertson* [1968] 3 All ER 557, CA) does not make someone unfit to plead and stand trial. Therefore, s.35(1) would appear to be a provision for defendants who have the capacity to give evidence on their own behalf but will probably not, as a result of their 'mental condition', act in their best interests. If this interpretation of the law is correct, these are complementary provisions. Alternatively, it is possible that Parliament intended to use s.35(1) to give a statutory basis for the inclusion of the undesirability of defendants giving evidence on their own behalf in the rules for fitness to plead and stand trial, in which case the interpretation of the law in the cases reported by Gray *et al* (2001) would suggest that these are one and the same issue.

Having regard to the wording of the statute, that is, 'undesirability' rather than 'inability' or 'incapacity', it would appear unlikely that they are the same issue, but until such a case goes to the Court of Appeal, it is likely that both approaches will be applied. The approach does matter: a defendant found fit to plead and stand trial but allowed to benefit from s.35(1) will either be found guilty or acquitted, and if acquitted, the court's powers will end there and then. However, if defendants are found to be 'under a disability', because it is undesirable for them to give evidence on their own behalf, they will be subject to the procedure under the CP(I)A and, if found to have done the act alleged, disposal of their case will be in the hands of the court (see p. 78). It is also worth noting that for the application of s.35(1) there is no requirement as to medical evidence. The court may apply it on the basis of the evidence of one doctor or a psychologist or even of its own motion. However, if the issue is held to fall within the criteria for fitness to plead and stand trial, there will need to be evidence from two registered medical practitioners, including one approved under s.12 of the MHA.

Regardless of the approach taken by the court, psychiatrists should be prepared to give reasons for their opinion and by reference to the factors that it is within their expertise to identify and describe. These are likely to include, for example, inappropriate behaviour resulting from the defendant as in Grubin's case, becoming anxious, frustrated, confused, irrational, angry or flippant. It is not enough to assert that the defendant would experience 'extreme difficulty' in giving evidence or that possibly (but put no higher than that) there would be an impact on defendant's mental health (*R v Ensor* [2010] 1 Cr App R 255).

Trial issues

Diminished responsibility

The defence of 'diminished responsibility' is a statutory defence in England and Wales under s.2 of the Homicide Act 1957 and in Northern Ireland under s.5(1) of the Criminal Justice Act (Northern Ireland) 1966 as substituted by s.52 of the CJA 2009 (Box 24) and, if successful, reduces the offence of murder to one of manslaughter ('on the grounds of diminished responsibility'). However, it has been a common law defence in Scotland for much longer. It came about in *HM Advocate v Dingwall* (1867) 5 Irvine 466 and was crucially defined by Lord Justice-Clerk Alness in *HM Advocate v Savage* (1923) JC 49:

Box 24 Diminished responsibility: legislative definition

Diminished responsibility according to the Homicide Act 1957 s.2 as substituted by s.52 of the Coroners and Justice Act 2009 is defined as follows:

A person ('D') who kills or is a party to the killing of another is not to be convicted if D was suffering from an abnormality of mental functioning which –

    (a) arose from a recognised medical condition
    (b) substantially impaired D's ability to do one or more of the things mentioned in subsection (1A) and
    (c) provides an explanation for D's acts or omissions in being a party to the killing.
(1A) Those things are –
    (a) to understand the nature of D's conduct
    (b) to form a rational judgment
    (c) to exercise self-control.
(1B) For the purposes of subsection (1)(c) an abnormality of mental functioning provides an explanation for D's conduct if it causes, or is a significant contributory factor in causing, D to carry out that conduct.

It is very difficult to put in a phrase, but ... some form of mental unsoundness; a state of mind ... bordering on, although not amounting to insanity; ... a mind so affected that responsibility is diminished ... there must be some form of mental disease.

It is not a defence against any charge other than murder: the psychiatrist who suggests that it should be pleaded as a defence to shoplifting will have a short or very uphill career as a psychiatric expert.

The defence has four ingredients: (1) abnormality of mental functioning; (2) the cause of any abnormality of mental functioning in the form of a recognised medical condition; (3) substantial impairment of ability to do one or more of three defined things (see Box 24, and below); and (4) an explanation for the killing.

'Abnormality of mental functioning' replaces 'abnormality of mind' in the Homicide Act 1957. Until case law provides a definition of 'abnormality of mental functioning' the courts may continue to rely, at least to some extent, on 'abnormality of mind' as it was defined by Lord Parker CJ in *R v Byrne* [1960] 2 QB 396 (Box 25). Furthermore, insofar as 'mental functioning' is a psychiatric concept, Ormerod (2011) has asked if there will be much for the jury to do if there is uncontradicted expert evidence as to the presence of abnormal mental functioning. Thus, although Lord Parker CJ made it clear in *Byrne* that, whereas 'medical evidence is of no doubt of importance' as to 'abnormality of mind', the jury is not bound to accept this evidence and the issue is 'in their good judgment', this may not apply to 'abnormality of mental functioning'.

So far as the cause of any 'abnormality of mental functioning' is concerned, the jury is likely to be asked to accept the evidence of the psychiatric expert as to the 'medical condition' from which the abnormality arose unless that evidence is questioned by other expert evidence. 'Medical condition' has replaced 'arrested or incomplete development of mind', 'inherent causes', 'disease' and 'injury' in the Homicide Act 1957, the so-called 'bracketed causes'. The term 'medical condition' has yet to be defined by case law but

---

Box 25 The 'abnormality of mind' test

Lord Parker CJ in *R v Byrne* [1960] 2 QB 396 set out the 'abnormality of mind' test as follows:

... a state of mind so different from that of ordinary human beings that the reasonable man would term it abnormal. It appears to us to be wide enough to cover the mind's activities in all its aspects, not only the perception of physical acts and matters and the ability to form a rational judgment whether an act is right or wrong, but also the ability to exercise will-power to control physical acts in accordance with that rational judgment.

it is likely that, within reason, any mental disorder listed in ICD-10 will be regarded as a 'medical condition'. It will also include non-psychiatric conditions such as epilepsy, thyroid disorders, sleep disorders and diabetes. It appears broader in scope than the 'bracketed causes' it replaces.

'Substantial impairment of ability' now replaces 'substantial impairment of mental responsibility' (although paradoxically the title of s.52 of the CJA 2009 still refers to 'Persons suffering from diminished responsibility'). Previously psychiatrists often tried to avoid giving an opinion on 'mental responsibility', because it related to a legal or moral concept. Furthermore, Lord Parker CJ, in *Byrne*, said that substantial impairment of mental responsibility was 'a question of degree and essentially one for the jury. Medical evidence is, of course, relevant ... but whether such an impairment can properly be called "substantial", [is] a matter on which juries may quite legitimately differ from doctors'. Now that the law has replaced 'mental responsibility for acts or omissions' with the 'ability' of defendants to: (1) understand their own conduct; (2) form a rational judgment; or (3) exercise self-control, it is likely that medical evidence will become more determinative of this issue. Ormerod (2011) has suggested that, as impairment of ability to do one of these three specified things is purely a psychiatric question, it would seem appropriate for the expert to offer an opinion on whether there is 'substantial' impairment, in which case arguably there will be greater influence from experts than previously. It remains to be seen whether the courts will continue to apply the two meanings of 'substantial' as approved in *R v Lloyd* [1967] 1 QB 175: (1) the broad, common-sense meaning; and (2) 'that the word meant more than some trivial degree of impairment but less than total impairment', but this seems likely and particularly so given the endorsement of both of these meanings by Judge LCJ in *R v R* [2010] EWCA Crim 194.

Mackay (2010, p. 751) has observed that, although these three 'abilities' can be traced to *Byrne*, 'by specifying what abilities need to be impaired [this] means that "abnormality of mental functioning" now seems narrower than "abnormality of mind", as the only mind's activities which are included are the three specified things in subsection (1A)'. Thus, however widely 'abnormality of mental functioning' is defined and however wide the range of recognised medical conditions, the defence now appears to be narrower. It is possible, for example, that personality disorders will be more likely to be excluded by the new formulation unless the defendant's ability to exercise self-control can be demonstrated to have been substantially impaired. Ormerod (2011, p. 533) has pointed out that if the ability 'to understand the nature of his own conduct' and the ability 'to form a rational judgment' are construed too narrowly, the criteria will be very similar to those for insanity and hence may be difficult to satisfy. He suggests that if these criteria are akin to those for insanity, the defendant might well plead that complete defence rather than the partial defence of diminished responsibility. It can also be argued that as 'ability' is more specific than 'mental responsibility' this leaves less leeway for the jury and so the defence will be harder to prove.

Medical evidence is also likely to be crucial in persuading, or dissuading, a jury that the abnormality of mental functioning has caused, or made a significant contribution to the cause of, the conduct that has led to the killing. This is a stronger causal requirement than previously, although it is arguable whether, in view of the requirement for the three specified things in subsection (1A), subsection (1B) adds to the clear linkage between the relevant substantial impairment and the homicidal conduct (Mackay, 2010). It does, however, make clear what may not have previously been as clear: that even when there is undoubtedly a mental condition present, unless this condition has a material bearing on the killing, this does not provide a defence.

With this new law in mind, it is reasonable to suggest that a psychiatrist preparing a report where there is an issue of 'diminished responsibility' should have in mind the questions set out in Box 26 and be aware that oral expert evidence will be more likely as the greater specificity of the defence will make it easier for the prosecution to contest the defence.

Homicides involving an alcohol-dependent defendant have been so problematic as to engage the Court of Appeal in issuing guidance on this issue (*R v Stewart* [2009] 2 Cr App R 500). This appeal did not take account of the then proposed changes to the law on diminished responsibility, and below the new terminology is in parentheses. It was held that whether or not the alcohol dependence syndrome constituted an abnormality of mind (*now* abnormality of mental functioning) would depend on the nature and extent of the syndrome and whether, looking at the matter broadly, the defendant's consumption of alcohol before the killing was fairly to be regarded as the involuntary result of an irresistible craving for, or compulsion to, drink.

It was held that the second question, that of causation, would normally follow from the answer to the first, so, if the alcohol dependence syndrome amounted to an abnormality of mind (*now* abnormality of mental functioning), it would be attributed to a disease or illness (*now* medical condition).

Box 26 Questions to be answered in a psychiatric report where 'diminished responsibility' is the issue

- Was there an abnormality of mental functioning at the material time?
- If so, did it arise from a recognised medical condition?
- Did the abnormality of mental functioning substantially impair D's ability to understand the nature of the conduct, form a rational judgment and/or exercise self-control?
- Did the abnormality of mental functioning cause, or make a significant contribution to, D's conduct in carrying out, or being a party to, the killing?
- Does the abnormality of mental functioning provide an explanation for D's acts and omissions in doing or being a party to the killing?

If the jury is satisfied that the defendant's alcohol dependence syndrome constituted an abnormality of mind (*now* abnormality of mental functioning) due to disease or illness (*now* a medical condition), the issue of 'substantial impairment of mental responsibility' (*now* substantial impairment of ability) is to be decided according to the conventional terms. But it was pointed out that the jury might be invited to reflect on the difference between defendants who failed to resist their impulses to behave as they actually did and an inability, consequent upon an alcohol dependence syndrome, to resist impulses to act as they did.

The judgment refers to the jury's consideration of the evidence of medical experts. Box 27 lists the issues likely to arise and on which the jury should be invited to form their own judgment. These issues, at least, should be covered in the psychiatric report.

There is the related issue of an abnormality of mental functioning occurring along with alcohol intoxication. The relevant authority is *R v Dietschmann* [2003] 1 AC 1209 HL. It is best illustrated by the appropriate judicial direction to the jury (italics and bracketed clauses are used below to reflect the new terminology of diminished responsibility):

Assuming the defence have established that the defendant was suffering from *an abnormality of mental functioning* … the important question is 'Did that abnormality substantially impair his *ability* [to perform the] acts or resisting the impulse in doing the killing?' You know that he had a lot to drink. Drink cannot be taken into account as something which contributed to his *abnormality of mental functioning* and to any impairment of *ability* arising from that abnormality. But you may take the view that both the defendant's *abnormality of mental functioning* and drink played a part in impairing his *ability* [in carrying out] the killing and that he might have killed if he had not taken drink. If you take that view then the question … to decide is this: 'Has the defendant satisfied you that, despite the drink, his *abnormality of mental functioning* substantially impaired his *ability* [in carrying out] his fatal acts.

The question posed is strictly a jury question but psychiatric experts are often asked to deal with it.

Box 27 Issues for the judgment of the jury where alcohol dependence is raised as a defence to a charge of murder

- The extent and seriousness of the defendant's dependency, if any, on alcohol
- The extent to which their ability to control their drinking, or to choose whether to drink or not, was reduced
- Whether they were capable of abstinence from alcohol, and if so,
  - for how long,
  - whether they were choosing for some particular reason to decide to get drunk or to drink even more than usual.

Infanticide

Infanticide is another partial defence to a charge of murder which, if successful, effectively reduces the offence to one of manslaughter. It is also an alternative to manslaughter. However, it differs from 'diminished responsibility' in that it can be charged from the outset and so it can avoid a woman being charged with the murder of her own child.

It is defined by s.1 of the Infanticide Act 1938 (as amended by s.57 of the CJA 2009). It is thereby limited to a woman who is charged with, or would otherwise be convicted of, the murder or manslaughter of her child under the age of 12 months. It is not a defence open to a man, to a woman who kills another woman's child or where the child is 12 months or older. It applies where the woman has caused her child's death by any wilful act or omission. In order for the defence to be successful, 'at the time of the act or omission' there has to be evidence that:

the balance of her mind was disturbed by reason of her not having fully recovered from the effect of giving birth to the child or by reason of the effect of lactation consequent upon the birth of the child....

The 'lactation' limb is now redundant given the lack of any evidence that lactation causes mental abnormality. On a strict interpretation of the law, the reference to 'giving birth to the child' means that if a mother kills her newborn baby and her 11-month-old child, when her balance of mind is disturbed by reason of giving birth to the newborn baby, she will not have a defence of infanticide to the killing of the 11-month-old child if she had by then recovered from giving birth to the older child.

The offence predates the defence of 'diminished responsibility' by half a century but, even though it serves a similar purpose, it has survived. This is partly because it can be charged as an offence at the outset. It is partly because, even though it is of more limited application, analysis of the successful cases suggests that it is an easier defence than 'diminished responsibility'. It is probably also because in 'diminished responsibility' the burden of proof is on the defence, whereas if the defence of infanticide is raised to a charge of murder the prosecution carries the more difficult burden of proving beyond reasonable doubt that it is not infanticide.

The difficulty for the psychiatrist is that disturbance of the balance of the mind is not a psychiatric concept, and whereas case law has defined 'abnormality of mind', there is no such definition of disturbance of the balance of the mind. Furthermore, as Mackay (1995) has pointed out, in the cases he reviewed, there was little analysis or discussion by the psychiatrists of this criterion. The nearest definition is in *R v Sainsbury* (1989) 11 Cr App R (S) 533, where the appeal court judges used the phrase 'left the balance of your mind disturbed so as to prevent rational judgment and decision'.

The cases reported by Mackay (1993) and the case reports of d'Orbán (1979) and Bluglass (1990) assist with the practical application of the law by the courts. Some of the cases analysed by Mackay were of women with fairly obvious mental disorders such as 'puerperal depressive illness', 'clinical depression' and a manic–depressive psychosis that manifest in command hallucinations, but his series also included a case of 'severe hysterical dissociation' and one in which the only abnormality was 'emotional disturbances'. This is consistent with that fact that a half of the women in the series reported by d'Orbán were not suffering from any identifiable mental disorder. Bluglass reported similar cases: a woman in whom no persisting psychiatric disorder was found other than her distressed state after the homicide; a woman who was depressed and distressed but showed 'no underlying disorder'; and a woman who gave birth to a baby with Down syndrome and for whom nothing more abnormal was reported than her shock, inability to accept the appearance of the baby and her sense of hopelessness about its future. The cases reported by Mackay and Bluglass therefore confirm the impression of d'Orbán that for infanticide 'the degree of abnormality is much less than that required to substantiate "abnormality of mind" amounting to substantially diminished responsibility'.

This matter was addressed by the College in its evidence to the Criminal Law Revision Committee (Bluglass, 1978). The College submission identified four circumstances which might in practice justify an infanticide verdict but might not be sufficient for a defence of diminished responsibility: (1) overwhelming stress from the social environment being highlighted by the birth of a baby, with the emphasis on the unsuitability of accommodation and so on; (2) overwhelming stress from an additional member to a household struggling with poverty; (3) psychological injury and pressures and stress from a husband or other member of the family from the mother's incapacity to arrange the demands of the extra member of the family; (4) failure of bonding between mother and child through illness or disability which impairs the mother's capacity to care for the infant.'

One of Bluglass's cases is particularly illustrative:

A 21 year old mother of a new baby, her first child, moved shortly after the child's birth to a new locality in another part of the country where she had no social contacts. She was left alone with her baby for long periods while her husband was establishing himself in a new job. She was a dull young woman (IQ 88) who became increasingly depressed and resentful in her attitude towards the child. One night in frustration and anger she threw the baby against the corner of his cot and killed him.... She was admitted to hospital for treatment of her depression and psychotherapeutic support. The child was aged 11 months ... and initially a defence of infanticide could not be supported as there appeared to be little connection between childbirth or lactation and her actions. There was widespread sympathy towards her by the court, which suggested that it could not be stated with certainty that there was no association with the effects of pregnancy and that a finding of infanticide was therefore appropriate. (Bluglass, 1990)

The role in this case of 'widespread sympathy' supports the view of Mackay that the criteria in the Infanticide Act 1938 have been used to ensure that leniency can be meted out in appropriate cases. However, whereas sympathy may move a jury to conclude that the prosecution has not proved beyond reasonable doubt that it is not infanticide, sympathy may not be enough to persuade the Court of Appeal to quash a murder conviction and substitute one of infanticide. In *R v Kai-Whitewind* [2005] 2 Cr App R 457 the Court acknowledged that this 'sad case' demonstrated the need for a re-examination of an unsatisfactory and outdated law but upheld the murder conviction.

In the meantime, notwithstanding the limited amendments by the CJA 2009, this unsatisfactory and outdated law remains on the statute book. The best advice to the psychiatrist in the case of a woman who has allegedly killed her own child aged less than 12 months is to set out, if it be so: (1) how the woman's mental state has changed since childbirth, and whether or not the changes could be regarded as amounting to an 'abnormality of mind' or recognisable mental disorder; (2) how this amounts to a disturbance of the balance of mind, if possible showing how it has affected rational judgment and decision-making; and (3), if possible, how this mental state can be attributed to the effects of childbirth. It is not necessary to identify a mental disorder within the meaning of s.1 of the MHA, albeit that this is now a broad definition, or show that the woman has an 'abnormality of mind'.

Although the maximum sentence for infanticide is life imprisonment, in 59 cases between 1979 and 1988 there were no custodial sentences and all disposals were by way of probation, supervision and hospital orders (*Sainsbury*), so reports in such cases are likely to need to give careful consideration to issues related to sentencing. Since then there has been at least one case where upon a plea of guilty to two offences separated by about four years, the defendant was sentenced to three years imprisonment.

Insanity

The defence of insanity is governed by the M'Naghten rules (*M'Naghten's Case* (1843) 10 Cl & F 200). The rules state that:

the jurors ought to be told in all cases that every man is to be presumed to be sane, and to possess a sufficient degree of reason to be held responsible for his crimes, until the contrary be proved to their satisfaction; and that to establish a defence on the ground of insanity, it must be clearly proved that, at the time of committing the act, the party accused was labouring under such a defect of reason, from disease of the mind, as not to know the nature and quality of the act he was doing; or, if he did know it, that he did not know he was doing what was wrong.

The presumption of sanity means that the burden of proving insanity is placed on the defence and the standard of proof is the civil standard, that is, the balance of probabilities.

The reference to 'the time of committing the act' means that what is at issue is the state of mind of the defendant at the material time.

Central to the defence is a 'defect of reason'. Whatever the popular notion of insanity, this is not a defence that is likely to be successful when the act is carried out on impulse or in a state of so-called loss of control or in a highly disturbed emotional state. It is necessary to show the defective process of reasoning that has resulted in the defendant either not knowing the nature and quality of the act he was doing (the first limb), or if he did, not knowing that what he was doing was wrong (the second limb), or both. This is a narrow, cognitive test. Thus, in *R v Clarke* [1972] 1 All ER 219, it was held that the momentary confusion and absent-mindedness of a depressed shoplifter, who retained her ordinary powers of reason, fell far short of a 'defect of reason'.

It is also of critical importance to identify a 'disease of the mind' that has resulted in the defect of reasoning. Although medical evidence is required (s.1. of the CP(IU)A), it is for the judge to decide what is a disease of the mind. The leading case is that of *R v Sullivan* [1984] AC 156 at 172, where Lord Diplock stated that:

'mind' in the M'Naghten Rules is used in the ordinary sense of the mental faculties of reason, memory and understanding. If the effect of a disease is to impair these faculties so severely as to have either of the consequences referred to in the latter part of the rules, it matters not whether the aetiology is organic … or functional, or whether the impairment is permanent or transient and intermittent, provided that it subsisted at the time of commission of the act.

This means that it is the role of the psychiatric expert to show that the impairment of faculties did occur and what the cause of the impairment was. The disease has to be 'internal'. Impairment of the faculties resulting from some external factor such as violence, drugs, including anaesthetics, alcohol or 'hypnotic influences' is held not to be due to disease (per Lawton LJ in *R v Quick* [1973] QB 910). In practice, in more than half of successful insanity defences the diagnosis is schizophrenia, the rest of the diagnoses being a large number of conditions each of which constitutes less than 10% of cases (Mackay, 1995).

It has been ruled that 'the nature and quality of the act' refers to the physical rather than the moral quality of the act. There are no published law reports which show how a successful defence based on the first limb operates. There are cases which show its unsuccessful operation (e.g. *R v Codère* (1916) 12 Cr App R 21). In fact, research, based in part on unpublished cases, has revealed that only about a quarter of successful insanity defences used the 'nature and quality' limb in a series of 52 cases between 1975 and 1989 (Mackay, 1995). Lord Diplock in *Sullivan* said that for jurors in the 1980s it could be put in the terms: 'He did not know what he was doing'. Standard (hypothetical) illustrations are of someone under the delusion that he was merely breaking a jar actually killing another, and a man cutting a woman's throat in the belief that he was cutting a loaf of bread (Ormerod, 2011: p. 285).

It has been ruled that not to know 'he was doing what was wrong' means *legally* wrong, or contrary to the law, and it does not mean *morally* wrong. Thus the defence was not available to Windle, who thought that it was morally right to kill his suicidal wife and yet knew that it was legally wrong – 'I suppose they will hang me for this' (*R v Windle* [1952] 2 QB 826). In Mackay's study, 56% of the cases relied on this second limb (and the reason that 56 plus 25 does not make 100 is that in the rest of the cases it was not possible to identify the basis for the defence in the psychiatric reports). Mackay is critical of the liberal fashion in which the psychiatrists approached the wrongness issue, that is, 'with little attempt made to distinguish between lack of knowledge of legal wrong ... as opposed to unawareness of moral wrong'. My own experience is of the defence being successful in cases of defendants with religious delusions. For example, a defendant, whose first name was Leo, believed that he was 'Leo, the Lion of Judah', that he was second only to God and that God's law required him to kill his next-door neighbour, for refusing to hand him the keys to Jerusalem; Leo believed this refusal gave him a legal right to kill him, notwithstanding that this was against the law of the land.

Automatism

The essence of the defence of automatism is involuntariness: the alleged act was carried out when the defendant was not in control of his or her mind or body. Automatism is defined by case law and three cases are of particular assistance to the expert:

The state of a person who, though capable of action, is not conscious of what he is doing ... it means unconscious, involuntary action, and it is a defence because the mind does not go with what is done. (*Bratty v Attorney General for Northern Ireland* [1963] AC 386 *per* Viscount Kilmuir LC)

and:

action without any knowledge of acting, or action with no consciousness of doing what is being done. (*R v Cottle* [1958] NZLR 999 *per* Gresson P)

and for the defence of automatism to succeed:

impairment of relevant capacities as distinct from total deprivation of these capacities [will not suffice].... It is fundamental to a defence of automatism that the actor has no control over his actions. (*R v Milloy* (1991) 54 A Crim R 340 *per* Thomas J)

The law distinguishes two forms of automatism: non-insane automatism (or sane automatism, *automatism simpliciter*) and insane automatism (i.e. automatism due to disease of the mind). The distinction is based on the cause of the automatism. Non-insane automatisms are caused by *external* factors, such as drugs, hypnosis or concussion. Insane automatisms are regarded as arising from an *internal* factor such as epilepsy, cerebrovascular disease or diabetes. If the trial judge decides that it is a case of 'insane automatism', he or she will direct the jury to decide whether the defendant is guilty or not guilty by reason of insanity (see above). The distinction is an important one. A successful defence of non-insane automatism results in acquittal. If it is a successful defence of insane automatism, disposal of the case will be under the CP(I)A.

From a medical perspective, the legal classification is unsatisfactory if not nonsensical:

For a violent act committed while the mind is disordered owing to an excess of insulin is a sane automatism if the insulin is injected, but an insane automatism if the insulin comes from an insulinoma of the pancreas. (Fenwick, 1990)

Furthermore, although sleep-walking arises from an internal factor, it is considered a non-insane automatism.

In relation to 'non-insane automatism' the evidential burden is borne by the defendant but the prosecution carries the burden of proving beyond reasonable doubt that it is not automatism. This means that the defence has to provide some evidence in support of automatism in order for the prosecution to attempt to rebut this evidence. The trial judge will decide if a proper evidential foundation has been laid before he or she allows the defence to be put to the jury.

Although the defence is ordinarily a defence to any criminal charge, including offences of strict liability, such as, in theory, driving over the prescribed speed limit, the defence is not open to those who have brought the state of automatism upon themselves, for example by becoming exhausted or through consumption of alcohol or use of drugs.

It follows that in a case where the defence of automatism is at issue, the psychiatrist should: (1) analyse the evidence as to the state of mind of the defendant at the material time so that, having regard to the legal definitions of automatism, the trial judge can decide whether or not the evidential foundation is laid; (2) identify the likely cause or causes for the abnormal state of mind; and (3) if psychiatric expertise is needed on this issue, consider the extent to which the defendant could be regarded as culpable for being in the state of automatism. If the evidential basis is laid for the defence, the trial judge will decide on the type of automatism, but in the event that he or she decides that it is an insane automatism the psychiatric expert should be prepared to assist the court as to the disposal of the case.

The psychiatrist is rather more likely to be instructed in a case of automatism caused by epilepsy or some other neurological condition than in the case of automatism resulting from psychiatric disorder. This is because such cases are more common and the CP(IU)A requires written or oral evidence from two registered and licensed medical practitioners, of whom at least one must be approved under s.12 of the MHA and few neurologists are so approved. Although, in such cases, the psychiatrist is likely to be heavily reliant on neurological opinion, often provided by a neurologist who has been instructed first, it is important that the psychiatrist heeds the advice of Fenwick (1990) as to the six points upon which to be satisfied before going to court to substantiate the diagnosis of epileptic automatism (Box 28).

Box 28 Fenwick's six points upon which the psychiatrist is to be satisfied for a defence of epileptic automatism

Fenwick (1990, p. 279) gives the following six points upon which the psychiatrist
should be satisfied before going to court to substantiate a defence of epileptic
automatism:

- The patient should be a known epileptic
- The act should be out of character for the individual and inappropriate for the
  circumstances.
- There must be no evidence of premeditation or concealment.
- If witnesses are available, they should report a disorder of consciousness at the
  time of the act (e.g. staring eyes, glassy look, stereotyped movements, con-
  fusion and evidence that the person was out of touch with the surroundings).
- A disorder of memory is the rule (but with no loss of memory antedating the
  event).
- The diagnosis of epilepsy can be substantiated on clinical grounds alone.

Intent

Except for offences of so-called strict liability, which do not require proof of
fault, such as driving over the prescribed alcohol limit, in order to convict
a person of a criminal offence, it is necessary for the prosecution to prove
beyond reasonable doubt two elements of the crime (Ormerod, 2011). The
first is that the person has caused something to happen, or is responsible
for a certain state of affairs, that is forbidden by the criminal law. This is
known as the *actus reus*. The second is that the person had a specific state
of mind in relation to the causing of the event or the existence of the state
of affairs. This is known as the *mens rea*. It is the mental element required
by the definition of the particular crime. Usually this means the intention
to cause the *actus reus*.

Psychiatric evidence is not admissible on the issue of whether or not an
accused person *had* the *mens rea* for a particular offence. This is an ultimate
issue for the jury to decide, either by reference to all the evidence, drawing
such inferences as appear to the jury, in the circumstances, to be proper, or
by the admission of the defendant. Psychiatric evidence may, however, be
admissible as to whether or not the accused had a condition that could affect
the *ability to form* the particular intent to commit the crime, that is, *could form*
the *mens rea*. The most common circumstance in which psychiatric evidence
may be sought as to the ability to form an intent is in cases where there is
evidence that an accused person was intoxicated with alcohol or drugs at
the material time.

There is a general rule that voluntary intoxication is not a defence. This is
usually expressed as 'A drunken intent is still intent'. It does not matter that
it is an intent that the defendant would not have formed if not intoxicated

93

and it does not matter if defendants were so intoxicated that they do not recall what their intent was or what they did.

Voluntary intoxication is, however, a defence to what are known as crimes requiring 'specific intent', which are distinguished from what are known as crimes of 'basic intent'. As the distinction is one of policy rather than principle, it is necessary to base the classification on the decisions of the courts. Thus, the following have been identified as crimes of specific intent: murder, wounding or causing grievous bodily harm with intent, theft, robbery, burglary with intent to steal, handling stolen goods, endeavouring to obtain money on a forged cheque, causing criminal damage where only intention to cause damage or endanger life is alleged, and an *attempt* to commit any of these crimes of specific intent. The following are regarded as crimes of basic intent: manslaughter, rape, malicious wounding or inflicting grievous bodily harm, kidnapping and false imprisonment, assault occasioning actual bodily harm, assault on a constable in execution of duty, common assault, taking a vehicle without the owner's consent, criminal damage where recklessness is alleged, and possibly an attempt to commit an offence where recklessness is a sufficient element in the *mens rea*, as in attempted rape.

A recent case (*R v Heard* [2008] QB 43) seems to have established that, whereas the offence of sexual assault requires intentional rather than reckless touching, it is not an offence of specific intent. This case adds to the difficulty in distinguishing crimes of specific and basic intent.

If you are instructed in such a case, first ascertain from the indictment, and if necessary by reference to the relevant act itself or a legal textbook, what the *mens rea* is for the offence. For example, it may be an allegation of burglary with intent, the particulars being that the accused entered, as a trespasser, a dwelling with intent to steal. The prosecution will need to prove that the accused entered with intent to steal. Second, ascertain from the witness statements what the evidence is that the accused was intoxicated and what the degree of intoxication was. The mere fact that the defendant has consumed alcohol or taken drugs is not enough. Third, the witness statements should be analysed for the presence or absence of evidence of the accused being able to act with forethought, form intentions and act on those intentions. To quote a typical summing up to the jury:

You look at his actions before, at the time of and, indeed, after the offence alleged. All these things, clearly, are capable you may think, of shedding a great deal of light upon what was on his mind at the time.... (Rix & Clarkson, 1994, p. 415)

For example, if there is evidence from the householder and from fingerprint evidence that the accused has moved aside a vase from the sill of the landing window by which he has entered the property, it may be difficult to argue that he was so intoxicated that he could not form the intent to steal. This means considering the evidence of witnesses as to what the defendant said and did before, at and after the material time. If the defendant has a recollection of what happened, or gave an account to the police or gives evidence at his trial, you also take into account what he told you or the police or says in evidence.

Pre-trial analysis usually allows 'intent' cases to be identified as belonging to one of three categories.

First, there are those in which there is such ample evidence of the accused acting intentionally and with forethought that, notwithstanding intoxication, it will not be possible to persuade a jury that the defendant was sufficiently intoxicated to lack the specific intent for the offence.

Second, there are those in which there is no evidence of the accused acting on intentions and with forethought and there is also evidence of behaviour that appears purposeless, pointless or confused. In such cases the psychiatric evidence may lead the prosecution to offer to accept a plea of guilty to a lesser offence, for example offering to accept a plea to unlawful wounding under s.20 of the Offences Against the Person Act 1861 instead of going to trial to try to prove the more serious offence of wounding with intent to cause grievous bodily harm under s.18, with the risk that the accused may be acquitted.

Third, there are cases in which the evidence does not point one way or the other. In such cases, be prepared to go to court and base your opinion not on the evidence as set out in the witness statements but on the evidence that these and perhaps other witnesses give in court.

Especially where defendants claim, or there is evidence, that they were under the influence of a drug with which it is assumed that most of a jury will be unfamiliar it is common to ask for a psychiatric opinion on the issue of intent, but many of these cases turn on the actual evidence from which the jury will infer intent rather than the pharmacology of the drug in question.

Psychiatric states which are particularly likely to give rise to issues as to the capacity to form an intent are depressive states, where there may be impairment of attention and concentration, such as 'the depressed shoplifter' (see p. 90), dissociation and depersonalisation.

Expert opinion needs to include an analysis of the psychopathology as well as consideration of the evidence. A man was charged with causing his estranged wife grievous bodily harm with intent following an attack with a ratchet spanner that he had fetched from the bottom of a cantilever tool box in the garage at 4 a.m.; in the course of this attack he struck between 20 and 25 blows, causing injuries that required 86 sutures, dislodging two teeth and fracturing her jaw (Rix & Clarkson, 1994). His defence, supported by psychiatric evidence, was that he was in a state of severe depersonalisation and derealisation in which his actions appeared to be elaborate but were not planned. The prosecution called a psychiatrist who explained to the jury the psychopathology of depersonalisation and whose opinion was summarised as: 'A depersonalised intent is nevertheless an intent'. By a majority verdict the defendant was convicted of causing grievous bodily harm with intent. The case illustrates the approach recommended in cases where dissociation is raised as a defence:

The courts should eschew any effort to discourage the defence of dissociation by interpreting it as evidence of insanity, or by withholding psychiatric evidence from the jury. The defence, if supported by medical evidence, should be adjudicated upon by the triers of fact, and if successful should result in an ordinary acquittal. But what is urgently needed is that the psychiatrist who deposes to dissociation in improbable circumstances should be subjected to skilled and deeply sceptical cross-examination, and that the Crown should, where possible, call counter-evidence. (Williams, 1983: p. 676)

Loss of control

The common law defence of provocation, which was only available as a partial defence to a charge of murder, and which achieved statutory recognition in s.3 of the Homicide Act 1957, was abolished by the CJA 2009. Section 3 of the Homicide Act 1957 and s.7 of the Criminal Justice Act (Northern Ireland) 1966 no longer have effect. Enter 'loss of control'.

Whether or not this brings to an end the period of judicial controversy and legal confusion that bedevilled the defence of provocation remains to be seen, as some of the controversy and confusion may re-emerge and loss of control may be but a rose by another name.

Instead of provocation there is, as a partial defence to a charge of murder, loss of control, which, if successful, reduces the offence to one of manslaughter. It does not apply where the defendant acted in a considered desire for revenge. This is because having time to think and to reflect, what is known as 'thinking time', is inconsistent with loss of control.

The defence bears the burden of proving that there was a loss of control. If, however, the judge finds that there is sufficient evidence to raise the issue, and upon which a jury properly directed could conclude that the defence might apply, the jury must assume that the defence is satisfied unless the prosecution proves beyond reasonable doubt that it is not.

Section 54(1) of the CJA 2009 states:

Where a person ('D') kills or is party to the killing of another ('V'), D is not to be convicted of murder if –
(a) D's acts and omissions in doing or being a party to the killing resulted from D's loss of self-control,
(b) the loss of self-control had a qualifying trigger, and
(c) a person of D's sex and age, with a normal degree of tolerance and self-restraint and in the circumstances of D, might have reacted in the same or in a similar way to D.

Section 54(2) provides that it does not matter whether or not the loss of self-control was sudden. This will assist, in particular, victims of prolonged domestic violence who kill their partner, as previously they had to prove a 'sudden and temporary' loss of control and were in difficulty in persuading the court that their 'slow burn' reaction to repeated violence nevertheless brought them within the scope of provocation (Rix, 2001).

For the psychiatric expert, the important provisions are those relating to the defendant's circumstances and the qualifying triggers. Subsection 3 states that 'circumstances' is a reference to all of the defendant's 'circumstances other than those whose only relevance' is that they bear on the defendant's capacity for tolerance or self-restraint. Ormerod (2011) has suggested that this opens up a broader range of subjective considerations than was allowed under previous case law. He has also observed that there is now no positive requirement that the defendant's individual circumstances have to affect the gravity of the triggering conduct in order for them to be included in the jury's assessment of what the person of the defendant's age and sex might have done.

The meaning of 'qualifying trigger' is set out in s.55. First, it can be the defendant's 'fear of serious violence from V against D or another identified person' (s.55(3)) (the fear trigger) and again this is an accommodation for victims of domestic violence who kill violent and abusive partners. Second, it can be a thing or things done or said (or both) which (1) constituted circumstances of an extremely grave character, and (3) caused the defendant to have a justifiable sense of being seriously wronged (s.55(4)) (the anger trigger). Third, it can be a combination of these two triggers (s.55(5)).

Three triggers are explicitly excluded (s.55(6)). First, it is not a qualifying trigger if it is serious violence that the defendant has caused by incitement in order to have an excuse to use violence. Second, it is not a qualifying trigger if the defendant has incited the victim to do what has seriously wronged the defendant in order to provide an excuse for violence. Third, sexual infidelity does not qualify as a trigger.

Psychiatric evidence was relevant and admissible in some cases where the defence of provocation was raised and it is likely that it will be relevant and admissible in some cases where the defence is one of loss of control. Insofar as the new law puts on a statutory footing the majority decisions of the Privy Council in *Attorney General for Jersey v Holley* [2005] 2 AC 580 and *Luc Thiet Thuan v The Queen* [1997] AC 131, PC, and the House of Lords in *R v Camplin* [1978] AC 705, they are likely to be of assistance to the psychiatric expert as they were in cases of provocation.

The new law appears to perpetuate, for loss of control, the requirement, for the defence of provocation, that the defence has to make out two conditions: (1) the 'subjective' condition that the defendant was actually triggered so as to lose self-control; and (2) the 'objective' condition that a person of normal tolerance and self-restraint would have done so (these two conditions being restated here in the language of loss of control).

The importance of *Camplin* was that the characteristics of the defendant could not be excluded; this qualified what, under the defence of provocation, the 'reasonable man' would have done, and what under the new law, a person of normal tolerance and reasonable restraint would have done. There is no reference to 'characteristics' in the new law but it is likely that 'circumstances' will be taken to include 'characteristics'. The following is an adaptation of the judgment in *Camplin* using a deletion and italic to reflect the terminology of the new law:

the gravity of *the trigger* may well depend upon the particular ~~characteristics or~~ circumstances of the person to whom a taunt or insult is addressed *or to whom any other trigger is directed*. To taunt a person because of his race, his physical infirmities or some shameful incident in his past may well be considered by the jury to be more offensive to the person, however equable his temperament, if the facts on which the taunt is founded are true than it would be if they were not....
... a proper direction to a jury ... [would be to] explain to them that the *person with a normal degree of tolerance and self-restraint* ... is a person having the *degree of tolerance and self-restraint* to be expected of an ordinary person of the sex and age of the accused, but in other respects sharing such of the accused's *circumstances* as they think would affect the gravity of the *trigger* to him; and that the question is not merely whether such a person would in like *circumstances* be *triggered* to lose self-control but also whether he would react to the *trigger* as the accused did.

This makes the distinction, which the new law now codifies, between factors affecting the gravity of the trigger, which are relevant, and factors affecting only those that bear on the accused's general capacity for tolerance or self-restraint, which have to be excluded.

Subsequently there were cases that blurred this distinction: *R v Humphreys* [1995] 4 All ER 1008, *R v Dryden* [1995] 4 All ER 987, *R v Thornton (No. 2)* [1996] 1 WLR 1174 and *R v Smith (Morgan)* [2001] 1 AC 146. They are now regarded as erroneous or wrongly decided. However, they shed light on the attempts to liberalise 'the reasonable man' test, reflecting that 'compassion to human frailty' which led Lord Diplock to take account of youth in *Camplin*. Insofar as there may be now more difficult attempts to liberalise the test within the straitjacket of the new law, these may remain important cases. Also, as observed in one authoritative legal text (Murphy, 1999), these cases, along with that of *R v Parker* [1997] Crim LR 760, suggest that the characteristics with which the reasonable man was (wrongly, as subsequently decided) invested could still be relevant because they affect the gravity of the provocation (trigger):

Thus an instance of abuse of a woman with battered woman syndrome can be regarded as more provocative than abuse of one not suffering from such a syndrome and a threat to evict a person who is possessive about his land (Dryden) may be more provocative than it would be to an ordinary person, even though each person would be expected to exercise the same level of self-control to a given level of gravity of provocation.

In the case of *Luc Thiet Thuan* the Privy Council ruled that the appellant's brain damage was not relevant to the objective test because it merely affected his powers of self-control rather than the gravity of the provocation. There was thus a direct conflict between the Privy Council in *Luc Thiet Thuan* and the House of Lords in *Smith (Morgan)*, where it was held that a characteristic such as Smith's severe depression was relevant not only to the gravity of the provocation but also to the standard of self-control expected.

The case of *Holley* provided the Privy Council with the opportunity to resolve the conflict and clarify the law. The conflict was resolved in favour of *Luc Thiet Thuan*. It was held that 'the sufficiency of the provocation ("whether the provocation was enough to make a reasonable man do as [the defendant] did") is to be judged by one standard and not a standard which varies from one defendant to another'.

Until the new defence has been deployed and there have been appeals, it is difficult to know what psychiatric evidence will be relevant and admissible where the defence of loss of control is raised. There may be less reliance on psychiatric evidence if, as Norrie (2010) suggests: 'Under the new law, defendants ... will be encouraged to portray themselves as ordinary people grievously harmed and acting out of a legitimate sense of anger at what has been done to them.'

The best advice meanwhile is to consider whether or not the defendant has any psychiatric disorder or syndrome, such as battered woman syndrome, and if so, to set out, if it exists, the evidence that the disorder or syndrome and history made the trigger appear more serious to the defendant and thus affected the perceived gravity of the trigger. For example, a particular look in the eye may be a qualifying trigger for the victim of domestic violence whose experience is that this look in the eye has always been the precursor of serious violence. Again in relation to domestic violence, there may be evidence of shameful incidents which contribute to the defendant believing, or being more sensitive to, some of the hurtful things said by the abusive partner and which might not otherwise be accepted as a qualifying trigger. Alternatively, psychiatric assessment may reveal a psychiatric condition that is associated with, or results in, an impairment of the defendant's general capacity for tolerance or self-restraint, in which case such evidence will be relied on by the prosecution to argue that the defence is not open to the defendant.

Duress and coercion

It may be a defence to a criminal charge, which if successful results in acquittal, to plead duress because:

> threats of immediate death or serious personal violence so great as to overbear the ordinary powers of human resistance should be accepted as a justification for acts which would otherwise be criminal. (*Attorney General v Whelan* [1934] IR 518 (Irish CCA))

Psychiatric evidence may be relevant and admissible because the mental state of the defendant, specifically 'the weak, immature or disabled person', may mean that they find the threats more compelling than 'a normal healthy person' but this defence does not apply if the defendant's will has been eroded by the voluntary consumption of alcohol or drugs. This is reflected in the direction (emphasis added) in *R v Graham* [1982] 1 All ER 801, 74 Cr App R 235, which was to require 'the jury [to be] sure that a sober person of reasonable firmness, *sharing the characteristics of [the defendant]*, would not have responded' as he did. Two problems emerge. The first is that characteristics that identify the defendant as not being 'of reasonable firmness' are problematic because, whatever the effects of such characteristics, the standard is the person of reasonable firmness ('the objective test'). Second, the psychiatrist needs to know what the law will admit as characteristics.

R v Emery (1993) 14 Cr App R (S) 394 perpetuates the problem. The Court of Appeal could find 'no scope for attributing to that hypothetical person one of the characteristics of the defendant a pre-existing mental condition of being "emotionally unstable" or in a "grossly elevated neurotic state"' but it was prepared to admit post-traumatic stress disorder as an admissible characteristic because it was a 'comparatively recent development … complex and … not known by the public at large'.

Likewise, in *R v Horne* [1994] Crim LR 584 the Court of Appeal upheld the refusal of the trial judge to admit psychiatric evidence on the basis that characteristics such as inherent weakness, vulnerability and susceptibility to threats were inconsistent with the requirements of the objective test because it 'would be a contradiction in terms to ask … them to take into account, as one of the characteristics, that he was pliant or vulnerable'. This contradiction in terms was also recognised in *R v Hurst* [1995] 1 Cr App R 82, where it was stated that the court found it hard to see how 'the person of reasonable firmness can be invested with the characteristics of a personality which lacks reasonable firmness'.

Judicial guidance comes from *R v Bowen* [1996] 2 Crim App R 157, which sets out five principles (Box 29). On the basis of these principles, even though the appellant in that case had, or may have had, a low IQ of 68, which inhibited his ability to seek the protection of the police, and he had been abnormally suggestible and vulnerable, the court held that:

We do not see how low IQ, short of mental impairment or mental defectiveness, can be said to be a characteristic that makes those who have it less courageous and less able to withstand threats and pressure.

This seems to suggest that 'mental impairment' or 'mental defectiveness' is an admissible characteristic but more than a low IQ is needed to make such a diagnosis. It also makes it clear that, notwithstanding the problem for people who are more pliable, vulnerable, timid or susceptible to threats than an ordinary person, 'medical evidence is admissible if the mental condition or abnormality of the defendant is relevant and the condition or abnormality and its effects lie outwith the knowledge and experience of laymen', as was held in *R v Hegarty* [1994] Crim LR 353.

Assuming that the mental state of the accused is relevant, it follows that psychiatric evidence is likely to be admitted if it satisfies the general test of falling outside the knowledge and experience of the lay person. Another case from around this time provides further information as to what the court might expect to find in the psychiatric report:

Box 29 Principles to be applied in a case of alleged duress

The ruling in *R v Bowen* [1996] 2 Crim App R 157 read as follows:

1 The mere fact that the accused is more pliable, vulnerable, timid or susceptible to threats than a normal person are not characteristics with which it is legitimate to invest the reasonable/ordinary person for the purpose of considering the objective test.

2 The defendant may be in a category of person who the jury think are less able to resist pressure than people not within that category ... recognised mental illness or psychiatric condition, such as post-traumatic stress disorder leading to learned helplessness.

3 Characteristics which may be relevant in considering provocation, because they relate to the nature of the provocation, itself will not necessarily be relevant in cases of duress.

4 Characteristics due to self-induced abuse, such as alcohol, drugs or glue-sniffing, cannot be relevant.

5 Psychiatric evidence may be admissible to show that the accused is suffering from some mental illness, mental impairment or recognised psychiatric condition, provided persons generally suffering from such conditions may be more susceptible to pressure and threats and thus to assist the jury in deciding whether a reasonable person suffering from such a condition might have been impelled to act as the defendant did. It is not admissible simply to show that, in the doctor's opinion, the accused, who is not suffering from such illness or condition, is especially timid, suggestible or vulnerable to pressure and threats.

---

the causes of the condition of learned helplessness, the circumstances in which it might arise and what level of abuse would be required to produce it; what degree of isolation of the person one would expect to find before it appeared and what sort of personality factors might be involved. (*Emery*)

Although this judgment focuses on 'learned helplessness', it gives an indication of the detailed evidence the court will expect from psychiatrists. Until the seeming inconsistencies of the law are resolved, the best advice to psychiatrists in cases of possible duress is to provide as detailed as possible evidence as to the mental condition and personality of the defendant and to explain as far as possible how these assist in understanding the ability of the defendant to resist threats of immediate death or serious violence, and to leave the court to decide on the admissibility of such evidence.

Failure to provide a specimen of breath or blood

In the case of a refusal to provide a specimen of blood or a specimen of breath required in the investigation of offences under the Road Traffic Act

101

1988, medical (Marks, 1995) and specifically psychiatric evidence (Rix, 1996b) may be admitted.

A phobia of needles, blood or AIDS is capable of being a medical reason for not supplying a specimen of blood. In *Johnson v West Yorkshire Metropolitan Police* [1986] RTR 77 the Court of Appeal found that a repugnance to the taking of a specimen was capable of being a 'reasonable excuse' for the failure to provide a specimen but 'only if the repugnance makes the suspect, not merely unwilling, but unable to comply with the request'. The Court also distinguished between 'repugnance' and 'phobia': 'Where repugnance is put forward as an excuse it will not provide a defence unless it amounts to a phobia recognised by medical science'. A phobia so serious that it manifests in symptoms such as light-headedness or fainting may be regarded as more compelling evidence of a 'medical reason' than one that is less serious (*Sykes v White* [1983] RTR 419). The role of the medical expert is to give an opinion as to the 'medical reason'; whether or not it amounts to a reasonable excuse is for the court to decide.

It is important, however, to have in mind the test of 'reasonableness' in this context and relate the opinion to the components of the test as formulated in a case of failure to provide a specimen of breath:

> In our judgment no excuse can be adjudged a reasonable one unless the person from whom the specimen is required is physically or mentally unable to provide it or the provision of it would entail a substantial risk to his health. (*R v Lennard* [1973] 57 Cr App R 542)

It is reasonable to draw attention to the risks of injury to arteries and veins, even by a doctor experienced in taking blood, and especially if the veins constrict as a result of anxiety or the suspect struggles to resist the needle.

A psychiatrist is likely to be instructed in cases involving failure to provide a specimen of breath when the defendant claims that, as a result of anxiety or a panic attack, they were unable to activate the breath-testing instrument or machine. This is an easy excuse to make but a difficult one to prove and courts take some convincing that it is a reasonable excuse. For a medical or psychiatric condition to be accepted as a reasonable excuse for not providing a specimen of breath the courts are unlikely to accept a condition that is not of 'an extreme nature' (Marks, 1995). Post-accident stress, unaccompanied by a mental or physical disability, does not constitute a reasonable excuse (*DPP v Eddowes* [1991] RTR 35). Cardiovascular or respiratory disease is sometimes an issue and in such cases the psychiatrist may report in tandem with a cardiologist or respiratory physician. It is also necessary to bear in mind that panic-like symptoms can occur in various medical conditions, including cardiovascular and respiratory disorders, but also phaeochromocytoma and hyperthyroidism.

The investigation of such cases includes careful analysis of the defendant's medical records. A needle or blood phobia to which there is no reference in the general practitioner records or an anxiety state or panic disorder that seems to have occurred for the first time when confronted by a police officer demanding a breath specimen is to be viewed with some suspicion. The medical records may indicate that blood tests have been taken, drugs administered by intravenous or intramuscular injection, advice given about overseas travel for which sometimes injections are needed and there may even be a history of intravenous drug misuse. The records may also include a comment from a general practitioner to the effect that he or she would not attempt to take blood again unless it was absolutely necessary. They may reveal a history of a panic disorder or some other psychiatric disorder of which panic is a symptom, but the absence of such a documented history can be overcome if there is convincing evidence from the defendant and witnesses.

The police Road Traffic Act documentation should be studied carefully. The police should record what the suspect says when refusing to provide a specimen. Of particular importance is a statement by the suspect that should or might have given the police officer 'reasonable cause to believe' that a specimen could not or should not be provided for medical reasons (*Davies v DPP* [1989] RTR 391). This is because the validity of the apparent medical reason has to be determined by a medical practitioner and the failure of a police officer to call a doctor to investigate the purported difficulty can be fatal to the prosecution case.

There will usually be witness statements from police officers in which they refer not only to what the suspect said but also the demeanour of the suspect. The custody record may include descriptions of the suspect's behaviour and what they have said. If an FME has attended, their statement should be studied along with their original notes unless all of their findings are recorded in the custody record.

A careful history should be taken of the condition which it is claimed prevented the defendant supplying the appropriate specimen and the defendants should be asked to describe exactly what happened when they were asked for the specimen of blood or what happened when they tried to blow into the breath-testing device. Care should be taken to distinguish what defendants spontaneously report as their experience and what symptoms had to be elicited by specific enquiry. As part of either a physical examination or a mental state examination, it is important to look for tattoos.

It is a good idea for the expert in breath specimen cases to have used a breath-testing instrument. Although what is critical is the difficulty that a person with an anxiety state or panic attack has using the breath-testing device and not the difficulty you would have, you may be asked in cross-examination, if you are called by the defence, whether or not you know how simple and easy it is, even for an intoxicated person, to comply with the instructions for providing a breath specimen. If you are asked, remember to point out that your familiarity is based on professional experience or otherwise wait for the inevitable joke about you having been breathalysed by the police.

Sentencing issues

The courts' requirements

Good Practice Guidance: Commissioning, Administering and Producing Psychiatric Reports for Sentencing (Her Majesty's Courts Service, 2010) sets out the courts' requirements of psychiatrists preparing reports for sentencing purposes. Although the guidance is directed at the courts which commission reports and the psychiatrists they commission, and does not refer to reports prepared at the request of defence solicitors, it is probably a good idea at least to have this guidance in mind when preparing reports for defence solicitors, as the expectations of the courts are likely to be increasingly influenced by this guidance.

It is particularly important to note that the guidance specifies a preference for the length of a sentencing report: two to four pages for a 'summary report' and up to eight pages for a 'full report'. Only a brief summary is needed of the defendant's personal background. Only a brief summary is needed of the psychiatrist's understanding of the event or events giving rise to the offence. Information is needed concerning: relevant psychiatric history; relevant family history; and current mental condition, including a mental state examination. 'Too much information' is identified in the guidance as a common problem because, 'Given the time constraints and focused nature of the sentencing context, only information relevant to the decisions at hand can be of practical value to the court'. It is stated that the court does not generally need an extended history, and collation of previous medical records in the report should be avoided. However, especially in more serious cases, such as where an indeterminate sentence may be passed, a very detailed report can provide an essential baseline for those considering the eventual release on licence of the prisoner many years later.

The guidance goes on to state: 'The court sentences; a psychiatrist can provide advice.' Such advice assists the sentencer to take into account treatment needs and balance the needs of the defendant with the management of risk to the public.

Box 30 suggests a format for the 'Opinion' section of a report prepared for sentencing and it is particularly based on the Scottish guidance.

Part III of the MHA

Part III of the MHA has provisions that may be utilised before sentence is imposed to inform sentencing decisions: remand to hospital for a report (s.35), remand to hospital for treatment (s.36) and an interim hospital order (s.38). Although it is the Ministry of Justice, and not the court, that makes a transfer direction under s.48, this provision is an important one for prisoners who have some form of mental disorder who are in urgent need of treatment in a psychiatric hospital and it is particularly important where s.36 does not apply, for example a summary case, and treatment is needed urgently before sentencing takes place.

Part III of the Act also gives the courts powers to make hospital orders (s.37), with and without restrictions (s.41), guardianship orders (s.37) and prison sentences with a hospital direction (s.45A).

Box 30 Issues to be addressed in a report for sentencing

In a report for sentencing, the Scottish Executive (2005, ch. 5, para. 71) indicates that the following points are to be covered:

Diagnosis

- Presence or absence of mental disorder as legally defined

Mental state at material time:

- Whether any mental disorder affected the behaviour giving rise to the offence

Treatment considerations

- Consent
- What treatment will involve
- What the components of treatment are
- Length of treatment
- Whether treatment should be under any particular order
- Availability of treatment/arrangements made
  - In-patient or out-patient/where the treatment will take place
  - Availability of bed
  - Under whose care will the person be
- Whether treatment will make a difference and, if so, how much
  - Distinguishing treatment which contains risk, prevents deterioration and reduces risk
- In the case of in-patient treatment, the likely circumstances of discharge

Prognosis considerations

- Effect of a custodial sentence on the disorder
- Effect of a custodial sentence on any possible treatment for the disorder
- Risk assessment
  - The kind(s) of violence the person is capable of perpetrating
  - The likely level of physical or psychological harm
  - The situation(s) in which the person is most likely to be violent
  - The likely victim(s) of that violence (e.g. self, public, known individuals, children, staff and fellow prisoners/patients)
  - The warning signs that the person may be at risk of being violent
  - The management strategies that need to be put into place to manage the risk of violence in the short term
  - The least restrictive environment in which the person's violence can easily be managed
  - Protective factors
  - Dynamic factors capable of change
  - The psychological, psychiatric or social treatments that may be given to help decrease the person's risk of violence in the long term
  - Risk of reconviction

With regard to hospital orders, note that there does not have to be a link between the mental disorder and the offence and a hospital order can be made even though the mental disorder has developed subsequent to the offence.

With regard to restriction orders, which can be attached only to a hospital order, the critical point is the risk of serious harm to the public in the event of a further offence being committed. It is not a serious risk of harm: 'serious' qualifies 'harm' and not 'risk' (Rix & Agarwal, 1999). The court has to have regard to: (1) the nature of the offence; (2) the antecedents of the offender; and (3) the risk of further offences if the defendant is set at large. Although 'antecedents' is likely to be taken to mean 'previous convictions', it is appropriate to draw attention to such matters as violence in institutional settings that has not resulted in criminal convictions. Although the court will have regard to the psychiatrist's risk assessment, it is the court that makes the ultimate assessment of the risk of serious harm. So, the court can make a restriction order where the medical recommendations have been for no restriction order and vice versa. A restriction order can be made where there is no history of violence. In *R v Golding* [2006] EWCA Crim 1965, where the appellant had been repeatedly convicted of burglary, he was considered to be at risk of causing serious harm because his psychosis was uncontrolled and he had a predilection for drugs that could lead him to react violently to confrontation by a householder.

Although the decision to impose a restriction order is for the judge, even if you have not specifically been asked for an opinion on a restriction order, it is helpful if the report indicates whether or not the court should consider a restriction order. No judge will object to an opinion on this point being offered and, as there is a requirement for the judge to hear oral evidence, it will assist in making arrangements for the hearing to have advance notice of the issue.

A report in such a case in Scotland should address the role of special restrictions in facilitating future management and this is a point of general application.

Criminal Justice Act 2003 provisions

In any case where the defendant is or appears to be mentally disordered, s.157 of the CJA 2003 requires that a medical report must be obtained before a custodial sentence is passed, other than one that is fixed by law, that is, upon conviction for murder. Paradoxically, in murder cases the court may dispense with such a report if the court considers it is not necessary. This seems somewhat confusing but at least it means that, probably, the sentencer has to make a conscious decision to dispense with the medical report and perhaps also give reasons. A medical report in this context is one prepared by a s.12 approved doctor. There is also a requirement to consider any other information on the defendant's mental condition and the likely effect of a custodial sentence on the condition and on any possible treatment for it. It is recognised that 'custody can exacerbate mental ill health, heighten vulnerability and increase the risk of self-harm and suicide' (Bradley, 2009, p. 7).

Mitigation

Section 166(1) and (5) of the CJA 2003 provides 'savings for powers to mitigate sentences and deal appropriately with mentally disordered offenders'. This allows the court, where appropriate, to be flexible in the sentencing of mentally disordered offenders. Furthermore, the Sentencing Guidelines Council (SGC) recognises 'mental illness or disability' as a mitigating factor, that is, one indicating lower culpability, and refers specifically to mental disorder being a mitigating factor in certain types of case. Thus, in the case of assaults on children and cruelty to a child, mental illness, specifically depression, is identified as a relevant area of personal mitigation and so are 'indifference or apathy resulting from low intelligence ... immaturity or social deprivation resulting in an inability to cope with the pressures of caring for children'; psychiatric illness is similarly a cause for mitigation. Mental disorder or mental disability is a specific mitigating factor for attempted murder. Where a defendant has a 'lower level of understanding due to mental health issues or learning difficulties' this can mitigate breach of an antisocial behaviour order. In the sentencing of children and young people, where the court is required under s.44 of the Children and Young Persons Act 1933 to consider their welfare, the courts are to have regard to the high rate of mental health problems and intellectual disabilities in young people in the criminal justice system, the impact of any speech or language difficulties on communication and the vulnerability of young people to self-harm, especially in custody. The SGC also suggests that a psychiatric report may be appropriate when sentencing for a sexual offence but in such cases the mental disorder may be such as to constitute an aggravating factor rather than a mitigating factor. This does not apply just to sexual offences. It was recognised in *R v Johnson and others* [2007] 1 Cr App R (S) 112 that the inadequacy, suggestibility or vulnerability of the defendants were characteristics capable of leading to, or reinforcing, the conclusion that they were dangerous.

Arson cases

Although there is no statutory requirement to obtain a psychiatric report in cases of arson, the courts usually follow the advice of Boreham J in *R v Calladine* (1975) *The Times*, 3 December, CA, that it would be unwise to sentence without a psychiatric report.

Community orders with specified requirements

Section 177 of the CJA 2003 makes provision for a mental health treatment requirement (s.207), a drug rehabilitation requirement (s.209) or an alcohol treatment requirement (s.212) to be added to a community order. Such an order should be considered for a defendant who does not, or does not any longer, need treatment as an in-patient, although it can include provision for in-patient treatment other than in a high-security hospital. Taylor & Krish (2010, p. 138) set out the further circumstances in which such an order may be made:

Such a disposal may be appropriate in a case where the custody threshold has been passed (as well as those cases in which it has not, but where the defendant's culpability is substantially mitigated by his mental state at the time of the commission of the offence, and where the public interest is served by ensuring he continues to receive treatment for his mental disorder). It is usually not suitable for a defendant who is unlikely to comply with treatment or who has a very chaotic lifestyle.

In order to make such an order with a mental health treatment requirement, the court must have a written or oral report from a s.12 approved doctor that the condition of the defendant is such as 'requires and may be susceptible to treatment', but it is not such as to merit a hospital or guardianship order. The report should indicate where the defendant is to be admitted, or where the defendant is to attend as a non-resident patient, or the registered medical practitioner or chartered psychologist by whom or under whose direction treatment is to be provided.

In order to make an order with a drug rehabilitation requirement, which includes drug treatment and testing, various criteria have to be met. The offender has to be dependent on, or have a propensity to misuse, a controlled drug. The propensity has to be such as requires and may be susceptible to treatment. Specifically, there has to be a realistic prospect of reducing the drug dependence (*Attorney General's Reference (No. 64 of 2003)* [2004] 2 Cr App R (S) 106). The court has to be satisfied that arrangements have been made or can be made for the proposed treatment. A probation officer needs to have recommended the requirement. The offender must express a willingness to comply and indeed there has to be clear evidence of the offender having a determination to free herself or himself from drugs (*Attorney General's Reference (No. 64 of 2003)*). The treatment can be as a resident in a specified institution or place, or as a non-resident. The treatment has to be by or under the direction of a specified person who has the necessary qualifications or experience. The CJA 2003 does not specify the nature of the offences for which an order with such a requirement should be made but *Attorney General's Reference (No. 64 of 2003)* indicates that it would generally be appropriate for an acquisitive offence committed to obtain money for drugs but rarely for an offence involving serious violence or threat of violence with a lethal weapon.

An alcohol treatment requirement requires the offender to submit to treatment, for a specified period, by, or under the direction of, a specified person who has the necessary qualifications or experience, with a view to the reduction or elimination of the offender's dependency on alcohol. The following criteria have to be met. The court has to be satisfied that the offender is dependent on alcohol and that the dependency is such as requires and may be susceptible to treatment. The court has to be satisfied that arrangements have been made or can be made for the proposed treatment. The offender must express a willingness to comply. The treatment can be as a resident in a specified institution or place, or treatment as a non-resident by or under the direction of a person who has the necessary qualification or experience.

Such requirements can be for up to a maximum of three years, which is the maximum length of a community order.

There are similar provisions for defendants aged under 18 years under s.1(1)(k) of, and Schedule 1 to, the Criminal Justice and Immigration Act 2008. However, instead of an alcohol treatment requirement, there is provision for an intoxicating substance treatment requirement, which includes alcohol as well as any other substance or product (but not a controlled drug) capable of being inhaled or otherwise used for the purpose of causing intoxication. It is similar in other respects to the alcohol treatment requirement for adults.

Suspended sentences with specific requirements

Under s.189 of the CJA 2003, when passing a suspended sentence, the court can make it a requirement to comply with mental health treatment, alcohol treatment or drug rehabilitation in terms identical to those that apply to a community order. However, the requirement cannot be for longer than two years and it cannot be longer than the period of time for which the sentence is suspended.

Imprisonment for life, imprisonment for public protection and extended sentences

The CJA 2003 provides for the imposition of indeterminate sentences of 'imprisonment for public protection' (IPP) (s. 225(1)) and extended sentences (s.227) when the defendant is convicted of one of a number of specified violent or sexual offences and, in the opinion of the court, there is a 'significant risk to members of the public of serious harm occasioned by the commission by him of further specified offences'. Harm is defined as 'death or personal injury whether that is physical or psychological'. 'Significant' is not defined in the CJA 2003 but it means more than a possibility – it must be 'noteworthy, of considerable amount or importance' (*R v Lang* [2006] 1 WLR 2509). The expectation was and still is that in most of these cases the courts would rely on the pre-sentence report, but *Lang* also established that in a small number of cases where 'the circumstances of the current offence or the history of the offender suggests mental abnormality' a medical report should usually be obtained. *Good Practice Guidance: Commissioning, Administering and*

Producing Psychiatric Reports for Sentencing (Her Majesty's Courts Service, 2010, p. 13) recognises that: 'Expert psychiatric evidence has an important role in supporting or challenging an inference of dangerousness'. In such cases defendants need to know that their assessment may lead to a longer than normal sentence. This is because 'Characteristics such as inadequacy, suggestibility or vulnerability of the offender might serve to mitigate the offender's culpability but they might also serve to produce or reinforce the conclusion that the offender was dangerous' (*Attorney General's Reference (No. 64 of 2006)* (2006) *The Times* 2 November).

Doing no harm may clash with justice. College guidelines may assist (Royal College of Psychiatrists, 2004). As the court is required to 'have in mind all the alternative and cumulative methods of providing the necessary public protection against the risk posed by the individual offender' (*Attorney General's Reference (No. 55 of 2008)* [2009] 2 Cr App R (S) 142) it is necessary to address what treatment, if any, may be available in the community as part of what the court terms 'the overall sentencing package'. The equivalent provision for a person aged under 18 years is a sentence of detention for life, a sentence of detention for public protection or an extended sentence under the PCC(S)A.

As Bickle (2008, p. 604) has observed: 'The law pertaining to indeterminate sentences has long embraced concepts of mental instability and dangerousness'. For example, in *R v Hodgson* (1967) 52 Cr App R 113, one of the requirements for an indeterminate sentence rather than a lengthy determinate sentence was that: 'The offender must be a person of mental instability who, if at liberty, will probably reoffend and present a grave danger to the public'.

It was stated in *R v S and Others* [2005] EWCA Crim 3616 that, as held in *Lang*, 'the cases in which a psychiatric report will be necessary on assessing risk are comparatively few. But in those cases where such a report is thought to be necessary, it will generally be essential for the psychiatrist to make an assessment with regard to seriousness for the guidance of the sentencing Judge'. Bickle's advice to the psychiatric expert at that time was to find out:

(1) whether on conviction, the index allegation would represent a specified or serious offence; (2) whether the defendant has been previously convicted for at least one relevant offence; (3) whether the defendant is 18 or over.... Expert witnesses should be aware that if all of these criteria are satisfied, there will be a statutory assumption of dangerousness in the event of conviction, and their evidence may be used in discussion of a rebuttal of this assumption. (Bickle, 2008: p. 110)

Legislative changes introduced by the Criminal Justice and Immigration Act 2008 have brought greater judicial discretion but they have not altered the reliance the courts place on psychiatric evidence and in *R v Reinaldo Rocha* [2007] EWCA Crim 1505 the Court of Appeal quashed the appellant's IPP, substituted a determinate sentence and criticised the trial judge for disregarding psychiatric evidence without explanation.

Risk assessment

Structured clinical or professional judgment is preferable to actuarial approaches in risk assessment but, either way, be prepared to explain and defend your approach, as there is an expectation that instruments will 'have proven validity for the category of people that the assessed person falls into (e.g. mentally disordered offenders, prisoners, sex offenders)' (Scottish Executive, 2005, ch. 5, para. 68). Also in Scotland, it is recommended best practice, and I suggest of general application, that the assessment should attempt to place the risk the person presents in the context of history and current offending, having regard specifically to the matters listed in Box 31 (drawn from the *Mental Health (Care and Treatment) (Scotland) Act 2003 Code of Practice*).

If the defendant is not suffering from any mental disorder, it is arguable that you should offer no opinion as to risk. It is also arguable that a formal training in risk assessment may qualify you to do so but in this case it must be clear that this is the basis of the opinion.

It is not enough to categorise risk as, for example, 'high'. The risk assessment section in Box 30 (p. 105) shows the information used in a risk formulation to identify the most likely risk scenario (the kind of violence, the severity of the harm, the situation in which the violence is most likely to occur, the likely victims and the warning signs), recognise the imminence of violence by warning signs, manage the risk in the short term, including an appropriate environment, and provide treatments aimed at reducing the risk of violence in the long term.

Treatment recommendations

The section on treatment has to be crystal clear, with unambiguous and clearly justified recommendations. It has to be an actionable opinion. If you

---

Box 31 Factors to be considered in risk assessment

The Scottish Executive (2005, ch. 5, para. 69) indicates that the following factors are to be considered in risk assessment:

- Personal and family history
- Criminal history and history of violence
- Substance misuse
- Psychiatric history
- Assessment of personality
- Other relevant risk factors for the population group into which the person falls (e.g. sex offender)

are not going to be responsible for the treatment, you must liaise closely with the people who are going to provide the treatment and ensure that you properly represent what they have to offer. This is vital. Your report will otherwise be of limited practical value. If you are recommending a community order you must liaise with the probation officer, preferably before finalising your report.

Witness issues

Vulnerable witnesses

Under the Youth Justice and Criminal Evidence Act 1999, special measures can be made available to provide effective support and assistance to vulnerable witnesses. Reports on such witnesses should address whether or not they have mental disorder (as defined in the MHA) or 'significant impairment of intelligence and social functioning'.

The absent witness

Section 116(1) of the CJA 2003 provides that if witnesses are unable to give evidence, their statement may be read to the court if they are 'unfit to be a witness' by reason of a 'bodily or mental condition'. A report in such a case should not only identify the witness's mental condition but explain clearly how it makes the person unfit to give oral evidence.

Credibility

It is not for the expert to tell the court whether or not a witness (or indeed a defendant) is credible. This is for the court to decide. However, a psychiatrist may be asked to give an opinion as to whether or not a witness 'is or was suffering from some recognised mental illness, disability or abnormality ... that undermines his credibility' (*Toohey v Metropolitan Police Commissioner* [1965] AC 595) or, for example, in the case of someone who is 'mentally handicapped' (*R v Barratt* [1996] Crim LR 495), to assist the court in an enquiry into their competence as a witness. Furthermore, in *S* [2006] EWCA Crim 2839 it was held that the court properly admitted the evidence of an expert witness that a complainant, who had autism, would not have been capable of inventing the evidence that she had given.

Most commonly, this issue arises in cases of adults alleging sexual abuse in childhood, in which case it is common to be asked to address the issue of 'false memory syndrome'. This is a highly specialised area and one where, in any event, it usually best to work collaboratively with a psychologist, especially if issues arise as to the genuineness of reported childhood memories. Where the evidence of a complainant is based on 'recovered memories' the psychiatrist should be familiar with the literature on this subject.

Occasionally there are cases in which the credibility is in question of an adult who has alleged sexual assault. Particularly where there is evidence of a form of personality disorder that manifests in dishonesty or exaggeration, medical records, particularly psychiatric records, should be carefully studied for examples of dishonesty or exaggeration.

It does not follow that everyone with a particular personality disorder lies or exaggerates. Even if there is expert psychiatric evidence that calls into question a witness's or complainant's credibility, it is important not to suggest that the person has not given or is not giving credible evidence. This is for the court to decide.

Just because someone suffers from a mental disorder, it does not follow that they are any more unreliable on matters unaffected by the mental disorder than any other witness. Thus, in *Barratt*, a witness had what had been described as 'fixed belief paranoia' and she had various bizarre beliefs about her personal life, but the court could see no reason not to rely on her evidence on matters unaffected by her mental condition.

If a person with mental disorder gives evidence as a witness, the jury will decide what weight to attach to the evidence. The authority for this is a case that has to be interpreted having regard to the concepts of the day: if the witness's evidence is so 'tainted with insanity as to be unworthy of credit', it is the proper function of the jury to disregard it and not act on it (*R v Hill* (1851) 2 Den CC 254).

Psychiatric harm

The courts have recognised that psychiatric illness or injury, including hysterical or nervous shock (*R v Morris* [1998] 1 Cr App R 368) (p. 139), can constitute harm that may form the basis of a charge of causing harm amounting to grievous bodily harm (*R v Ireland* [1998] AC 147; *R v Dhaliwal* [2006] 2 Cr App R 348) or amounting to actual bodily harm (*R v Chan-Fook* [1994] 1 WLR 689) under the Offences Against the Person Act 1861. In order to prove that such harm exists, the prosecution needs psychiatric evidence as to cause and effect, that is, whether or not the defendant's conduct resulted in the injury. Distress, grief, anxiety or other psychological harm that does not amount to a recognisable psychiatric illness is not bodily harm for the purposes of the Offences Against the Person Act 1861 (*Dhaliwal*).

Propensity

Under ss.101 and 103 of the CJA 2003, evidence of the defendant's bad character is admissible if 'it is relevant to an important matter in issue between the defendant and the prosecution' (s.101(1)(d)) and such matters include 'the question whether the defendant has a propensity to commit offences of the kind with which he is charged' (s.103(1)(a)). This means the propensity to act in a particular way. Thus, evidence of previous convictions, which would usually be withheld from the jury, may be admitted. Also, in the case of a defendant with a psychiatric history, a psychiatric expert might be instructed to consider the defendant's psychiatric and other records in order to identify any evidence which might indicate a propensity to commit the offence with which the defendant is charged. In such a case, there needs to be a careful analysis of the evidence relating to the alleged offence, as any evidence obtained by the psychiatrist from the records will have to be compared with the facts of the alleged offence.

Thus, in a case of alleged murder, there may be evidence of similar but non-fatal violence in the form of attacks on fellow patients or staff in psychiatric institutions. In a case of alleged murder, where the defendant was under the influence of certain intoxicants, the records may contain evidence of similar behaviour when under the influence of such drugs. It may be relatively easy to pick out episodes in the defendant's history that bear a similarity to the alleged offence, but, in order to address the issue of propensity, it is also necessary to take careful note of evidence that may be inconsistent, as cross-examination will be likely to focus on this in order for the defence to argue that there was no such propensity. For example, fatal injuries may have been inflicted with a weapon but the defendant, although with a history of violent attacks on members of the public, patients and staff, may never have used a weapon. Alternatively, it may have been in only a minority of recorded incidents of misuse of a particular drug that the defendant has behaved the way that it appears that the assailant acted.

It is important to restrict opinion to the matter of propensity. Do not offer an opinion as to whether or not, in the light of the evidence subjected to psychiatric analysis, the defendant was responsible for the offence alleged. This is for the court.

In any event, even if there is evidence of propensity, it is for the court to decide whether the issue is of substantial importance in the whole case and whether or not the evidence has substantial probative value. In deciding on the probative value of the psychiatrist's evidence the court will have regard to such factors as the nature and number of events.

Appeals

A person convicted can appeal on the basis either that the conviction was unsafe or that the sentence was too severe. Under the Criminal Appeal Act 1968 the court must give 'leave to appeal' or what is now known under CrPR as 'permission to appeal'. A person who has served a notice to appeal but has not been granted permission to appeal is an 'applicant' and a person who has been granted permission is an 'appellant'. An application to appeal should be made only where there are grounds that indicate a real prospect of success.

Where the appeal depends on the admission of fresh evidence, there has to be a reasonable explanation for the failure to adduce the evidence at trial. Such was found in *R v Gilbert* [2003] EWCA Crim 2385, where the appellant appealed against his conviction for murder. He had given evidence at the trial that voices in his head made him kill his victim but the defence advanced was provocation and no medical evidence was called. A psychiatrist prepared reports for the Criminal Cases Review Commission (CCRC) and indicated that the appellant was seriously mentally ill before, during and after the offence and his condition was such that he would very likely have succeeded with a plea of diminished responsibility. He relied on statements from the appellant's daughters and several references in the appellant's probation records to 'voices'. Although the Crown argued that there was no reasonable explanation for not adducing evidence in support of diminished responsibility at the trial, the court allowed the application to adduce evidence on the basis that there was a chance that the appellant did not advance the true facts because he was ill.

Moyle is a similar case. The appellant had been convicted of murder following a fight outside a public house. At his trial there was evidence from a consultant psychiatrist that his responsibility was to some extent impaired by illness but it was not 'substantial' impairment. The appellant had refused to see the psychiatrist instructed by the prosecution. In one of the psychiatric reports prepared for his appeal it was asserted that the appellant had been concealing his symptoms and he had refused to see the second psychiatrist because he felt that he was part of a conspiracy to have him hung, drawn and quartered. He felt that if he had disclosed his symptoms at the time he would have been convicted of witchcraft. He believed that Satan had all the court and jury under his influence and they were possessed. The court accepted that the appellant's decisions at the time of his trial were affected by the illness itself, quashed the conviction and substituted a conviction for manslaughter on the grounds of diminished responsibility.

Thus, in appeal cases it is important for the psychiatrist to consider the effects of the appellant's illness on his thinking and behaviour at the time of the trial.

The evidence of a further expert which is to the same effect as that of an expert at the trial is not likely to be regarded as fresh evidence and it is regarded as a potential subversion of the trial process to allow at appeal another and supposedly more persuasive expert to give the same opinion evidence that was unsuccessfully given at the trial or to present an alternative expert opinion based on the same factual evidence that was available at the trial (*R v Meachen* [2009] EWCA Crim 1701).

Reports for the Parole Board and discretionary lifer panels

The word 'parole' is derived from the French expression for 'word of honour', so the implication is that, if released, the prisoner is honour bound not to commit further offences.

The Parole Board (Parole Commission in Northern Ireland) makes decisions on the applications for parole of prisoners serving sentences of between four to seven years and in the case of prisoners serving seven or more years it makes a recommendation to the Home Secretary. The Parole Board reviews the cases of prisoners serving a mandatory life sentence and the first review is usually about three years before the expiry of the tariff, which is the minimum period they are ordered to serve before becoming eligible for parole, and it reviews, as a 'discretionary lifer panel', the cases of prisoners serving a discretionary life sentence as soon as they have served their tariff. The primary concern of the Board is the risk to the public of a further offence being committed when the prisoner would otherwise be in prison. The Parole Board can recommend a transfer to open conditions.

The Parole Board also makes decisions about those who were aged under 17 years on the date of the commission of the offence and who have been detained during Her Majesty's pleasure. This is known as an HMP panel.

Parole Board members are advised to take into account 'medical or psychiatric considerations' and so an up-to-date psychiatric report is likely to be requested for the hearing. The report should deal with any psychiatric history, including responsiveness to treatment and the relationship between the psychiatric disorder and offending, any requirement as to psychiatric treatment that might be made a condition of release and the likelihood of cooperation with and a response to such treatment. Insofar as they fall within the expertise of the psychiatrist, which will depend on the nature of the case, the report should address: any risk to the victim or other persons; attitude and behaviour in custody; remorse; insight into offending behaviour; steps taken to achieve any treatment objectives; and the likelihood of cooperation with supervision in the community. The report should be based on study of the parole dossier and it should pay particular attention to the psychology reports.

The report will form part of the final parole dossier, which will be made available to the prisoner in advance of the hearing. However, exceptionally the report could be withheld if, on psychiatric grounds, it is felt the mental and/or physical health of the prisoner could be impaired by disclosure. Alternatively, the prisoner could be provided with a redacted version. It is the governor who decides on withholding and redaction.

Legal commentators and advocates have been critical of the psychiatric reports that form part of the parole dossier.

These are generally very poor reports consisting of little more than a recitation of the prisoner's history. Where conclusions about current risk are set out reasons in support do not usually accompany them. In the face of these reports it is often helpful for the prisoner's representative to commission an independent report from a consultant forensic psychiatrist and to apply to the Panel for a direction that the expert can attend as a witness. (Livingstone & Owen, 1999, p. 426)

The message is clear. Provide a psychiatric analysis of the prisoner's case, not a mere recitation of the history, consider the risk to others and give the reasons for the particular statement as to risk. If the prisoner is going to need psychiatric supervision in the community, set this out in as much detail as possible, even though the area to which the prisoner may be released is uncertain. This may require liaison with the health and probation services in the relevant area.

If called to give evidence, remember that although s.32(3) of the Criminal Justice Act 1991 adds an inquisitorial quality to Parole Board proceedings, the judges who chair them come from an adversarial tradition and will often conduct hearings as if they are adversarial.

Discussions between experts

The criminal courts are rapidly catching up with the civil and family courts in making use of experts' meetings (CrPR Rule 33.6). In *Henderson* the court stated that experts' meetings should take place well in advance of the trial and should be attended by all significant experts, including the defence experts; a careful and detailed minute should be prepared, and a statement made of the areas of agreement and disagreement. The court stated that it was preferable that others, including legal representatives, should not attend.

Further reading

Taylor, C. & Krish, J. (2010) *Advising Mentally Disordered Offenders: A Practical Guide* (2nd edn). Law Society.

CHAPTER 6

Reports in personal injury cases

I cannot leave this case without expressing my profound gratitude to counsel on both sides … for the deep humanity with which they have conducted this tragic case. (Hirst J in *Aboul-Hosn v Trustees of the Italian Hospital and Others: Kemp & Kemp* A4 101)

Psychiatrists who prepare reports in criminal cases will sooner or later be asked to prepare reports in personal injury cases. Personal injuries are 'any disease and any impairment of a person's physical or mental condition' (s.38, Limitation Act 1980).

These are most likely to be reports on the psychiatric injuries suffered by the victims of road traffic accidents or industrial accidents. They may be reports on the psychiatric injuries suffered by patients who allege that they have been harmed by medical negligence. In these cases, the psychiatric evidence is necessary in order to quantify the injuries suffered and to allow the parties to agree, or the court to decide, how much money ('quantum'), if any, to award the claimant ('claimants' in England and Wales, 'pursuers' in Scotland, 'plaintiffs' in Ireland). In some of these cases, the psychiatric evidence may be needed to assist as to 'causation' issues. This means assisting with regard to whether or not the injury sustained, specifically the psychiatric injury, is indeed a psychiatric injury attributable to the accident or the allegedly negligent medical care or an injury caused other than by the person against whom the case is brought ('the defendant') or is perhaps not a psychiatric injury as such but a psychiatric disorder that already existed, or would have occurred in any event.

The psychiatrist may also be instructed in cases where the allegation is of negligent psychiatric care. Most psychiatrists preparing reports in personal injury cases are likely to be a consultant for some time before they are instructed in such cases, usually because they are regarded as requiring a certain level of seniority and experience.

In most cases the expert is instructed by solicitors acting for one party, either the claimant or the defendant. An expert may be jointly selected but instructed only by a single party; the expert is still a party expert. It is also possible for the expert may be jointly instructed by the solicitors acting for two or more defendants; an expert so instructed is a party-appointed expert. The party-appointed expert is under a duty to provide the report to, and communicate only with, the instructing solicitors unless the instructing solicitors agree, or the solicitors for the opposing party put questions to the expert under Rule 35.6 of the CPR, or the court orders it. Occasionally the expert is instructed by the opposing parties on a joint basis. An expert so instructed is known as a single joint expert (SJE) (see p. 138).

The pre-action stage

A personal injury case starts when someone believes that they have been wronged and they consider seeking a remedy through the civil courts. The wrong they have suffered is a 'tort' and the law dealing with such wrongs is known as 'tort law'.

A patient may believe that she has been treated for years for schizophrenia when the diagnosis was bipolar affective disorder. The widow of a man who has hanged himself in a psychiatric ward may believe that his care was not up to standard. The victim of a road or industrial accident may believe that he is entitled to financial compensation for the injuries sustained. A patient who has suffered post-operative complications may believe that her surgery was carried out negligently and that she is entitled to financial compensation for the psychological as well as physical harm she has suffered.

The purpose of civil proceedings in such cases is to use financial compensation to put people back to where they would have been but for the wrong that they have suffered. This is the principle of the law of tort. This is the law's best response. The law cannot, of course, often offer complete restitution – the hand that has been mangled in an industrial accident cannot be replaced – so a sum of money is given that is proportionate to the suffering and loss of function that the injury involves. The categories of damage and the usual amounts of compensation they attract are set out in the Judicial Studies Board's *Guidelines for the Assessment of General Damages in Personal Injury Cases* (2010) (the JSB Guide). The intention is that the parties should agree, or the courts should award, similar amounts for similar sorts of injury. Such damages are known as 'general damages' for pain, suffering and loss of amenity. There may also be general damages for future loss and expense such as 'loss of earnings' and 'care', and these are usually called 'special damages', although, strictly speaking, this is the term for money spent or liabilities accrued up to the date of settlement or trial. The size of a settlement or award can depend very much on the damages for loss of earnings and care. A brain-injured barrister who was tipped to become a QC will have a larger loss-of-earnings claim than a retail assistant. A child born with multiple disabilities resulting from obstetric negligence may have a claim for care that runs into millions of pounds.

In a personal injury case, the first stage is for the potential claimant to consult a solicitor. How the solicitor proceeds at this stage, before any action is taken on behalf of the potential claimant ('the pre-action stage'), is governed by one of the pre-action protocols. The CPR introduced pre-action protocols in order to reduce the costs and delays associated with litigation. They may be produced by a variety of bodies but are all held by the Ministry of Justice (and available on its website, http://www.justice.gov.uk). There are protocols for personal injury, clinical negligence and professional negligence. Although the protocols govern the steps to be taken before litigation starts, they are also intended to resolve as many as possible disputes without recourse to litigation.

There are three elements in the tort of negligence: a duty of care must be owed by the defendant to the claimant; there has to be a breach of that duty; and there has to be damage that results from the breach of duty. Thus, in a psychiatric negligence case, the potential claimant's solicitor will need, at an early stage, an advisory report from a psychiatrist dealing at least with the issue of liability, that is, breach of duty and usually also causation. This is because potential claimants need to prove that the alleged negligence has contributed to their present condition, that is, prove causation. In many such cases, and in, for example, an accident case, an opinion will also be needed on condition and prognosis in order to know whether or not any significant injuries or damage can be attributed to the allegedly negligent care or the accident. In short, the role of the expert is to help the solicitor decide whether or not the client appears to have a case and whether or not it should be pursued.

A report prepared at the pre-action stage is not governed by the CPR because these apply only to cases that are subject to civil proceedings. However, the conduct of the cases at this stage should comply with the pre-action protocols and there may be penalties for parties, when proceedings are issued if they have not complied with the relevant pre-action protocol.

The liability (breach of duty and causation) report

In cases of alleged psychiatric negligence, for example, most breach of duty and causation reports are reports on papers or 'desktop' reports, although some, sooner or later, require a consultation with the potential claimant. In such cases, the psychiatrist may be supplied with little more than the medical records and, in some cases, a draft witness statement from the potential claimant or family members and a sudden untoward incident report. In a fatal case, the documents provided may also include reports and statements prepared for the inquest, and if it has concluded, a note of the inquest proceedings. Sometimes the psychiatric report is requested before the inquest, in order to assist with questions to be asked and issues to be explored at the inquest.

The first stage in preparing a breach of duty and causation report, in a case of alleged psychiatric negligence, is to construct, from the medical records, a careful and sufficiently detailed chronology of the case. It will have to be particularly detailed for the period of allegedly negligent care. At this stage, the amount of historical detail will depend on the nature of the allegations. If what was done, or not done, should have taken into account what happened in earlier episodes of illness or care, these episodes will need to be set out in sufficient detail to explain how they are relevant.

It is important to start out having in mind the fact that satisfactory care is the norm. Even in cases where negligence may be admitted or proved, not all of the care will have been negligent. It is therefore necessary for the assumed facts of the case, derived from the medical records, to be set out so that the day, and usually the time, when it can be clearly established that the standard of care fell below the accepted standard is demonstrated.

The chronology has to be constructed usually from multiple sources of information. Especially when patients are in the community, there will be information in general practitioner records, hospital out-patient clinic records, the records of various community teams and various non-medical professionals, at the least. Even where in-patient records are multiprofessional, there may be other relevant records.

Computers and word-processing have now made it unnecessary for the psychiatric expert to use a roll of ceiling paper, as Dr Neville Gittleson did in the benzodiazepine litigation, with one end at the front door and the other end at the back door, upon which he set out, by hand, the chronology of the case, usually finding that, at one or more points, he still could not squeeze all of the relevant information into the space he had allowed. With computerisation a paragraph can be created in which, with information from multiple sources, an account is set out of all the relevant information about what happened to the patient over the course of several hours or even minutes. Where information does come from multiple sources, it is important that the source of each piece of information or quotation can be found in the records, so such a paragraph is likely to include a number of page references in parentheses. If you do not include them in the first draft, you will spend hours trying to track a single elusive reference at a later stage. If the medical records are not paginated, ask the claimant's solicitors to provide paginated records. This is because the model practice direction for clinical negligence cases requires that all references to medical notes in any report should be made by reference to the pages in the paginated bundle of records prepared by the claimant's solicitors.

If there is non-contemporaneous information, such as the evidence of the potential claimant or family members, information taken from statements or reports prepared for a sudden untoward incident enquiry, an inquest or evidence given at the inquest, the next step is to incorporate this information in the body of the report. It has to be distinguished from the information in the medical records, because it is non-contemporaneous, and the most convenient convention is for this to be set out in *italic* type. For obvious reasons, the evidence of the potential claimant or family members and the evidence of the doctors, nurses and others employed by the defendant may not be consistent with what is recorded in the medical records. This approach best allows comparison of the assumed facts and consideration of the significance of any inconsistencies or discrepancies.

Having constructed such a chronology, with all of the available information, your task is to go through the chronology, day by day, hour by hour or even minute by minute, looking for any evidence that care has fallen below the standard expected of a psychiatrist, or other mental health practitioner, acting with ordinary care. This criterion reflects the case law on negligence. This and other formulations of negligence are set out in Box 32. Where

---

Box 32 Three tests for negligence

In *Hunter v Hanley* (1955) SLT 213 it was ruled that:

'In the realm of diagnosis and treatment there is ample scope for genuine difference of opinion and one man is clearly not negligent merely because his conclusion differs from that of other professional men.... The true test for establishing negligence in diagnosis or treatment on the part of a doctor is whether he has been proved guilty of such failure as no doctor of ordinary skill would be guilty of if acting with ordinary care.'

In *Bolam v Friern Hospital Management Committee* [1957] 1 WLR 582 it was ruled that:

'The test is the standard of the ordinary skilled man exercising and professing to have that special skill. A man need not possess the highest expert skill at the risk of being found negligent. It is well-established law that it is sufficient if he exercises the ordinary skill of an ordinary competent man exercising that particular art ... he is not guilty of negligence if he has acted in accordance with a practice accepted as proper by a responsible body of medical men skilled in that particular art.... Putting it the other way round a doctor is not negligent if he is acting in accordance with such a practice, merely because there is a body of opinion that takes a contrary view.'

In *Bolitho v City and Hackney Health Authority* [1998] AC 232 it was ruled that:

'The use of these adjectives ("responsible", "reasonable", "respectable") all show that the court has to be satisfied that the exponents of the body of opinion relied upon can demonstrate that such opinion has a logical basis. In particular in cases involving, as they so often do, the weighing of risks against benefits, the judge before accepting a body of opinion as being responsible, reasonable or respectable, will need to be satisfied that, in forming their views, the experts have directed their minds to the comparative risks and benefits and have reached a defensible conclusion on the matter.'

you are critical of what was done at a particular point in time, address the risk:benefit ratio so as to justify subsequently, if it be so, your conclusion that there was a breach of the duty of care. Vague expressions as to poor or inadequate care will not suffice. The more fully and specifically the criticisms are set out, the greater will be the likelihood that the defendants will appreciate the thoroughness with which the claim has been investigated. This will reduce the likelihood of the case being delayed by a request for further details of the claim and it will increase the likelihood of the defendant making or agreeing an offer to settle.

In such a report, in answering specific questions or responding to a general question as to breach of duty, the 'Opinion' section should then set out detailed opinions as to the occasions when care fell below the expected standard. This means detailing what care fell below the requisite standard, what the requisite standard was, including what treatment should have been provided, how the course of the potential claimant's condition would have been different but for the failing, and what effect, if any, this failing has had on the patient's condition (that is, causation).

If experts do not employ such an approach, they should expect that counsel will employ such an approach in conference. At various points, the psychiatrist will be asked: 'Did the care/treatment fall below the standard expected of mental health professionals/psychiatrists acting with ordinary care?' and 'Was this a breach of duty?' If so, counsel will want to know what should have been done and the outcome thereof and what has been the consequence of the failure identified (that is, causation).

As indicated, these questions will assist counsel in the consideration of causation. This is because, in personal injury cases in general, not just negligence cases, even if claimants can establish a breach of duty, they have to show on a balance of probability that this caused injury. This is because liability means breach of duty and causation. This means: (1) that the injury would not have occurred but for the defendant's negligence (the 'but for' test); (2) that the defendant's negligence made a material contribution to the injury; (3) where relevant, that the defendant's negligence materially increased the risk of future injury; and/or (4) if consent is at issue, whether, had the claimant been adequately informed, he or she would not have accepted the treatment at that time.

The matter of 'material contribution' is important because there are often cases where there is, as it were, a 'negligent component' and a 'non-negligent (unavoidable) component'. The courts' approach in these cases, in short, is that, provided the negligent component made a 'material' (i.e. not negligible) contribution to the harm, and that provided its contribution is scientifically indivisible and 'unapportionable', the claimant will recover in full. Alternatively, where apportionment is legitimate and scientifically possible the court must adjust the damages accordingly. Psychiatrists should be wary of apportioning causation, for example x per cent to the previous psychiatric history, y per cent to the accident or breach of duty and z per cent to some unrelated life event or circumstance, lest they are asked to provide the legitimate and scientific proof for the percentages quoted.

Very commonly, the psychiatrist will identify what appears to be inadequate care by other mental health professionals. If so, it is important to indicate that expert evidence may be needed from other mental health professionals, such as a nursing expert, in order to be able to substantiate such allegations. This is not the expert stepping outside their area of expertise. It is assistance to the potential claimant's legal representatives, who might not otherwise recognise this feature of the case. This is an example of the difference between a pre-action 'advice' or 'advisory report' and a 'report' prepared under the CPR.

It is also usual for the expert to be asked, in an advisory report, to anticipate what responses the defendant may make to the allegations and to set out what the expert's responses would be to these if they were put in cross-examination. This enables the lawyers to form a preliminary view as to the likely success of the case. This will influence their response to any offer by the defendant to settle at the pre-action stage and it will influence the decision to issue proceedings and how to respond to an early offer to settle. In this section of the report, it is important to have in mind that the test for negligence is a two-stage one: first, apply the direction of McNair J in *Bolam* (Box 32) – Is there a body which would have done the same? If there is, apply the judgment in *Bolitho v City and Hackney Health Authority* [1998] AC 232 (Box 32).

Instructing solicitors and counsel need to know how likely it is that the defendant will find an expert, regarded as a responsible and respectable psychiatrist, who will argue that it was reasonable or logical, having regard to the potential risks and benefits, to have done what it is alleged should not have been done or not to have done what it is alleged should have been done. It does not matter that this expert may represent a minority position. The defendant needs only one such responsible and respectable psychiatrist.

This report should be identified as a 'Draft – for discussion with solicitors and counsel only (Not to be disclosed)'. If the case proceeds and proceedings are issued, a subsequent version of this report may be disclosed but, other than exceptionally, not the pre-action draft report. However, any expert's report, however it is titled or headed, may be exposed in cross-examination.

Before you sign your report and post it, remind yourself of the following:

It is worth emphasising that claimants' lawyers do not want to be given a case simply to please them, whether out of sympathy, or a natural inclination to oblige, or because that is perceived as the way to more cases and fees. It is easy enough to offer a finding of substandard treatment at a distance and in writing; but it is quite another to defend it under cross-examination. It does the patient no favours if a case initially supported by the expert has to be discontinued at a later stage when he realises what he is up against. (Lewis, 2006: p. 127)

The letter of claim

If making a claim rather than (or in addition to) pursuing other remedies is the course recommended by the solicitor, and the (potential) claimant wishes to do so, the solicitor may send a 'letter of claim' setting out the grounds for the claim. As the pre-action protocol in clinical negligence cases advises that this should include a clear summary of the facts on which the claim is based, including the alleged adverse outcome, the main allegations of negligence, the potential claimant's injuries and present condition and prognosis, the psychiatrist should prepare the report bearing in mind that it will be used in order to set out a letter of claim dealing with these points. In practice, in clinical negligence cases, it is common for the solicitors to rely on a records-based report that assists as to the main allegations of negligence and which does not deal with condition and prognosis in much more detail than is necessary to show that the potential claimant has suffered significant injury. However, as a 'condition and prognosis' report will be needed if proceedings are issued, the psychiatric expert, or perhaps another expert such as a neurologist, will be instructed, if this has not happened already, to prepare a 'condition and prognosis' report.

The condition and prognosis report

The condition and prognosis report will require a consultation with the potential claimant who has allegedly suffered injury, or in a case of allegedly negligent care, where the case relates to a patient who has died, it will be a 'report on papers' providing expert opinion on what the patient's diagnosis was and what the prognosis would have been but for the alleged failings in care. If the latter, there may be a claim under the Fatal Accidents Act 1976, in which case the opinion should include when the deceased could have been expected to return to work and, if so, what this work might have entailed.

Unless otherwise directed, for example to prepare a 'draft' report, most condition and prognosis reports that are prepared prior to the issue of proceedings are nonetheless prepared as if proceedings had been issued. They are produced as the report which will be relied upon in the proceedings and so they have to comply fully with the requirements of the CPR. They will refer to 'the claimant' (hereinafter in this section 'the claimant' rather than 'potential claimant') even though no claim has yet been made.

In the case of alleged psychiatric negligence the consultation will be used, along with the medical records, to decide whether or not the claimant has suffered any psychiatric damage over and above their underlying disorder or whether or not the course of the underlying disorder has been changed for the worse. If compensation is offered or awarded, it will be for the injury sustained as a result of the alleged negligence and not for psychiatric damage that would have been suffered in any event.

In a case of alleged medical negligence, where it is alleged that psychiatric injury has resulted, or in the case of a road traffic or industrial accident, the task will be similar: to identify any psychiatric injury that has resulted and answer detailed questions about the condition and prognosis of the claimant.

You must list all the documents you have seen (see also p. 43). However, you may be sent documents that it is not intended to disclose until later in the proceedings; if they are listed in your report and you have, or appear to have, relied on them, this may lead to an application by the other side for their disclosure. This is not usually a problem. If there is information in the claimant's draft witness statement that is of relevance, use the witness statement to guide you in eliciting the information from the claimant, but rely on what the claimant tells you and not on what is in the draft witness statement. In a case of alleged medical negligence you may have been sent the expert surgeon's liability and causation report as well as a condition and prognosis report, but the former will not be disclosed until later in the proceedings and probably not in its initial form. It may be problematic for the relationship between you and your instructing solicitors if they say that you can list the condition and prognosis report but you should not mention the liability and causation report. If the latter deals with a point to which you need to refer, you can do so in general terms (e.g. 'If it is the case that …/If the parties agree or the court finds that…)', though strictly you should list the report if you have seen it, whether or not you have relied on it.

Structure and content of the report

In most personal injury cases where a report is needed on condition and prognosis, there is a standard set of issues: any relevant medical history; the psychiatric injury sustained, if any; treatment received; present condition; prognosis; any recommendations as to treatment. Additionally, it is central to the assessment of the claimant's injuries to establish the extent and duration of any continuing disability. Thus, you have to comment specifically on any areas of continuing complaint or disability or impact on daily living. If there is such continuing disability, you have to comment upon the level of suffering or inconvenience caused and, if possible, in the prognosis section (see below), give your view as to when or whether the complaint or disability is likely to resolve.

Any relevant medical history

Two aspects of a claimant's medical history are particularly likely to be relevant in personal injury litigation. These are a history of psychiatric disorder and a history of physical illness that has, in the past, been complicated by psychiatric symptoms or might be so complicated in the future.

A history of psychiatric disorder may be relevant because if it is alleged that psychiatric disorder has resulted, for example, from an accident, there will be the issue of whether a disorder that has been present only since the accident is nevertheless unrelated to it, that is, it was either present at the time of the accident or would have occurred in any event. A history of psychiatric disorder is also relevant because it may indicate a predisposition, or what the law recognises as a vulnerability, to psychiatric disorder.

Likewise, where previous physical ill-health has been complicated by psychiatric symptoms and especially if, with recurrence, chronicity or deterioration, the psychiatric symptoms have become more frequent or more severe, there will be the question of whether or not psychiatric symptoms subsequent to the accident are related to the pre-existing and on-going physical ill-health and not the accident.

Psychiatric injury

Set out the psychiatric diagnosis or diagnoses, if any. In straightforward cases, a paragraph on each diagnosis may suffice. It is common convention to use ICD-10 or DSM-IV-TR™ diagnoses and to include code numbers. This is not necessary for those personal injury lawyers and judges who have their own copies of ICD-10 and DSM-IV-TR™, but it makes their jobs easier. However, one judge, who does not have copies of these, said that between one case and another he forgets what the acronyms stand for. He also commented that there is too much emphasis on attaching a label to the claimant's condition and it is the contents of the jar, not the label, that matters. He reported his experience of psychiatrists who agree about everything relevant to the claim but vehemently disagree only as to the diagnosis. He echoes Gunn & Taylor (1993, pp. 102–103):

The term 'positive psychiatric illness' can embrace the whole range of morbid emotional responses as well as the ordinary form of neurotic and psychotic disorders. The doctor thus must attempt to determine the existence of any psychiatric disorder and its relation to the incident. The court is more concerned with the existence of disorder in itself, its attribution, and its consequences than with niceties of diagnosis and classification. Diagnostic terms should be used simply and conventionally, but it is unnecessary to follow slavishly definitions from textbooks and glossaries such as DSM III or ICD.

Justify the diagnosis by reference to symptoms and signs. Indicate the extent to which the evidence from the medical records supports the diagnosis. Indicate to what extent there is other corroborative evidence. Make clear if the diagnosis is based entirely on self-report.

If diagnoses have been suggested by other experts and these are not supported, indicate this and say why.

Commonly there may be a range of reasonable opinion as to diagnosis. State what other diagnoses may reasonably be made and indicate why your diagnosis is to be preferred.

Treatment received

In a straightforward case, having set out in some detail, in the body of the report, the treatment received, on the basis of both the records and the claimant's report, this section can often be brief. Set out the form or forms of drug therapy and the form or forms of psychological therapy that have been employed. Make it clear if treatment has been insufficient, such as an inadequate dosage of an antidepressant or too short a course of cognitive–behavioural therapy. Make it clear if there is treatment that ought to have been given that has not been given.

If the claimant has not complied with treatment, it is important to explain why. This necessitates asking about such matters as failure to attend appointments, discontinuation of medication, or a frequency of repeat prescriptions which suggests that medication has been missed. The importance of this is that a claimant is under a duty to mitigate the loss. A distinction has to be made, by the parties or the court, between the claimant who is simply uncooperative with treatment and the claimant whose failure to comply with treatment is understandable. Instances of the latter include misunderstandings, appointments at genuinely inconvenient times or places, intolerable drug side-effects, and a failure to engage with the therapist.

Present condition

'Present condition' means the severity of the potential claimant's injury in terms of the degree of suffering and impairment of functioning or functional deficit. Although the categories of damage in the JSB Guide mix up condition and prognosis, it is usually helpful to consult the JSB Guide and ensure that information under this heading is provided as to matters that are taken into account by lawyers and the courts in deciding the severity of the damage sustained. These are: (1) the injured person's ability to cope with life and work; and (2) the effect on the injured person's relationships with family, friends and those with whom he or she comes into contact. Further, some experts take into account such matters as: (3) the extent to which treatment would be successful; (4) future vulnerability; (5) prognosis; (6) whether medical help has been sought; and (7) whether the injury results from sexual and/or physical abuse and/or breach of trust, and if so, the nature of the relationship between victim and abuser, the nature of the abuse, its duration and the symptoms caused by it.

It is then possible to grade the claimant's condition by reference to the categories of severity in the JSB Guide but this is not essential and it can be argued that this is for the parties or the court to decide, having regard to their evaluation of all of the evidence. Experts have been criticised for not using the classification, and experts have been criticised for doing so! Criticism may be avoided by using the classification and adding that you acknowledge that this is an ultimate issue 'for the parties to agree or for the court to decide' (which is often a helpful phrase in any medico-legal report). The categories of psychiatric damage generally (including for post-traumatic stress disorder) are 'severe', 'moderately severe', 'moderate' and 'minor', but the criteria differ slightly.

It may be helpful, in this section, to include a rating of the claimant on the Global Assessment of Functioning Scale (Luborsky, 1962). This is particularly helpful as many psychiatrists who use DSM-IV-TR™ do so, thus facilitating comparison and detection of change.

The effect of the claimant's condition on their capacity for work or their 'earning capacity' is usually of particular importance because in many cases the loss of earnings claim is a major element of the sum of compensation claimed or awarded.

It is also helpful to indicate whether or not the claimant has a disability within the meaning of the Equality Act 2010 (see p. 187), as this has implications for how damages are calculated.

Treatment recommended

If there are outstanding requirements as to treatment these have to be set out with sufficient detail for the treatment to be costed, as it may need to be obtained privately, and for it to be arranged.

An action for negligence was brought against a psychiatrist who reported on a victim of the Hillsborough football disaster (*Hall v Egdell* (2004 unreported)). The psychiatrist had diagnosed reactive depression and the claimant called experts, whose evidence was that he had failed to diagnose post-traumatic stress disorder. The judge found that the expert had been negligent in gathering the data to found his conclusion but he also found that, as the expert was the first doctor consulted by the claimant since the disaster, he had an obligation to the claimant as a patient and he should have informed the claimant's general practitioner of his recommendation as to treatment. So, if recommendations are made for treatment, incorporate a request in the report that such recommendations are passed on to the claimant's general practitioner or private doctor and ask to be advised if this recommendation is not acted upon. In the event that the recommendation is not acted upon, consider writing directly to the doctor. If those instructing you object or threaten to object, at least discuss the matter with a colleague or colleagues first and document their advice, but better still also, or instead, take the advice of your medical defence organisation (MDO).

Do not send your report to the claimant's general practitioner or private doctor without the written authority of your instructing solicitors. Take note of the case of *Cornelius v de Taranto* [2000] EWCA 2381, where a claimant was awarded £3000 for breach of contract. The action was against a psychiatrist who had prepared a medical report on the claimant in connection with an allegation of constructive dismissal. In order to arrange treatment for the claimant, the psychiatrist sent the report, which contained material defamatory of the claimant, to her general practitioner and another psychiatrist. The psychiatrist was found liable and on appeal the finding was upheld. However, the judge at first instance had ordered the psychiatrist to pay £45,000 towards the claimant's costs. Because the claimant had lost a substantial part of her claim, the Court of Appeal quashed this order, no doubt much to the relief of the psychiatrist and his MDO.

Prognosis

Cases cannot go on forever, although some may appear to do so. Cases have to be settled by the parties or decided by the court on the basis of a prediction as to the course and outcome of the claimant's condition, including the award of damages for what might happen in the future. This is often one of the most difficult parts of a condition and prognosis report. It is difficult enough in many cases to predict the course and outcome of a psychiatric disorder in clinical practice; it is more difficult and complicated in the case of patients who know that the level of damages will take into account the duration and outcome of their condition.

A further matter that sometimes has to be addressed in relation to prognosis is the risk of deterioration. This is because judges can award 'provisional damages' where the evidence persuades them that, although the chances of deterioration in the claimant's condition are less than 50%, there is nevertheless a real risk that a substantial deterioration may occur in the future, in which event the award will allow the claimant to return to court to seek further damages.

In this section, also indicate whether or not the claimant has been rendered more vulnerable to psychiatric disorder in the future.

The response to the letter of claim

In a potential negligence case, in response to the letter of claim, solicitors acting for the National Health Service Litigation Authority (NHSLA) are likely to commission an overview report. In order to respond quickly, and in order to avoid the cost of further negotiations or even civil proceedings in a case that ought to be settled quickly and without dispute, the NHSLA now has a scheme for obtaining brief overview reports within a short timescale.

An expert so instructed is asked to prepare a short report, without a detailed recitation of the facts of the case. However, the task is the same as for the expert instructed by the potential claimant's solicitors. The only difference is that little or nothing of the chronology is expected to be set out in the body of the report.

Upon receipt of this report the NHSLA may admit the claim. If the potential claimant's solicitors have already made an offer to settle, the NHSLA may then make its own offer to settle. The NHSLA can also make an offer to settle of its own motion, that is, without waiting for the report from the potential claimant's solicitors. If the case is so settled, no further expert opinion is likely to be needed. If the claim is admitted, but there remains an issue as to condition and prognosis, the potential claimant's solicitors will need to provide the 'condition and prognosis' report.

In accident cases, solicitors acting for the insurers of the defendant may seek to settle the claim upon receipt of a letter of claim and without proceeding to litigation. In such cases, the defendant's solicitors may instruct their own psychiatric expert to prepare a report on the claimant.

Sometimes they include in their instructions a copy of the report prepared at the request of the claimant's solicitors and sometimes they prefer their expert to prepare their report 'blind'.

Serving proceedings

If the claim cannot be settled, or the dispute otherwise resolved, it is open to the potential claimant's solicitors to 'issue proceedings'. From this point onwards the CPR apply and the potential claimant is now a claimant.

Within four months of the issue of proceedings, the 'claim form' must be served and if the 'particulars of claim' are not served at the same time, they must be served within 14 days of the service of the 'claim form'.

The 'particulars of claim'

The 'particulars of claim' has to include a concise statement of the facts on which the claimant relies. It has to be accompanied by a medical report regarding the alleged personal injuries. Previously, the report had to substantiate the alleged injuries and this was sometimes interpreted as meaning that the report had to confirm causation. Where causation issues may be complicated, a further report dealing with causation, condition and prognosis may be requested at a later stage in the proceedings.

A psychiatrist who has been instructed in a potential case of psychiatric negligence will usually be sent a draft particulars of claim for comment. There may be some urgency, as the particulars of claim have to be served either with the claim form no more than four months after proceedings are issued or within 14 days of service of the claim form (see above).

It is likely that the draft particulars of claim will reflect closely the 'Opinion' section of the draft liability report, especially if you have responded with sufficient clarity and precision to the questions that were put to you, but as this report is a draft, pre-action document, it will not be disclosed with the particulars of claim.

Check the accuracy of the summary of the medical history. Do not expect to see the whole medical history or even as detailed a history as you have set out in your report. The factual section of the particulars of claim has to be concise. However, when setting out the allegedly negligent acts or omissions, it will be necessary to rely on the facts and matters in this section. So make sure that the appropriate parts of the medical history have been summarised.

Be sure that you can support all of the allegations of negligence. If not, you need to point this out at this stage. Make sure that all of the criticisms of the claimant's care are reflected in the particulars of claim. If they are not, point this out, though there may be good reason for not including some, not least if it is clear that, albeit that they relate to failings, they do not amount to a breach of duty or they are not failings that have been causative of damage.

Cooperation between expert and barrister at this stage can avoid the defendant making a preliminary request for further information or clarification to which the claimant's barrister and solicitor may be unable to respond without your assistance and which will necessitate you having to go back not just to your report but perhaps even to the case records to provide the necessary answers.

The defence

If a defence is going to be served, this has to be served no more than 56 days after receipt of the particulars of claim.

Where you are instructed by the defendant's solicitors, it is likely that the defence will reflect some of the points you have made in your overview report.

Where you are instructed by the claimant's solicitors, you are likely to be sent the defence and asked to comment on it. It may be apparent, from the points made, that the defendant's solicitors have an opinion from a psychiatrist who has taken a very different view of the case to that which you have taken. Do not feel you have to prepare for action stations and a duel to the death. The system may be adversarial but you and the other expert are not adversaries. The defence may fairly make some points that undermine the allegations of negligence that you have supported. Where you consider that some of your opinions are going to be undermined or that your position on certain points may not after all be tenable, you need to point this out at this stage. Time and money may be wasted and justice delayed if this does not emerge until the experts' meeting. Even more may be lost, particularly your reputation, if this emerges only when you are under cross-examination. On the other hand, it is not surprising to find that points made in the defence do not take into account information of which you are aware in the medical records or they may be only the most favourable, for the defendant, of a number of interpretations of what happened. So, assist those instructing you to decide what points in the defence may have to be conceded and what points are going to become trial issues.

Exchange of lay witness statements

The next stage, and by a date fixed by the court, is the exchange of lay witness statements. In many straightforward personal injury cases, these will not be relevant and they will probably not be sent to the psychiatric expert. In, for example, a complicated 'employment stress' case and especially in a case of alleged psychiatric negligence, they may be of critical importance and the Court of Appeal has repeatedly stated that expert reports must take into account witness statements served by the other party (e.g. *Johnson v John and Waltham Forest Health Authority* [1998] MLC 0224, CA). This is not surprising, as it is often only at this stage that the parties appreciate the full evidential basis for each other's position. As the exchange of witness statements usually precedes by several months the exchange of expert reports on breach of duty, liability and causation, it will usually be necessary to amend your report in the light of this further evidence and to do so having regard to the date on which the court has ordered the exchange of expert reports.

Covert surveillance

Such is the level of fraud in civil litigation that solicitors acting for defendants and insurance companies sometimes employ private investigators to carry out covert surveillance on claimants.

The story is told of an Australian case in which a severely disabled, wheelchair-bound claimant was invited to his solicitor's offices and shown a film that appeared to be of him standing on top of a wagon and catching sacks which were being thrown up to him and which he was stacking neatly on the wagon. He was quick to point out that the film was not of him but of his identical twin brother. He was told, in no uncertain terms, that if his twin brother did not provide a statement and come to court, his claim was in difficulty. His twin brother was located, he came to court and he won his case. As he was leaving court, his barrister turned to him and commented that he was very lucky that his twin brother had come to his rescue. The claimant commented that he was lucky indeed because if the camera had panned down to ground level the investigator would have filmed him standing there, throwing the sacks up to his brother!

Should the expert advise covert surveillance? I think not. A positive recommendation to carry out covert surveillance makes the expert a hostage to fortune, because it might lead to a very obvious cross-examination suggesting inappropriate involvement in the litigation process. If there are reasons to doubt the credibility of the claimant and they derive from the application of the psychiatrist's expertise, they should be set out in the report. Genuinely held opinions should be expressed in the report and can be acted upon by the solicitors if they see fit. If the report has been requested by the defendant's solicitors, they may well respond by organising covert surveillance. If it has been requested by the claimant's solicitors, they may well respond by warning their client about covert surveillance! Some experts might highlight this part of the report in a 'side letter' but that might lead to the same cross-examination.

Experts are commonly asked to comment on covert surveillance evidence but seldom as interesting as in the Australian case. Most commonly it is hours of supermarket shopping, which is enough to make any psychiatrist or lawyer 'paranoid' about supermarkets. Commonly it is views of a house in the dark, curtains closed and reaching the stunning climax that the subject had not been observed that day. Occasionally it is miles and miles of driving but rarely as interesting as reality television programmes about 'traffic cops'. I have yet to see anything like the covert surveillance that *Kavanagh QC* had in evidence when his client was filmed in his wheelchair being pushed in and out of the sex shops and massage parlours in Soho – or was it Amsterdam?

Experts instructed by defendants' solicitors and insurance companies will usually be asked to comment on the covert surveillance after they have prepared their report, even though some or all of the covert surveillance predates their instruction and/or consultation with the claimant. This is in order to avoid experts being influenced by the covert surveillance in their approach to claimants and in order to avoid experts having to conceal from claimants the fact that they have seen this evidence, which usually will not yet have been disclosed to the claimant's solicitors. It is certainly unsatisfactory and arguably unethical for the expert to see the surveillance evidence, not disclose this to the claimant, not list it as evidence they have considered and to try to ignore it when reaching their opinions. As it may be difficult not to be influenced by such evidence, it will be misleading not to list it as evidence upon which the opinions are based. Experts instructed by claimants' solicitors are likely to see this evidence much later in the proceedings, as it is not usually disclosed to the claimants' solicitors earlier. Trial by ambush may be long past but defendants' solicitors will try to keep their ammunition dry for as long as possible.

Most of the evidence obtained by covert surveillance that is of significance is evidence of claimants apparently being less disabled than they have claimed to be: expert analysis of such evidence is best provided by other experts. For example, an orthopaedic expert is best placed to point out that a claimant's arm movements are not as limited as the claimant has reported them to be and as they have been on examination. Such evidence may, however, cast doubt on the claimant's credibility and this may have implications for reliance on the claimant's self-reported and otherwise largely, or entirely, uncorroborated psychiatric symptoms. In such a case, a useful formula for the psychiatrist is along the following lines:

Insofar as the parties may agree or the court may find, on the basis of this covert surveillance evidence, that the claimant has been unreliable in his claim that he cannot do x, y and z, it is necessary to point out that if the claimant has also been unreliable in the report of his psychiatric symptoms, there must necessarily be some doubt as to whether or not the claimant has suffered any psychiatric disorder, or if the claimant has, how severe his condition is.

Less commonly, the covert surveillance will reveal evidence of direct relevance to the psychiatric expert. In some cases, there will be evidence of claimants living a more active and potentially fulfilling life than they have reported. In a case where a claimant who has presented with, say, a depressive syndrome and a loss of interest in football and is shown by the covert surveillance attending football matches week after week, this will have implications for the psychiatric diagnosis and for the assessment of the severity of the claimant's condition.

Often it will be difficult to establish the mental state of a claimant from covert surveillance, but occasionally, for example, there may be evidence of a claimant socialising, laughing, joking and conversing at length in a manner that contrasts strongly with a depressive presentation at consultation and the reported history of depressive symptoms.

In any case, it may be fair and sensible for the expert to ask for the claimant's comments on the surveillance before offering an opinion on its significance.

Exchange of expert reports

Expert reports are usually exchanged simultaneously.

Written questions to experts

Rule 35.6 of the CPR permits a party to put questions to an expert instructed by another party for the purpose of clarification of their opinions. This does not prevent a party putting questions to its own expert (*Stallwood v David* [2007] 1 All ER 206), although in substantial litigation (or what might be termed 'a big case') it is almost always preferable to discuss issues in conference or on the telephone.

Such questions must be put within 28 days of the service of the report on the other party. Often they arrive after a much longer interval because the court has given permission or the other party has agreed to their late commission.

Experts are not expected to answer questions that are not properly directed to clarification of the report, or are disproportionate or are asked out of time. In what may be such cases the expert should discuss the questions with the instructing solicitors and, if appropriate, the party asking the questions. As a last resort, the expert can file a written request to the court for directions (see p. 138).

If the expert does not answer the questions, the court may order that the party may not rely on the evidence of that expert and/or the party may not recover the fees and expenses of that expert from another party.

Experts' answers to questions automatically become part of their reports. They are covered by the statement of truth and form part of their expert evidence. Some solicitors expect that answers will conclude with the statement of truth; others consider it unnecessary.

The expert's instructing solicitors are responsible for payment of fees for answering the questions and not the party putting the questions.

Discussions between experts

At any stage the court may direct a discussion between the experts for the purpose of identifying and elaborating the issues in the proceedings and, where possible, reaching an agreement on those issues or at least narrowing the issues, and identifying what action, if any, may be taken to resolve outstanding issues. The court can also direct that, following such a discussion, the experts must prepare a statement for the court 'setting out' the issues on which they agree and those on which they disagree with a summary of the reasons for disagreement. Previously the experts had to 'show' the issues on which they agreed and disagreed and the change to 'setting out' reflects a need for clarity.

Arrangements for discussions have to be proportionate to the value of the case. So, in many cases, 'meetings' by letter, email or telephone should suffice. Face-to-face meetings will be more likely in high-value cases, where there are several experts and where, for example in a case of alleged psychiatric negligence, the experts are going to have to look together at, and refer to, many documents, which are likely to be sorted and numbered differently. The parties' lawyers may be present only if the parties agree or the court orders it; if in attendance, they should not normally intervene other than to answer questions put to them by the experts or to advise on points of law. Nowadays they are rarely present, as the courts have long since decided that their attendance is inappropriate. However, if it is a large and potentially complicated experts' discussion with a number of experts or a number of parties, it may be appropriate for it to be chaired by a lawyer, such as a barrister, who is independent of the parties.

The *Protocol* (Civil Justice Council, 2005) assumes that there will be an agenda. Some High Court judges and masters have expressed surprise that experts have discussions without an agenda. The *Protocol* states at 18.4:

The parties, their lawyers and experts should cooperate to produce the agenda for any discussion between experts, although primary responsibility for preparation of the agenda should normally lie with the parties' solicitors.

The *Protocol* (18.6) also refers to the court giving directions if the parties cannot agree the agenda promptly or if a party is unrepresented.

In practice, agendas are the exception rather than the rule, especially in simpler and lower-value cases. However, in high-value claims with complex negligence and causation issues, they are almost always required.

When experts ask for an agenda they may be asked if one is necessary, or solicitors may even tell the experts that they are the ones who know what the issues are. If pressed, solicitors may simply tell the experts to draw up their own agenda. There is nothing in the *Protocol* about experts asking the court for directions for the drawing up of the agenda when the parties' solicitors fail in what is described as their primary responsibility. There are many cases in which the experts' opinions are so close and the issues so straightforward that an agenda is unnecessary. There are other cases in which the opinions are far apart and the issues are complex. In such cases, if there is no agenda, the statement will often not assist as much as it ought and one or both parties may have to come back to the experts with questions to clarify the statement or belatedly produce an agenda that then calls for a second joint statement. There can be no complaint about experts not answering the questions if the questions were not put to them.

If you have an agenda and decide to depart from it, be careful that the further issues are relevant to the issues between the parties and that the time spent dealing with them is proportionate.

Preparation for a discussion between experts must include comparing the materials that each expert has seen – usually reports, records, DVDs/videos and statements. Your instructing solicitors should have told you which of your reports, addenda, letters and so on have been disclosed. You should not refer in your meeting to documents that have not been disclosed. You should not be in the position of finding out, after you have signed the joint statement, that you have referred to, and relied upon, covert surveillance that has not been disclosed, for example.

It is very important that the experts should have had access to the same materials. Significant differences of opinion may disappear or change in their significance once both experts have seen the same materials. If one expert has not seen documents that the other expert has seen, it is best to adjourn until they can both rely on the same body of evidence.

Usual practice is for one expert to prepare a draft and then send it to the other expert. Some solicitors are critical of this practice and may threaten to ask the court to order disclosure of the first draft. It is, however, a practice of which judges generally approve. The expert who writes the draft usually finds that its preparation powerfully concentrates the mind on the issues. Often it will be clear that there is close agreement on a number of the issues. Areas of disagreement may also be clear but usually there will be some difficulty identifying the reasons for disagreement. Identifying reasons for your own disagreement with the other expert is often easier than identifying reasons for their disagreement with your opinion. If an expert significantly alters his or her opinion, the joint statement has to include a note or addendum by that expert explaining the change of opinion.

The report has to be signed by both experts within 7 days of the conclusion of the discussion and copies have to be provided to the parties within 14 days of signing.

It is important to realise that it is not the job of the experts to assist in resolution of the case by seeking to agree on everything. Their job is to identify the issues which remain at issue and not to strain to reach agreement. It is for the parties, or if they fail, the court to resolve the dispute. 'Trial by expert' must not replace 'trial by judge'. Also, an expert must not accept instructions from instructing solicitors to avoid, or defer, reaching a conclusion.

The single joint expert

The CPR encourage the use of SJEs. An SJE is an expert who is instructed jointly by both the claimant and the defendant(s). Unless otherwise ordered by the court or agreed by the parties, the parties are jointly and severally liable to pay the expert's fees.

Sometimes a party informs the other side whom it proposes to appoint as its party-appointed expert and the other side has the opportunity to object. The expert then appointed by the party, albeit being one approved by the other side, remains a party-appointed expert. They are not thereby an SJE. However, if there has been no objection to their appointment, the other side will have to make out a case to the court if they want to appoint their own party-appointed expert.

The parties are encouraged to try to agree joint instructions but the default position is that each party can give instructions. If instructions are received from only one, the expert can give notice that unless the other instructions are received within, normally, seven days the expert will begin work without them. If the instructions are received before the report is completed, the expert will have to decide whether or not it is practicable to comply with them without adversely affecting the timetable or incurring what may be further disproportionate expense. Inform the parties if you are not going to comply with the late instructions; they may seek guidance from the court. If instructions are late, or not received at all, this must be made clear in the report.

Like any experts, SJEs owe their first duty to the court. However, the requirements of independence, impartiality and transparency call for special measures. All correspondence should be copied to both parties, at the same time. This includes a letter of appointment sent to the claimant. Telephone conversations with solicitors on either side are best avoided. If unavoidable, remind the solicitor of your joint status, advise that you will make a record of what is discussed, make such a record and send a brief 'minute' of the discussion to both parties. Do not attend any meeting or conference which is not a joint one without the agreement of the parties in writing or an order from the court. Also, ascertain who will be paying the fee for your attendance. Ensure that the report is sent simultaneously to both parties.

The SJE ploughs a lonely furrow and although it is rare for an SJE to give oral evidence it really is a 'Billy no mates' experience. You cannot leave that lonely furrow to go to either side for advice or support. If neither party is satisfied with the opinion or the outcome of the case, you may be blamed by both parties, who may feel that trial by expert has replaced trial by judge.

Asking the court for directions

The CPR allow experts to file a written request for directions to assist them in carrying out their function as an expert. This will usually be a last resort, after discussions with instructing solicitors have not resolved the matter. The request should be in the form of a letter to the district judge of the relevant court and it should begin with a reference to the title of the claim, the claim or case number, full details of why directions are sought and copies of any relevant documentation.

A draft should be sent to the instructing solicitors at least seven days before the request is filed at the court and to all other parties at least four days before it is filed. This gives the parties a last opportunity to take steps to avoid the court having to deal with the matter.

Circumstances in which an expert might ask the court for directions are where an SJE is provided with incompatible instructions by the opposing parties or where the expert has identified some particular document or records as being of critical importance and one party or the other refuses to make them available. Other circumstances are where grossly inappropriate or disproportionate questions are put by the opposing side and for which your instructing solicitors are going to have to pay.

Report requirements

The declaration should include at least the following:

I understand that my overriding duty is to the court, both in preparing reports and in giving oral evidence. I understand, have complied and will continue to comply with that duty. This report is addressed to the court.

I am aware of the requirements of Part 35 and Practice Direction 35, the *Protocol for the Instruction of Experts to Give Evidence in Civil Claims* and the Practice Direction for pre-action conduct.

The statement of truth is:

I confirm that I have made clear which facts and matters referred to in this report are within my own knowledge and which are not. Those that are within my own knowledge I confirm to be true. The opinions I have expressed represent my true and complete professional opinions on the matters to which they refer.

Particular issues in, and types of, personal injury action

Nervous shock

Someone who suffers injuries in a road traffic accident or complications as a result of allegedly negligent surgery, say, is a 'primary victim'. However, the 'primary victim' does not necessarily have to be the person injured by the event itself. Thus, the mother who labours and gives birth to a baby in an asphyxiated and brain-damaged state is considered by the law herself also to be a 'primary victim', albeit that the directly injured party is her baby. Likewise, a physically uninjured passenger in a car in which other occupants suffer horrendous injuries in an accident will also be treated as a primary victim for the purposes of nervous shock damages.

Policy decisions of the courts limit the extent to which 'secondary victims', such as a bystander who witnesses a car accident, or parents whose child dies following negligent medical care or a rescuer, can recover damages for psychiatric injury. The reasons for the policy are obvious, but the reasoning in some of the decisions is odd, to say the least. Lord Steyn has referred to 'a patchwork quilt of distinctions which are hard to justify' (*Frost v Chief Constable of South Yorkshire Police* [1998] QB 254).

Psychiatric damage, so caused, equates with what the law calls 'nervous shock' and there are two leading cases that provide definitions of it (Box 33). Both indicate a requirement for a psychiatric illness, albeit *Alcock* only implicitly (by excluding psychiatric illness of gradual onset) or what Lord Bridge described in *McLoughlin v O'Brian* [1983] 1 AC 410, HL, as a 'positive psychiatric illness'. Shock, on its own, and in the lay sense of the term, anxiety or depression as symptoms but not amounting to psychiatric illness, disappointment or grief, unless pathological, does not amount to 'nervous shock' as defined. There has to be something more than what are regarded as normal or ordinary emotional responses to events. As Lord Denning said in *Hinz v Berry* [1970] 2 QB 40:

In English law no damages are awarded for grief and sorrow caused by a person's death. No damages are to be given for worry about the children, or for the financial strain or stress, or the difficulties of adjusting to a new life. Damages are however recoverable for nervous shock, or to put it in medical terms, for any recognisable psychiatric illness caused by the breach of duty of the defendant.

It can be seen that the term 'nervous shock' is somewhat unfortunate. At first glance it seems to refer to the actual experience of being shocked.

Box 33 'Nervous shock'

There are two leading cases that provide definitions of 'nervous shock':

'I understand "shock" in this context to mean the sudden sensory perception – that is, by seeing, hearing or touching – of a person, thing or event, which is so distressing that the perception of the phenomenon affronts or insults the claim-ant's mind and causes a recognizable psychiatric illness'. (Brennan J in *Jaensch v Coffey* (1984) 155 CLR 549)

'"Shock" in the context of this cause of action, involves the sudden appreciation by sight or sound of a horrifying event, which violently agitates the mind. It has yet to include psychiatric illness caused by the accumulation over a period of time or more gradual assaults on the nervous system.' (Lord Ackner in *Alcock v Chief Constable of South Yorkshire* [1992] 1 AC 310)

The legal definitions, however, demonstrate that in law it refers to the psychiatric illness that is a consequence of the shock, which may not in all people cause psychiatric illness, rather than the shock itself. Judges now more often use terms such as psychiatric injury and mental injury.

Evolving case law has established that nervous shock claims can be made where the claimant has been put in fear of immediate personal injury (*Dulieu v White & Sons* [1901] 2 KB 669), where the shock results from a fear of imminent injury to others (*Hambrook v Stokes Brothers* [1925] 1 KB 141, CA), where the claimant witnesses a shocking event (*Hinz v Berry*) and where the shock is caused by sight or hearing of the immediate aftermath of a shocking event (*McLoughlin v O'Brian*).

Case law provides guidance on what is meant by the immediate aftermath. Relatives of victims of the Hillsborough football stadium disaster who arrived eight hours later to see their loved ones at the hospital or mortuary were held not to have witnessed the 'immediate aftermath' (*Alcock*) but arriving within one hour to find children dead and seriously injured is within the immediate aftermath (*McLoughlin v O'Brian*). There has to be close contact in the immediate aftermath: it is not enough for the parents to follow the ambulance transferring their son from one hospital to another, for the father to glimpse him briefly in the ambulance and for the mother to see him as he is being rushed on a trolley to intensive care, however shocking his appearance a few hours later and however distressing the subsequent two-day vigil before their son's life support machine is switched off (*Taylorson v Shieldness Produce Ltd* [1994] PIQR P329, CA).

Case law also provides guidance, albeit not entirely clear, on what is meant by 'sudden' (see Box 33). Lord Ackner in *Alcock* excluded psychiatric illness that was caused by the accumulation of more gradual assaults on the nervous system over a period of time. In *Sion v Hampstead Health Authority* [1994] 5 Med LR 170, the claimant failed because the psychiatric report did not provide evidence of 'shock' and instead described a continuous process starting with the claimant's arrival at the hospital following his son's road traffic accident, proceeding through what it was subsequently alleged was negligent medical treatment and culminating in his not unexpected death two weeks later. However, as has been observed (Lewis, 2006), there did appear to have been some discrete, 'shocking' events, including a sudden deterioration, sudden respiratory difficulties, cardiac arrest and transfer to the intensive-care unit. The judgment here is to be contrasted with that in *Tredget and Tredget v Bexley Health Authority* [1994] 5 Med LR 178, where the judge held that the two-day period beginning with the traumatic birth of a fatally injured baby and culminating in the baby's death was a single, frightening and harrowing event. Likewise, in *North Glamorgan NHS Trust v Walters* [2002] EWCA Civ 1792; [2003] PIQR P316, it was held that the relevant 'event' comprised a series of events, in this case beginning with the negligent delivery of a baby, being told first that brain injury was unlikely, then being told that there had been brain damage and life

141

support was needed and culminating in the baby dying in its mother's arms upon withdrawal of life support. What Lewis (2006: p. 291) describes as 'a seamless tale lasting a period of 36 hours which for the mother was undoubtedly one drawn-out experience' was accepted by the court as being one 'horrifying' event, albeit that it was also made up a series of blows, each of which was a sudden assault.

There is an additional requirement, the proximity test. This is a twofold test: the relationship between the claimant and the victim has to be based on sufficiently close ties of love and affection; and the claimant and the event have to be proximate. It is not sufficient merely to be informed of the death of a loved one, however sudden and unexpected the news. However graphic television reporting of an event, such as the Hillsborough disaster, the viewer has no claim because this is removed from witnessing the event itself.

Causation is often problematic in many of these cases. It is easy for defendants to argue, and difficult for claimants to disprove, that the psychiatric illness has been caused by the death of the loved one, children in particular, and it would have occurred in any event, whether or not the parent had witnessed the tragedy or its immediate aftermath. Causal analysis depends in part on knowing what the normal reactions are, for example, of parents to a stillbirth, an early neonatal death, the sudden accidental death of a 2-year-old child or the death of an 18-year-old child. It depends in part on understanding the unique history of the claimant so as to explain, if possible, why they have reacted the way that they have.

A psychiatric report in a case of alleged 'nervous shock' sustained by a secondary victim should include the following. The claimant's previous psychiatric history and personality have to be explored in order to say whether or not the claimant was of normal fortitude; for primary victims it does not matter whether or not they are of normal fortitude but secondary victims have to show that they are not unusually susceptible to psychiatric harm of the kind in question (*Bourhill v Young* [1943] AC 92). The section on diagnosis should make a clear distinction between positive psychiatric illness and states of anxiety, depression, stress, grief and so on that do not amount to a psychiatric disorder. There should be a careful analysis of the experience of the claimant. The factual basis for this should be set out in the body of the report. There should be a detailed and strictly chronological account of the claimant's reported experience or experiences, with careful attention to what the claimant appreciated, by sight, sound or through other senses, at the time rather than what was later learned. The documentation of the experience should include how the claimant felt at various points in time so as to identify what it was that violently agitated, affronted or insulted the mind. In answering questions as to causation it should then be possible to identify one or more sufficiently shocking or horrifying events. If part or all of the psychiatric injury would have occurred even in the absence of the shocking event or events, this needs to be made clear. However, it may be sufficient for the claimant to show no more than that the event or events made a material contribution to the psychiatric illness.

Mere mental or emotional distress

There are a number of circumstances in which compensation may be awarded for what has been termed 'mere mental or emotional distress' (Handford, 2006). The torts of trespass to the person – battery and false imprisonment – can attract compensation for the mental distress occasioned. Examples are: anger and indignation at unnecessary dental treatment (*Appleton v Garrett* [1997] 8 Med LR 75); the reaction to being forcibly ejected from the Harrods department store on account of the shopper's appearance (*Corr v Harrods Ltd* [1999] EWCA 2381 Civ); manhandling and assault by police officers followed by wrongful detention in a police cell for four hours (*Thompson v Commissioner of Police for the Metropolis* [1998] QB 498); and a ship's steward wrongly accused of indecently assaulting a child and locked up until the *Queen Elizabeth* docked in New York (*Hook v Cunard SS Co Ltd* [1953] 1 WLR 682). The hurt feelings of tenants wrongly evicted by their landlords can attract damages (*Drane v Evangelou* [1978] 1 WLR 455). In *Khodaparast v Shad* [2000] 1 WLR 618 damages were awarded to an Iranian woman whose former lover caused her distress by using photographs of her in advertisements in pornographic magazines. In *Batty v Metropolitan Property Realisations Ltd* [1978] QB 554 damages were awarded for injury to a householder's peace of mind caused by the imminent collapse of the house.

Damages can also be awarded for mental distress resulting from a breach of contract. Thus in *Jarvis v Swans Tours Ltd* [1973] QB 233, a solicitor was compensated for the injured feelings brought about by a disappointing holiday. A Scottish case in which a photographer failed to turn up to take photographs of the pursuer's wedding led to a successful award for mental distress (*Diensen v Samsom* (1971) SLT 49). Damages have even been awarded for the distress caused by selling someone a faulty car (*Bernstein v Pamson Motors (Golders Green) Ltd* [1987] 2 All ER 220).

The Protection from Harassment Act 1997 (PHA) provides for an award for any anxiety caused by what is now the tort of harassment.

It is arguable that when it comes to ordinary feelings, hurt or upset or 'mere mental or emotional distress', the courts should not turn to experts in psychiatry. Arguably these are matters within the experience of judges (and juries) or, if an expert is needed, it should be a psychologist who is an expert on normal human behaviour. However, these are cases in which expert psychiatric evidence may be necessary if only to make the distinction between mere mental or emotional distress and actual psychiatric illness.

Limitation issues

There is a three-year limitation period in most personal injury actions. In historic child abuse cases, where the personal injuries have resulted from deliberate conduct, and where there has been no systematic negligence by the defendants, it is a six-year non-extendable period. The limitation period is the period during which the claim must be brought. It begins in theory when the cause of action, that is, the accident or allegedly negligent treatment, occurs. Section 33 of the Limitation Act 1980 provides the court with a discretion to allow a case to proceed 'out of time'.

In cases such as those of historic child abuse and medical negligence the limitation period begins when the claimant has the relevant 'knowledge'. First, this is knowledge that the injury was significant, which means that a reasonable person with the claimant's knowledge would have considered the injury sufficiently serious to justify suing a defendant who did not deny liability and had the means to pay. This is an objective test for which the impact of the claimant's injuries on the ability to issue proceedings is not a relevant consideration (*A v Hoare* [2008] UKHL 6). Second, this is knowledge that the injury is attributable in whole or part to the act or omission which constitutes the alleged negligence or breach of duty; the meaning of 'attributable' comes from *Spargo v North Essex Health Authority* [1997] MLC 0651, where Brooke LJ said that it meant 'capable of being attributed to' or 'a real possibility'. Third, it is knowledge of the identity of the defendant.

This leads to questions as to when claimants acquired actual knowledge and whether or not they had constructive knowledge (defined below) at an earlier date. In a case of alleged negligence, a potential claimant may not acquire actual knowledge until the solicitors receive a report from a medical specialist who is able to attribute significant physical or mental injuries to a specific breach of duty. In a case of alleged historic child abuse, the potential claimant may not acquire actual knowledge until the solicitors have a report from a psychiatrist or a psychologist that attributes significant psychiatric damage to the alleged abuse.

What constitutes 'actual knowledge' will depend, in part, on the 'particular patient', as was established in *Nash v Eli Lilly & Co* [1993] 1 WLR 782, CA:

Whether or not a state of mind for these purposes is properly to be treated by the court as knowledge seems to us to depend, in the first place, upon the nature of the information which the claimant has received, the extent to which he pays attention to the information as affecting him, and his capacity to understand it. There is a second stage at which the information, when received and understood, is evaluated. It may be rejected as unbelievable. It may be regarded as unreliable or uncertain. The court must assess the intelligence of the claimant; consider and assess his assertions as to how he regarded such information as he had; and determine whether he had knowledge of the facts by reason of his understanding of the information.

These considerations are most likely to arise in people with intellectual disabilities and in people with personality abnormalities or a disorder that may have resulted from child abuse.

'Constructive knowledge' refers to the circumstance in which a claimant would have had 'actual knowledge' if he or she had asked the right questions or sought the right advice earlier. Section 14(3) of the Limitation Act 1980 refers to 'knowledge which he might reasonably have been expected to acquire – ... from facts observable or ascertainable by him'. It includes 'facts ascertainable with the help of medical or other appropriate expert advice which it is reasonable for him to seek'. Although the words 'reasonably' and 'reasonable' represent an objective test, as with 'actual knowledge', the personal or individual characteristics of the claimant can be taken into account, so again psychiatric evidence may be needed as to their nature and potential effects. What amount to relevant characteristics can be problematic. In *Adams v Bracknell Forest Borough Council* [2004] UKHL 29 an intelligent man with severe dyslexia had not sought any advice about his literary difficulties because he did not want to talk about them. However, even though he had a social phobia, which arguably could have accounted for, or been connected with, his shyness and embarrassment, Lord Scott, on the basis that others with a similar dyslexia would not be inhibited by shyness or embarrassment from asking the right questions or seeking expert help, ruled that his shyness and embarrassment should be disregarded. Baroness Hale agreed that such characteristics were not relevant as they were strictly personal characteristics.

This case went all the way to the House of Lords and there are likely to be further cases that require judicial decisions on the eligibility of characteristics. Therefore in such a case the psychiatrist should do the following. Ensure that characteristics are specified with clarity. Refer to the evidence for their existence. Make it clear whether or not the characteristics are a feature of a recognised mental disorder, thus allowing a distinction to be made between, for example, shyness as an ordinary personality characteristic and shyness which is a feature of Asperger syndrome. Explain how the characteristic affects such processes as the ability to pay attention to personally relevant information, the capacity to understand the information, the ability to evaluate the information and the ability to make reasonable enquiries. You may not have any better idea as to whether or not the court is going to take into account the characteristics, but you will make the lawyers' jobs easier and be better able to understand the decision reached.

In certain cases, such as cases of historic child abuse where, for example, the claimant has sought and received treatment of a psychological or psychotherapeutic nature that has involved making a connection between early life experiences and difficulties in adult life, the psychiatric expert may need to assist in the interpretation of records that may shed light on when the claimant became aware of a psychiatric injury attributable in whole or in part to the abuse or when they should have asked their therapist or another suitable person whether or not they had suffered psychiatric damage as a result of the abuse. Where the claimant has suffered a multitude of adverse events and circumstances and where the therapy is not for what has been diagnosed at the outset as a specific psychiatric disorder, it cannot be assumed that seeking therapy in itself is proof of 'actual knowledge' or receipt of therapy that 'makes the links' is proof of 'constructive knowledge'.

The limitation period does not begin to run if the potential claimant is under a 'disability'. Section 28(1) of the Limitation Act 1980 provides that 'if the person was under a disability, the action may be brought before the expiration of three years from the date when he ceased to be under a disability or died, whichever first occurred, notwithstanding that the limitation period has expired'. Section 38(2) defines 'disability': 'a person shall be treated as under a disability while he is an infant or of unsound mind' and s.38(3) defines someone of 'unsound mind': 'a person who by reason of mental disorder ... is incapable of managing and administering his property and affairs'. For the purposes of s.38(2), for 'of unsound mind' is to be substituted 'lacks capacity (within the meaning of the Mental Capacity Act 2005) to conduct legal proceedings'.

There is also provision under s.33 of the Limitation Act 1980 for the court to exercise discretion and allow a case to be brought that would otherwise be barred by statute. This is the fall-back position for claimants in historic child abuse cases who fail the objective test as to their date of knowledge because the impact of their injuries on their ability to issue proceedings is regarded as a relevant consideration for the court in deciding whether to exercise discretion under s.33.

Therefore a psychiatric report that addresses limitation issues should have regard to some of the circumstances to which the court is particularly directed. The statute includes: factors which have influenced the claimant's decision to come forward at the stage at which he or she did so and the corollary, which is reasons for delay on the part of the claimant; the duration of any disability of the claimant arising after the date of accrual of the cause of the action; the extent to which the claimant acted promptly and reasonably once he or she knew whether or not the act or omission of the defendant, to which the injury was attributable, might amount to a cause of action; the steps, if any, taken by the claimant to obtain medical advice and the nature of such advice as may have been received; and the effect of the claimant's psychiatric injuries on the ability to issue proceedings. Case law has also established the potential relevance of an impairment of health that falls short of a 'disability' (*Davis v Jacobs and Camden and Islington Health Authority* [1999] Lloyd's Rep Med 72, CA). Where psychiatric evidence has a bearing on any of these, this should be made clear. The psychiatric expert does not have to decide, or give an opinion on, the exact date of knowledge.

Employment stress

The case of *Walker v Northumberland County Council* [1995] IRLR 35 established that an employer could be held liable in damages for psychiatric injury caused by employment stress. When four employers appealed against findings of liability for psychiatric illness caused by stress at work, the Court of Appeal had the opportunity to set out clear guidance for the lower courts in such cases (*Hatton v Sutherland* [2002] ICR 613). The effect of *Hatton* was to limit the employer's liability for causing psychiatric harm, thus making it difficult for employees wishing to bring employment stress cases against their employers. The pendulum has now swung back. In *Dickins v O2* [2008]

EWCA Civ 1144, the court widened the boundaries, making it easier for employees to bring employment stress claims and with the prospect of being awarded damages for the whole of their psychiatric injury and not just for the proportion attributable to the employer's breach of duty.

Box 34 sets out the issues that usually have to be addressed in employment stress cases based on the relevant guidelines of Hale LJ in *Hatton* and as modified by *Dickins*. The following points should be noted. The test is the same whatever the nature of the employment, as no occupations should be regarded as intrinsically dangerous to mental health. It is necessary to take into account the nature and the extent of the work done by the employee, for example whether the workload is more than is normal for that particular job, whether the work is particularly intellectually or emotionally demanding, and whether demands are being made of the employee that are unreasonable compared with the demands made of others in the same or comparable jobs. These, however, may be matters about which the parties disagree and the court may have to decide. Until *Dickins*, the psychiatrist had to make a thorough analysis of the various factors (employment-related and non-employment-related) that contributed to the psychiatric injury because under *Hatton* employers were liable only for the proportion of the harm

---

Box 34 Likely issues in an employment stress case

Guidelines on the issues that usually have to be addressed in employment stress cases were given by Hale LJ in *Hatton v Sutherland* [2002] ICR 613, subsequently modified by *Dickins v O2* [2008] EWCA Civ 1144:

- Has the claimant suffered an injury to health (as distinct from occupational stress)?
- Is the psychiatric injury attributable to stress at work?
- If there are other causes for the employee's psychiatric injury, can it be obviously inferred that the employer's breach(es) of duty made more than a minimal contribution to the psychiatric injury?
- Is there evidence that the employer knew of some particular problem or vulnerability such that they were not entitled to assume that the employee could withstand the normal pressures of the job?
- Is the workload much more than is normal for the particular job?
- Is the work particularly intellectually or emotionally demanding for the employee?
- Are the demands being made of the employee unreasonable when compared with the demands made of others in the same or comparable jobs?
- Has the employee already suffered from illness attributable to stress at work?
- Have there recently been frequent or prolonged absences which are un-characteristic of the employee, or something such as a request for a sabbatical, and, if so, is there reason to think that these are attributable to stress at work, for example because of complaints or warnings from the employee to others?
- Having regard to any pre-existing disorder or vulnerability, would the employee have succumbed to a stress-related disorder in any event?

attributable to their wrongdoing, but now it has to be proved only that the employer's breach of duty made a minimal contribution to the employee's injury, and nonetheless the employer will be responsible for the whole injury. An aetiological formulation will be necessary but the psychiatrist will avoid difficult questions of apportionment of causes on a fractional or percentage basis.

At common law, in contrast to the position under the PHA and the Equality Act 2010 (see p. 187), the claimant must prove that the defendant reasonably foresaw psychiatric damage (*Hatton*) and where reasonable foreseeability is required the psychiatric expert may have to address the issues of vulnerability or predisposition to psychiatric injury. If employers knew or ought to have known of an employee's vulnerability to stress, they owe a greater duty of care to the employee (*Walker*), but if they were not made aware of it, they are entitled to assume that the employee can cope with the normal stresses and strains of working life.

It should be noted with regard to foreseeability that an employer cannot be said to have been in a position to foresee psychiatric injury where an employee had disclosed information about a mental condition in confidence to the occupational health department, as no other employee has a right of access to that information without the employee's consent (*Hartman v South Essex Mental Health and Community Care NHS Trust* [2005] ICR 782).

Exaggeration and malingering

In view of the high rates of fraudulent claims (see for example *Guardian*, 2009), particularly in road traffic accident cases, it is necessary to give some careful consideration to issues of exaggeration and malingering when assessing claimants in personal injury actions. These issues are often ignored completely.

However, psychiatrists and psychologists are extremely poor at detecting deception (Hickling *et al*, 2002). Practitioners underestimate the knowledge, preparation and skills of some malingerers (Faust, 1995) and the ability to detect malingering is unrelated to experience and qualifications (Faust *et al*, 1988). Some lawyers have been known to advise their clients about the symptoms of post-traumatic stress disorder.

So far as the law is concerned, the credibility of the claimant, indeed any witness, is a matter for the court to decide. If it is going to be the defendant's case that a claimant is fabricating or exaggerating, the claimant's solicitors have to be put on notice that this is an issue. The courts do not allow it to be raised only at the trial.

So far as medicine is concerned, it is important to realise that 'malingering' is not a diagnosis or mental disorder as such. It is listed in DSM-IV-TR™ not as a diagnosis but as an additional condition that may be a focus of clinical attention. Furthermore, I agree with Dr Ian Bronks (who has kindly commented on this section for me) that the suggestion that malingering should be strongly suspected if any combination of the four circumstances set out in DSM-IV-TR™ is present goes too far, is badly thought out and is poorly worded. The notion that malingerers are likely to have antisocial personality disorder is outdated and flies in the face of the obvious facts.

Psychiatrists have no special skills that enable them to tell whether or not someone is genuine and there is no reason to suppose that psychiatric consultation is an effective means of detecting malingering, exaggeration or misrepresentation. So it is wise to avoid describing the claimant in the mental state examination as appearing genuine or commenting that she or he did not seem to be exaggerating. To state, as some experts do, that the claimant has endorsed symptoms and psychological problems in a manner which is highly consistent with individuals honestly reporting their difficulties may be no more than testimony to the claimant's skills in deception.

Never underestimate the acting ability of people in any walk of life. It is just that not all of them have gone to Hollywood or won Oscars or even been the backbone of the amateur dramatic society. Sooner or later in the medico-legal field you will be provided with conclusive evidence that what may have appeared to be a genuine case is nothing of the sort, where perhaps incontrovertible covert surveillance evidence identifies as a malingerer a claimant described by other medical experts as genuine.

The particular expertise of the psychiatrist is to help the court decide whether or not a psychiatric disorder is manufactured or exaggerated. The psychiatrist's task is more difficult than that of other experts as, in the case of psychiatric disorders encountered in personal injury litigation, most depend for their diagnosis entirely or mainly on reported symptoms rather than objective signs. There are no objective tests that can be used to diagnose a psychiatric condition or measure its severity. Psychiatrists, however, do have expert knowledge and experience of the natural history of psychiatric disorders, in particular the evolution, onset and course of symptoms, the typical and atypical presentations of particular conditions, patterns of symptoms and comorbidity, the relationship between symptoms and signs and the usual impact of disorders on personal, social and occupational functioning.

In his reports, Dr Ian Bronks refers to the need to have regard to evidence in four areas. First, consider whether the symptoms of which complaint is made are inherently improbable. Second, look for discrepancies between the statements made by the claimant and the facts or probable facts as revealed by other evidence. Third, look for discrepancies between statements made by the claimant at different times about the condition. Fourth, consider the claimant's demeanour on interview. He points out that this last area is probably the least important.

Similar, and to some extent overlapping, points are made by Rogers (2008), who identifies six empirical indicators that would typify a dissimulated (that is, exaggerated or fabricated) presentation of a claimant. (1) Claimants attempting to dissimulate exhibit a tendency to endorse more blatant than subtle symptoms. (2) Similarly, they tend to endorse an unlikely number of symptoms with extreme and unbearable severity. (3) They often have difficulty distinguishing symptoms that are infrequent in psychiatric populations from those that are more common and they often endorse many rare symptoms. (4) They are often unaware of the incongruities between their actual presentation and reported impairment. This is similar to the point in DSM-IV-TR™ about a 'Marked discrepancy between the person's claimed stress or disability and the objective findings'. (5) They often manifest an eagerness to discuss, and elaborate upon, symptoms or an obvious response set. (6) They often have difficulty remembering symptoms they previously endorsed and their severity, so repeating a set of clinical enquiries, even in the course of a single consultation, measures the stability of the response set.

Other suggested indicators are lack of cooperation with assessment, particularly if there is a significant difference between how claimants cooperate with their own and the defendant's experts, failure to accept treatment offered and failure to comply with treatment recommended or prescribed. However, the vast majority of those who exaggerate or misrepresent their psychiatric condition are, in every other respect, respectable, law-abiding members of the community with no indication of personality disorder, and they are just as pleasant and cooperative with assessment and treatment as others. Furthermore, allowance has to be made for the attitude of an expert, which can persuade a claimant to be awkward, and also for the effects of brain damage.

Reliance on the demeanour of the claimant can be problematic in other respects. Some experts rely on the following: hostility from the claimant; refusal to answer simple questions; responses in history-taking that are defensive or unelaborated; frequent 'don't know' answers; disparaging remarks; and a refusal to attempt certain tests. However, there is no evidence to justify reliance on these.

Malingerers' responses are sometimes defensive or unelaborated, particularly if they are not sure of the 'correct' reply for the impression they are trying to make. A hostile claimant is not necessarily exaggerating or malingering; the litigation process and particularly some experts instructed by defendants can make claimants hostile, but this is infrequent, even in cases in which the claimant subsequently complains that the expert was hostile. Some claimants may be unable to answer simple questions, at least in the circumstances of a medico-legal consultation. Test conditions, or the claimant's mental state at the time of testing, may lead to more frequent 'don't know' answers, or a refusal to attempt certain tests, than in more optimal test conditions. Again, the litigation process or the expert's attitude, rather than exaggeration or malingering, may be the explanation for defensiveness or disparaging remarks. An expert instructed by the defendants should be mindful of the fact that the non-verbal behaviour associated with a prejudged opinion of disbelief can induce in a claimant hostility, defensiveness and lack of cooperation.

There may be evidence from other experts that assists, in particular from psychologists. Psychological testing may include symptom validity tests, tests with internal symptom validity indicators and tests of effort and malingering. It is important to recognise, however, that performance on some of these tests can be adversely influenced by such factors as genuine memory impairment, dementia, education, IQ and age. Psychological expertise is necessary to interpret such test results and it is important that the psychiatrist does not 'cherry-pick' from the results of psychological testing and give an opinion as to exaggeration or malingering that is not made by the expert psychologist. Leave to the psychologists the tests which only they are qualified to administer, score and interpret. It is quite appropriate, however, to refer to the opinions of other experts as being consistent, if they are, with your own psychiatric opinion on the evidence as to fabrication and exaggeration.

It is important to conclude any opinion as to fabrication or exaggeration by pointing to the subjectivity and fallibility of such an opinion and with an acknowledgment, if fabrication or exaggeration is identified, that this will be an ultimate issue for the parties or the court and the role of the expert is to analyse and form an opinion so as to assist the parties or the court.

What you cannot do is to ignore the issue or side-step it, as many orthopaedic surgeons do, by stating baldly that it is a matter for the court. Ultimately all facts, inferences and opinions are a matter for the court. However, some of these require expert assistance.

Further reading

G v Central & North West London Mental Health NHS Trust [2007] EWHC 3086 (QB).
Blom-Cooper, L. (ed.) (2006) *Experts in the Civil Courts.* Oxford University Press.
Bryant, G. (2003) Assessing individuals for compensation. In *Handbook of Psychology in Legal Contexts* (2nd edn) (ed. D. Carson & R. Bull), pp. 89–107. Wiley.
Handford, P. (2006) *Mullany & Handford's Tort Liability for Psychiatric Damage* (2nd edn). Lawbook Co.
Lewis, C. J. (2006) *Clinical Negligence* (6th edn). Tottel.
Powers, M. J., Harris, N. H. & Barton, A. (2008) *Clinical Negligence* (4th edn). Tottel.

CHAPTER 7

Reports for family proceedings relating to children

[I]f your work is conscientiously undertaken, your report and oral evidence honest, fair and well-reasoned, and provided that you have worked within the area of your expertise, you have nothing to fear, and much to gain from participating in family proceedings as an expert witness. (Wall, 2007, p. 1)

The nature of family proceedings

Family proceedings principally relate to children. They comprise: (1) care, placement and adoption proceedings ('public law proceedings') and (2) family proceedings held in private which (a) relate to the inherent jurisdiction of the High Court with respect to children, (b) are brought under the Children Act 1989 in any family court, or (3) are brought in the High Court and county courts and 'otherwise relate wholly or mainly to the maintenance or upbringing of a minor' ('private law proceedings').

Public law proceedings

Public law proceedings, sometimes also known as care proceedings, usually involve an application by a local authority to take a child (or children) temporarily or permanently into its care. In order to do so, two threshold conditions have to be met. The court has to be satisfied that the child was suffering, or was likely to suffer, 'significant harm' at the hands of the parent(s). If so satisfied, it has to be better for the child for the court to make an order than to make no order, and it has to be in the child's best interests.

Private law proceedings

Private law proceedings are mainly concerned with disputes between separated parents about their children, such as with whom they should live or contact arrangements. Usually there is no local, or other public, authority involvement. In such cases the Children and Family Court Advisory and

Support Service (CAFCASS) may be invited to provide evidence. The inherent jurisdiction of the Family Division of the High Court is a power to override the parents so as to safeguard children who are incapable of caring for themselves. Most often this occurs when the parents and child are in disagreement as to whether or not the child should have some particular medical treatment.

As some of these proceedings take place in public, in response to a preliminary enquiry about being instructed experts should make any representations they wish to be made to the court about being named or otherwise identified in any public judgment given by the court.

The role of the expert

Expert evidence in such cases is often integral to the safeguarding of children. In these cases, the courts rely heavily upon the objectivity, professional competence and integrity of experts. The courts expect careful and balanced opinions. Clinical judgment has to be soundly based and objectively justified.

Eligible experts

Opinion may be sought from perinatal psychiatrists, child and adolescent psychiatrists, forensic psychiatrists and general adult psychiatrists. Often their opinions are sought along with the opinions of other related professionals, such as psychologists, psychotherapists and social workers. Some professionals in the field work as teams and reports are commissioned from a team rather than an individual expert. This work can be difficult, time consuming, intellectually gruelling and emotionally demanding.

The duties of the expert

The overriding duty of an expert in family proceedings is similar to that in other legal fora: it is to the court and this takes precedence over any obligation to the person from whom the expert has received instructions or by whom the expert is paid. It is also important to bear in mind that in cases under the Children Act 1989, if not in all family proceedings, the interests of the child or children are paramount. It is for this reason that in family proceedings parents cannot tell you anything 'off the record'. They need to be aware that any information that you regard as relevant to interests of the child will be shared with the other parties, at least through the report, and may be given as evidence in court. If, in the course of the assessment, you learn something which, in your opinion, should be disclosed as a matter of urgency to the police or any child protection agency, rather than only putting it in the report, the confidentiality of the proceedings does not preclude such action, but it is advisable to discuss this with instructing or lead solicitors, and if they disagree with your course of action it is advisable to seek the advice of your MDO.

Several of the duties of the expert are similar, or identical, to their duties in other fora. The following are particular duties laid upon experts in family cases that are also applicable in other legal fora. The expert has a duty to provide advice to the court that conforms to the best practice of the expert's profession. If it is recommended that a second opinion be sought on a key issue (a rare occurrence), the expert's duty includes advising, if possible, what questions should be put to the second expert. It is the expert's duty, in expressing an opinion, to take into consideration all of the material facts, including any relevant factors arising from ethnic, cultural, religious or linguistic contexts at the time the opinion is expressed, identifying not only the facts upon which the opinion is based but also any literature, research or other material upon which reliance is placed. There is a particular requirement to identify materials that have not been supplied to the expert or which are not medical or other professional records, as they may raise issues as to standard of proof, admissibility of hearsay evidence or other important legal issues. Requests to third parties for information and their responses should be identified. When advancing a proposition, a distinction is to be made between a hypothesis, in particular if controversial, and an opinion deduced in accordance with peer-reviewed and peer-tested technique, research and experience accepted as a consensus in the scientific community.

Adversarial or non-adversarial?

Family proceedings are regarded as non-adversarial, and therefore more inquisitorial, insofar as the court is concerned not with deciding which side wins but in deciding what is best, or what is the least unacceptable outcome, for the child. However, it may still feel adversarial for the expert because one or more parties may seek, through questions put following disclosure of the expert report or through cross-examination at the hearing, to undermine the expert's opinion in the interests of the party they represent. If you feel that pressure is being put on you by the solicitors acting for one of the parties, either by restricting your investigations or as to your opinion, this should be resisted and a careful note made. For example, experts may be asked to assess parents who are recently separated and when the expert says that it will be necessary to interview the parents together, a solicitor may refuse.

Court control

In family proceedings, the court must give permission for the instruction of an expert, the court decides what documents can be disclosed to the expert, the court alone has the power to authorise any examination of a child, and if an assessment has taken place without the court's permission, the court decides whether or not evidence arising out of such an assessment can be adduced. The court may order that there is only one psychiatric examination of the child.

Instructions

Instructions will usually come from the solicitor instructed by the children's guardian in a public law case or on a joint basis by each of the parties in a private law case. If you receive instructions as a party expert, you can invite the instructing solicitors to consider whether joint instruction would be feasible.

Instructions to an SJE must be through a jointly agreed letter. A party cannot independently instruct the SJE unless the court so directs. If the parties cannot agree the instructions, they have to write to the court, which will then compile the instructions.

In keeping with the less adversarial proceedings, all instructions to experts are disclosable. They are not legally privileged.

Official guidance

The use of expert evidence in family proceedings is now governed by the Family Procedure Rules 2010 (SI 2010/2955) (FPR). This is due to be accompanied by a Practice Direction and it is worth noting that the previous Practice Direction also applied to expert reports commissioned before the commencement of proceedings, because the expert might in due course be reporting to the court.

Experts in family proceedings should be more in the picture about the proceedings than in some other courts because, where an order or direction requires experts to do something, or otherwise affects experts, they have to be served with a copy of the order.

Discussions

If, in addition to your assessment of the child or parent, you discuss the case with any of the solicitors, professionals or other experts, there should be a record of the discussion:

What the court is anxious to prevent is any *unrecorded* informal discussions between particular experts which are either influential in, or determinative of, their views and to which the parties to the proceedings (including perhaps other experts) do not have access. This also applies to any documentary evidence to which you have access. (Wall, 2007, pp. 45–46)

If your discussion is with a professional or another expert, make your own record and decide who will produce an agreed note of the discussion. If your discussion is with a solicitor, he or she will make an 'attendance note' but you must still make your own note. Ask the solicitor to send you a copy and if you disagree with it, write to the solicitor and keep a copy of your letter. Such notes and records have the potential to become the subject of examination or cross-examination in court and if not volunteered at the time on account of their importance, they must be disclosed if so requested.

The court's timetable

The introduction to the guidance on the content of the report (para. 3.3 in the Practice Direction *Experts in Family Proceedings Relating to Children*) emphasises that the report should be prepared and filed in accordance with the court's timetable. Of course, this is important in any legal forum – justice delayed is justice denied – but the more so in cases involving children, as the court's timetable has to have regard to the speed of childhood development and the potential impact of the court's decisions at different stages of the child's development. This urgency is reflected in the very short period of time during which, following service of the expert's report, the parties can put questions to the expert.

Compliance and truth

The report has to include the statement 'I [the expert] understand and have complied with my duty to the court'. It should end with the statement of truth:

I confirm that insofar as the facts stated in my report are within my own knowledge I have made clear which they are and I believe them to be true, and that the opinions I have expressed represent my true and complete professional opinion.

Issues in family proceedings

Experts in family proceedings may be asked to address one or more of the following issues. There may be an issue as to whether or not an adult party, or intended party, to the proceedings lacks capacity, within the meaning of the MCA, to 'conduct' the proceedings (that is, to instruct the solicitor and so on). An adult who lacks capacity is a 'protected party' and must have a representative such as a 'litigation friend', 'next friend' or guardian. There may be a related issue as to whether or not a protected party who is competent to give evidence should give evidence, having regard to both their 'best interests' and the implementation of any 'special measures' to assist them.

Similarly, in the case of a child who is nearing 18 years of age and who is a party to the proceedings, but not subject to them, there may be an issue as to capacity to conduct the proceedings.

The court may require an assessment of a child or children in terms of health, development and functioning (Box 35). Where there are problems or difficulties, the court needs to know their aetiology and their prognosis, the latter having regard to whether or not their problems or difficulties are addressed. The short-term and long-term needs of the child or children have to be considered with regard to the nature of caregiving, education and treatment.

Parents (or primary caregivers) may need to be assessed (Box 36). Such assessment can include: factors and mechanisms that would explain any harmful or neglectful interactions with the child or children; interventions that have been tried and the results thereof; the ability of the adult to meet the child or children's needs; what other assessments are indicated (e.g. adult mental health assessment, forensic assessment, cognitive assessment); whether or not interventions, such as parenting work, support, family therapy, are needed; how these interventions would relate to the time-scales for the child/children; the likelihood of such interventions resulting in change; how alternatively the child/children's needs can be met. These are all matters that should usually be addressed by a perinatal or child or adolescent psychiatrist or should be so addressed in tandem with a consultant in adult mental health.

A consultant in adult mental health may be specifically instructed to address issues of mental illness, personality disorder and substance misuse in parents or other caregivers. When addressing the issue of treatment, response to treatment and timescales, it is important to bear in mind that therapeutic optimism, if not justified, can lead to a child or children staying longer with a parent who has a mental illness, or personality disorder or substance misuse and suffering more harm before the court decides that their interests are best met by removing them from the care of the parent. It is such therapeutic optimism that has probably resulted in the caution urged upon the courts 'in receiving supportive testimony from adult psychiatrists called on behalf of patients, who may be unused to the child-focused, as opposed to patient-focused, approach of the court' (Hershman et al, 1991, p. C-314).

In family cases, experts should expect to receive, in their letter of instruction, a synoptic view of the proceedings, the background to them and a set of specific questions that are within the ambit of their expertise, do not contain unnecessary or irrelevant detail, are kept to a manageable number and are clear, focused and direct. The letter should identify any other expert instructed and other relevant people such as a treating clinician. You have a right to talk to these people provided that you keep an accurate record and indicate in your report that such discussion has taken place.

Box 35 Questions in letters of instruction to a child mental health professional or paediatrician in Children Act 1989 proceedings

A. The child(ren)

1. Please describe the child(ren)'s current health, development and functioning (according to your area of expertise), and identify the nature of any significant changes which have occurred

- Behavioural
- Emotional
- Attachment organisation
- Social/peer/sibling relationships
- Cognitive/educational
- Physical
  - Growth, eating, sleep
  - Non-organic physical problems (including wetting and soiling)
  - Injuries
  - Paediatric conditions

2. Please comment on the likely explanation for/aetiology of the child(ren)'s problems/difficulties/injuries

- History/experiences (including intrauterine influences, and abuse and neglect)
- Genetic/innate/developmental difficulties
- Paediatric/psychiatric disorders

3. Please provide a prognosis and risk if difficulties not addressed above.

4. Please describe the child(ren)'s needs in the light of the above

- Nature of caregiving
- Education
- Treatment – in the short and long term (subject, where appropriate, to further assessment later).

Box continues opposite

The documentation that accompanies the letter should be indexed and paginated. If you receive an unsorted bundle of papers, you can send them back to your instructing solicitors and direct their attention to *Re CS (Expert Witness)* [1996] 2 FLR 115. With very few exceptions, unless the court gives permission, the documents cannot be disclosed to third parties. This does not preclude the expert from using them in discussions with other experts or professionals in the case. Nor does it preclude the expert from making them available to an expert who is peer-reviewing the expert's report or evidence.

If there is an issue upon which you have not been asked for an opinion, but which you consider relevant, you have two options: you can go back to

Box 35 *continued*

B. The parents/primary caregivers

5. Please describe the factors and mechanisms which would explain the parents' (or primary caregivers') harmful or neglectful interactions with the child(ren) (if relevant)

6. What interventions have been tried and what has been the result?

7. Please assess the ability of the parents or primary caregivers to fulfil the child(ren)'s identified needs now.

8. What other assessments of the parents or primary caregivers are indicated?

- Adult mental health assessment
- Forensic risk assessment
- Physical assessment
- Cognitive assessment

9. What, if anything, is needed to assist the parents or primary caregivers now, within the child(ren)'s timescales and what is the prognosis for change?

- Parenting work
- Support
- Treatment/therapy

C. Alternatives

10. Please consider the alternative possibilities for the fulfilment of the child(ren)'s needs.

- What sort of placement?
- Contact arrangements

Please consider the advantages, disadvantages and implications of each for the child(ren).

your instructing solicitors and seek their advice; or you can express your opinion. What you must avoid is wasting time and money on issues that are not relevant. However, some letters of instruction allow for an opinion on 'any other issue which you feel to be relevant'.

Documents seen

The information that you have taken into account in the preparation of your report is of critical importance in the court's understanding of your

---

Box 36 Questions in letters of instruction to adult psychiatrists and applied psychologists in Children Act 1989 proceedings

- Does the parent/adult have – whether in his/her history or presentation – a mental illness/disorder (including substance misuse) or other psychological/emotional difficulty and if so, what is the diagnosis?
- How do any/all of the above (and their current treatment if applicable) affect his/her functioning, including interpersonal relationships?
- If the answer to Q1 is 'yes', are there any features of either the mental illness or psychological/emotional difficulty or personality disorder which could be associated with risk to others, based on the available evidence base (whether published studies or evidence from clinical experience)?
- What are the experiences/antecedents/aetiology which would explain his/her difficulties, if any, (taking into account any available evidence base or other clinical experience)?
- What treatment is indicated, what is its nature and the likely duration?
- What is his/her capacity to engage in/partake of the treatment/therapy?
- Are you able to indicate the prognosis for, timescales for achieving, and likely durability of, change?
- What other factors might indicate positive change?

It is assumed that this opinion will be based on collateral information as well as interviewing the adult.

---

opinion. Either produce your own list all of the documents you have seen or, where possible, simply reproduce the list of documents as provided upon instruction; the list should appear as an appendix to your report.

The standard of proof

The standard of proof in family proceedings is the civil standard – on a balance of probabilities. Your opinions should be given on this basis. Sometimes it is more appropriate to say that something is *consistent* with a particular set of facts. Bear in mind that the court will decide the facts and, depending what facts the court finds, your conclusion may be weakened. Sometimes it is necessary to give more than one opinion, depending on which set of facts is accepted by the court.

For example, a parent with a history of substance misuse denies having used drugs for some time but there is witness evidence that the parent has recently been using drugs. The parent denies this. The court will decide whether or not the parent has continued to use drugs but it needs alternative opinions to match its alternative findings. Do not say which set of facts you prefer unless you are using your psychiatric expertise to suggest that one version is more likely than the other. It is not enough for you to say that you believe the parent in preference to the witness. The credibility of parties and witnesses is for the judge to decide. If, on psychiatric grounds, you have a view, say, as to the parent's lack credibility you can say so, but you must be thorough and balanced in your reasoning and, even if you think that your argument is compelling, as it ought to be, you should be prepared for the parent's advocate to challenge your opinion in court. Beware of psychometric testing, as the Court of Appeal has made it clear that it has no place where the credibility of an adult witness is an issue (*Re S (Care: Parenting Skills: Personality Tests)* [2004] EWCA Civ 1029; *Re L (Children)* [2006] EWCA Civ 1282).

Delivery of the report

Send your report to your instructing solicitors or, if jointly instructed, to the lead solicitors. They will make copies and distribute them as appropriate. This will happen irrespective of which party has commissioned the report and what your opinion is. Even if your opinion is detrimental to the case of your instructing party, the report will be disclosed to the other parties and to the court.

Questions to the expert

Questions must be put to the expert within ten days of the service of the report on the court by the instructing party. The requirement that questions be put only once, be put within ten days and be just for clarification can be waived *only* by the court or where a Practice Direction permits.

Experts' meetings and discussions

Experts' meetings

Experts' meetings may be directed by the court. Attendance may be by telephone or video-link. These meetings differ from experts' meetings in civil and criminal cases in that the court directs a solicitor or other professional to make arrangements for the meeting and chair the meeting. Generally this is the solicitor for the child or children. They also differ in that they usually involve experts from different disciplines and so there may be a global discussion relating to those questions that concern most or all of the experts. This does not preclude separate discussion between or among experts of the same or related disciplines. A further difference is that the parties do not have to agree in order for the content of the discussion to be referred to at trial and there is no rule that the parties cannot be forced to accept the agreement reached by the experts.

Not less than two business days before the meeting, the expert should receive an agenda; only in exceptional circumstances will questions be added within the two-day period and under no circumstances are extra questions allowed at the meeting. The statement of agreement and disagreement has to be signed, served and filed at court not less than five days after the meeting.

Jointly instructed experts should not attend experts' meetings unless all of the parties have agreed in writing or the court has ordered it, if there is an agreement or direction as to who is to pay the expert's fees and such attendance is proportionate to the case.

Discussions

In public law Children Act proceedings the court can direct a meeting between the local authority and any relevant experts in order to assist the local authority in the formulation of plans and proposals for the child. The court directs the arrangements, nominates the chair and the minuting. However, experts should make their own detailed notes of the meeting.

If the parties' solicitors are present at the meeting, they will be partisan and their questions will seek to advance their client's position. Restrict your answers to the questions on the agenda. This is not a mini-trial. Your answers to their questions will be 'on the record', whether the meeting is in person or by telephone, and subsequently you may be cross-examined on them. This makes it essential that there is a proper record of the meeting.

Going to court

Notwithstanding the speed with which family proceedings ought to take place, experts are expected to have substantial notice of any hearing at which they are expected to give evidence and the date and time should, if possible, be at their convenience. The court will attempt to be accurate about the time and duration of the expert's evidence so as to avoid delay. Arrangements may be made for the evidence to be given by telephone conference or video-link.

In preparation for the hearing, as well as checking that it is going ahead on the date notified and that your evidence is still needed, make sure that you have been kept up to date with any developments in the case and supplied with any further documents that have become available. If you are attending court, make sure that you know what the issues are that you are going to be required to address in your oral evidence.

Outcome

At present, the guidance in the 2008 Practice Direction represents a counsel of perfection, insofar as, within ten days after the final hearing, the solicitor instructing the expert should inform the expert of the outcome of the case and the use made of the expert's opinion. Furthermore, within ten days of receiving the court's written reasons for its decision, the instructing solicitor or lead solicitor should send the expert a copy. Experts, however experienced, ought to find much to learn and much that shapes practice if these two directions are strictly followed.

Further reading

Wall, N. (2007) *A Handbook for Expert Witnesses in Children Act Cases.* Jordan Publishing.

CHAPTER 8

Reports in cases involving capacity

Autonomy entails the freedom and the capacity to make a choice. (Baroness Hale in *R v C (Respondent) (On Appeal from the Court of Appeal (Criminal Division))* [2009] UKHL 42)

The MCA has codified a considerable amount of case law relating to capacity but interpretation of the new statutory law continues to be informed by the earlier case law. The expert who gives evidence as to capacity therefore has to be familiar not only with the statute but also with the case law that paved its way. Common law, as to such matters as the capacity to make a will and to marry, has not been affected.

It is a fact, and not just rumour, that soon after the MCA came into force, a psychiatric hospital created a form for doctors to complete, on admission of all patients, on which they had to indicate whether or not the patient had capacity. Requests to find out for what decision the patient's capacity was being certified were met initially with silent puzzlement and then the response that it did not matter, as the issue was only whether the patient had capacity. Another hospital was still using the same form in October 2010.

Capacity, however, is issue specific and time specific: 'in law capacity depends on time and context ... inevitably a decision as to capacity in one context does not bind a court which has to consider the same issue in a different context' (*Masterman-Lister v Brutton & Co and Jewell & Home Counties Dairies* [2002] EWCA Civ 1889) and 'the Court must focus on the matters which arise for decision now, and on the Claimant's capacity to deal with them now' (*Saulle v Nouvet* [2007] EWHC 2902 (QB)). A person may lack the capacity to make a gift at one time and have the capacity to make the same gift at a later date. A person may have the capacity to marry at 11.30 a.m. (*In the Estate of Park deceased, Park v Park* [1954] P89) but not have the capacity to make a will early in the afternoon of the same day (*In re Park, Culross v Park* (1950) *The Times* 2 December). The test of mental capacity is not monolithic but tailored to the task in hand (*Perrins v Holland and Anor* [2009] EWCA Civ 1398). It is also tailored to the gravity of the decision: a person need only have such capacity as is 'commensurate with the gravity of the decision' (*Re T* [1992] 2 FCR 861).

The statute law

The MCA begins with (1) the principle that people must be assumed to have capacity unless it is established that they lack capacity (s.1(1)); (2) the principle that people are not to be treated as unable to make a decision unless all practicable steps have been made to help them to do so without success (s.1(3)); and (3) the principle that people are not to be treated as unable to make a decision merely because they make an unwise decision. The MCA applies only to persons aged 16 years and over.

Section 2(1) indicates that people lack capacity in relation to a matter if, at the material time, they are unable to make a decision for themselves in relation to the matter because of an impairment of, or disturbance in the functioning of, the mind or brain.

The 'test' for capacity is set out in section 3(1):

A person is unable to make a decision for himself if he is unable:
to understand the information relevant to the decision,
to retain that information,
to use or weigh that information as part of the process of making the decision, or
to communicate his decision (whether by talking, using sign language or any other means).

The court has the power to make 'declarations' as to whether a person has or lacks capacity to make decisions on such matters as are described in the declaration (s.15(1)a). (A declaration is a statement regarding a person's legal status, rights or obligations; it is not enforceable but it is used to clarify an issue such as capacity.) The court has the power to make a decision or decisions on a person's behalf in relation to his or her property and affairs (s.16(2)a) and to appoint a deputy to make decisions on the person's behalf in relation to such matters (s.16(2)b). It appears that the need for a deputy to be appointed to manage the person's property and affairs is likely to arise in the same circumstances that governed the appointment of receivers under Part VII of the MHA.

The powers under s.16 (but detailed in s.18) with respect to a person's property and affairs include: the control and management of the person's property (s.18a);, the sale, exchange, charging, gift or other disposition of the person's property(s.18b), (3) the acquisition of property in the person's name or on the person's behalf (s.18c); the settlement of any of the person's property (s.18h); the conduct of legal proceedings in the person's name or on the person's behalf (s.18k). This largely reproduces the list which applied to the Court of Protection under s.96 of the MHA.

For the purposes of s.38(2) of the Limitation Act 1980, for 'of unsound mind' is to be substituted 'lacks capacity (within the meaning of the Mental Capacity Act 2005) to conduct legal proceedings' (CPR 21.1(2)).

The standard of proof is the balance of probabilities (s.2(4)).

Irresponsibility and vulnerability

The issues that have probably troubled experts the most are 'irresponsibility', in the sense of the risk of the person making rash or irresponsible decisions, and 'vulnerability', in the sense of the person being at risk of exploitation. In *Masterman-Lister*, the trial judge rejected the submission that a finding of incapacity was required 'if the effect of the injury to his brain renders [the plaintiff] vulnerable to exploitation or at the risk of the making of rash or irresponsible decisions' and Chadwick LJ in the Court of Appeal confirmed this, stating that: 'It is not the task of the courts to prevent those who have the mental capacity to make rational decisions from making decisions which others may regard as rash and irresponsible'. In *Lindsay v Wood* [2006] EWHC 2895 (QB) it was acknowledged that medical practitioners understood this to mean that vulnerability to exploitation is irrelevant to questions of capacity and must be ignored when deciding on the issue of capacity. However, the court did not regard this as a correct understanding of the judgment of Chadwick LJ in *Masterman-Lister*: while 'vulnerability to exploitation does not *of itself* lead to the conclusion that there is lack of capacity … [the] issue is … whether the person has the mental capacity to make a rational decision' (emphasis added).

Nor did Chadwick LJ regard it as a correct understanding of what he said about the significance of rash and irresponsible decisions when I made the same point when I was addressing a group of pupil barristers. I did not realise that Chadwick LJ was one of the other speakers and in the audience until he corrected my interpretation of his judgment. Furthermore, other cases have confirmed the relevance of vulnerability. In *Mitchell v Alasia* [2005] EWHC 11 reliance was placed on qualities such as impulsiveness and volatility when deciding whether the claimant was, by reason of mental disorder, incapable of managing and administering property and affairs.

Irresponsibility and vulnerability *are* relevant, so psychiatrists and psychologists should take them into account, but recognise that, on their own, they are not determinative of capacity. The test is about comprehension and decision-making, not about wisdom, and if irresponsibility or vulnerability can be attributed to faulty comprehension and decision-making caused by an impairment of the functioning of the mind or brain, their relevance is obvious.

Capacity issues

It would be impossible to list, let alone consider, all of the decisions about which a capacity issue might arise. Thus, the following is not an exhaustive treatment but includes many of the decisions in relation to which issues of capacity commonly arise. Over the years, I have learned a lot from my instructing solicitors and from the advice of counsel about what decision-making requires for different decisions. This is reflected in the rest of the chapter. If any solicitors or barristers recognise some of what I have written, I hope that they will forgive me for not having kept a record of what I have learned from which cases and which lawyers.

Appointment of an appointee to act in respect of Department for Work and Pensions proceedings

Whether or not a person requires an appointee in Department for Work and Pensions proceedings calls for consideration of their ability:
- to understand the basis of probable entitlement to benefits
- to understand and complete the claim form
- to respond to correspondence relating to social security benefits
- to collect or receive benefits
- to manage the benefits in the sense of knowing what the money is for
- to choose whether to use it for that purpose and if so how.

Making a will

Testamentary capacity has a long history in common law. *Banks v Goodfellow* (1870) LR QB 549 remains the leading case. John Banks was a bachelor in his 50s and he lived with his teenage niece, Margaret Goodfellow. He had paranoid schizophrenia and he believed that a grocer, long since dead, was pursuing and persecuting him. He also believed that he was being chased by evil spirits. In his will, he left his entire estate of 15 properties to his niece. On his death, his testamentary capacity was challenged because, in the meantime, his niece had died and so the properties were passed to her half-brother. It was held that, as there was no connection between his delusions and the disposition of his property, he was not incapable of validly disposing of his property by will:

It is essential ... that a testator shall understand the nature of the act and its effects; shall understand the extent of the property of which he is disposing; shall be able to comprehend and appreciate the claims to which he ought to give effect; and, with a view to the latter object, that no disorder of mind shall poison his affections, pervert his sense of right, or prevent the exercise of his natural faculties – that no insane delusion [sic] shall influence his will in disposing of his property and bring about a disposal of it which, if the mind had been sound, would not have been made.

On the other hand, in *Smee & Others v Smee and the Corporation of Brighton* [1879] LR 5 PD 84, where the testator (wrongly) believed that he was the son of George IV, who had built Brighton Pavilion, and therefore left a reversionary interest in his estate to fund a free library for the people of Brighton, it was held that his delusion had drastically affected his testamentary wishes and his will was pronounced invalid.

In such cases the psychiatric expert should therefore assess the ability of testators to understand the nature of a will, that is, that they will die, the will shall come into operation on their death, but not before, and that they can change or revoke their will at any time subject to having the capacity to do so. Also to be assessed is testators' understanding of the effects of making a will and making choices with regard to: who the executors should be and, perhaps also, why they should be appointed; who gets what under the will; whether a beneficiary's gift is outright or conditional, such as the right to occupy a property only during their lifetime; that if the testator spends the money or gives away or sells properties, the beneficiaries might lose out; a beneficiary might die before the testator; and whether they have already made a will, in which case they need to understand how the new one differs from the old one.

The testator must comprehend broadly the extent of the property (that is, what the will will 'bite' on) and so must the expert. This is not the same as the value of the property, which can change rapidly in unstable economic times, and which can change in the lifetime of the testator. It may be that there is property that is jointly owned and will pass to the joint owner irrespective of anything that is said in the will. There may be benefits payable, such as pension rights, that the will cannot determine. There may be debts and the testator should understand how these are to be paid.

In order to understand the claims to which the testator ought to give effect, the expert also has to be able to identify the testator's family members, along with others who might have a claim on the estate. 'A testator with a complex estate and many potential beneficiaries may need a greater degree of cognitive ability than one with a simple estate and few claimants' (*Parker and another v Felgate and Tilly* (1883) 8 PD 171). The testator should be able to take into account the extent to which possible beneficiaries may already have received adequate provision, be better off financially than others, have been more attentive and caring, or may be in greater need of assistance on account of their particular circumstances. The expert will need to be informed about such matters by the instructing solicitors. However, it is important to bear in mind that there is no requirement that the testator should behave 'in such a manner as to deserve approbation from the prudent, the wise or the good' (*Bird v Luckie* (1850) 8 Hare 301) and indeed this was put on a statutory basis in s.1(4) of the MCA.

Sometimes obvious incapacity supervenes after a will has been made and before it is executed. In *Parker* the testator's condition deteriorated between her giving instructions and the will being signed in her presence and at her direction (its execution). It was held that there were three questions to be answered:

1   When the will was executed, did she remember and understand the instructions she had given to her solicitor?
2   If it had been thought advisable to stimulate her, could she have understood each clause of the will when it was explained to her?

3   Was she capable of understanding, and did she understand, that she was executing a will for which she had previously given instructions to her solicitor?

As these questions have to be answered in sequence and a positive response to any or all of them indicates that the will is valid, it follows that the bottom line is that the testator should understand that she was executing a will for which she had previously given her solicitors instructions. This is an important point in cases in which there was clearly a deterioration in the testator's condition between giving the instructions and signing the will. *Perrins v Holland* established that no more is required than that the testator believes that it gives effect to the instructions. *Clancy v Clancy* [2003] EWHC 1885 Ch is worth reading to see how a modern-day court tests the psychiatric evidence in such a case.

It is important to bear in mind that a testator can still act in an unorthodox way: 'But the law does not say that a man is incapacitated from making a will if he proposes to make a disposition of his property moved by capricious, frivolous or even bad motives' (*Boughton v Knight* [1873] LR 3 PD 64).

The case of *Kostic v Chaplin* [2007] EWHC 2909 is illustrative. Zoran Kostic's father left most of his £8.2 million estate to the Conservative Party. Zoran Kostic's challenge to the two wills made by his father was on the basis that he suffered from an undiagnosed and untreated mental illness which had resulted in a delusional belief that there was a worldwide conspiracy of dark forces and that he was included in the conspiracy. In pronouncing against the wills, the court held that, as a result of his mental illness, Kostic was unable to appreciate his son's claims on the estate. The court also had regard to the fact that, as the experts agreed, it was also possible for the testator 'to hold ordinary conversations with people unaffected by the delusional system and to have ordinary relationships with them without his delusions becoming apparent'.

Likewise in *Ritchie, Ritchie and Others v National Osteoporosis Society and Others* [2009] EWHC 709, where the deceased left nothing to her children on the basis of their maltreatment of her, the court found that these allegations were untrue and, as the medical evidence suggested that she may have omitted her children from her will on account of paranoid delusions, her will was declared invalid.

Also in *Walters v Smee* [2008] EWHC 2029, the court found that the dispositions of the testatrix in her 2004 will, made a month before she died, were motivated largely, if not wholly, by 'misapprehensions' that were the result of her dementia and its effect on her cognitive faculties.

Related to testamentary capacity is the matter of 'undue influence'. *Wingrove v Wingrove* (1885) 11 PD 81 established that, in law, 'undue influence' could be summed up in one word – 'coercion' – and:

The coercion may ... be of different kinds ... [a] person in the last days of life may have become so weak and feeble, that a very little pressure will be sufficient to bring about the desired result.

It will be for the court and not the expert to decide whether undue influence was brought but the expert may be needed to identify the nature and cause of a state which renders the testator vulnerable to coercion and to give an opinion as to the likelihood of the undue influence alleged being sufficient coercion.

Revoking a will

It was established in *Re Sabatini* (1970) 114 SJ 35 that capacity to revoke a will requires:

- understanding the nature of the act of revoking a will
- understanding the effect of revoking a will (including perhaps a greater understanding of the intestacy rules than is necessary for the making of a will)
- understanding the extent of the property
- comprehending and appreciating claims to which the testator ought to give effect.

Capacity to make a lasting power of attorney

Under s.9(1) of the MCA, a lasting power of attorney (LPA) is a power of attorney under which the donor confers on the donee(s) authority to make decisions about all or any of the following: the donor's personal welfare or specified matters concerning his or her personal welfare; and the donor's property and affairs or specified matters concerning their property and affairs, including the authority to make such decisions in circumstances where the donor lacks capacity.

In relation to this particular decision, the donor has to be able to answer the following questions:

- What is a lasting power of attorney?
- Why do they want to make a lasting power of attorney?
- Who are they appointing as attorney(s)?
- Why have they chosen that/those person(s) as attorney(s)?
- What are the nature and scope of the powers being given to the attorney (the attorney will be able to assume complete authority over the donor's property and finances and will be able to do anything with them that the donor could have done)?

Donors will also need to appreciate that their attorney's authority to make decisions will apply as soon as the lasting power of attorney is registered (unless they specify that it should only apply when they lack capacity to make a relevant decision), but they can revoke the lasting power of attorney at any time if they have the capacity to do so. This contrasts with a power of attorney as to welfare, rather than property, where the attorney can make decisions on welfare only if the donor lacks capacity. Also, donors will need to understand the reasonably foreseeable consequences of making or not making the lasting power of attorney or of making one on different terms or appointing different attorneys.

Capacity to make a personal injury trust

Personal injury trusts have an important place in the settlement and resolution of personal injury claims because they ensure that the funds or property are used for the claimant's benefit. They are important where the claimant has no experience of handling a large sum of money. They can protect the claimant from exploitative relatives. They relieve the claimant of the responsibility of financial administration. They allow the claimant to retain means-tested benefits, or, if eligible for them in the future, to qualify for them.

Personal injury trusts are sometimes called special needs trusts. They are but one form of special needs trusts. A special needs trust set up by or for someone who has received a large inheritance can afford them similar benefits.

For claimants to have the capacity to create a personal injury trust, they need to be able to answer the following questions (which the expert should assess):

- What is a personal injury trust?
- Why does the claimant want to create a personal injury trust?
- Whom is the claimant appointing as trustee(s)?
- Why has the claimant chosen that/those person(s) to act as trustee(s)?

Capacity to marry

The issue of capacity to marry is particularly likely to call for evidence from experts in cases involving a person with an intellectual disability. The leading case is that of *Sheffield City Council v E and S* [2004] EWHC 2808 (Fam), where the local authority began proceedings as it had responsibilities for E and it had concerns about her relationship with an older man, S. E was aged 21 years but she was said to function at the level of a 13-year-old. There were concerns that E was at risk of domestic violence and sexual exploitation, as S was aged 37 years and he had a substantial history of sexually violent crimes.

Munby J held that: (1) the question was about the capacity to marry and not, specifically, the capacity to marry a particular person; (2) it was not necessary to show that the person had capacity to take care of their own person and property; (3) the issue of whether it is wise to marry or wise to marry a particular person was not relevant; (4) it was capacity to marry that was at issue and not whether it was in the best interests of the person to marry or to marry a particular person; (5) the test remained that set out in *Park v Park* [1954], which is that the person is mentally capable of appreciating the responsibilities that normally attach to marriage; (6) it is not enough to understand that they are taking part in a marriage ceremony, as there must also be an understanding of the duties and responsibilities that normally attach to marriage.

After quoting and relying upon cases going back 120 or more years, Munby J set out a modern view of marriage, including the duties and responsibilities that ordinarily attach to marriage:

> Today both spouses are the joint, co-equal heads of the family. Each has an obligation to comfort and support the other. It is not for the husband alone to provide the matrimonial home or to decide where the family is to live. Husband and wife both contribute. And where they are to live is, like other domestic matters of common concern, something to be settled by agreement, not determined unilaterally by the husband. Insofar as the concept of consortium – the sharing of a common home and a common domestic life, and the right to enjoy each other's society, comfort and assistance – still has any useful role to play, the rights of husband and wife must surely now be regarded as exactly reciprocal.

> To have the capacity to marry one must be mentally capable of understanding the duties and responsibilities that normally attach to marriage. What then are the duties and responsibilities that in 2004 should be treated as normally attaching to marriage? In my judgment the matter can be summarised as follows: Marriage, whether civil or religious, is a contract, formally entered into. It confers on the parties the status of husband and wife, the essence of the contract being an agreement between a man and a woman to live together, and to love one another as husband and wife, to the exclusion of all others. It creates a relationship of mutual and reciprocal obligations, typically involving the sharing of a common home and a common domestic life and the right to enjoy each other's society, comfort and assistance.

Consent to marriage must include the capacity to consent to sexual intercourse (see below), which is regarded as an ordinary consequence of the celebration of marriage (*KC & NC v City of Westminster Social and Community Services & Another* [2008] EWCA Civ 198).

Notwithstanding a person's capacity to give valid consent to marry, it is a ground for annulment of a marriage, under ss.11–13 of the Matrimonial Causes Act 1973, that, as a result of mental disorder (as defined in the MHA), the party was unfitted to marriage, which means being incapable of living in a married state and being unable to carry out the duties and obligations of marriage. It is not enough that it is difficult to live with the spouse (*Bennett v Bennett* [1969] 1 WLR 430).

Capacity to separate, divorce or dissolve a civil partnership

There have been no reported court decisions in the UK concerning the capacity to separate, divorce or dissolve a civil partnership. The courts are likely, however, to have regard to the Canadian case of *Calvert (Litigation Guardian) v Calvert* (1997) 32 OR (3d) 281, in which the judge ruled:

Separation is the simplest act requiring the lowest level of understanding. A person has to know with whom he or she does or does not want to live. Divorce, while still simple, requires a bit more understanding. It requires the desire to remain separate and to be no longer married to one's spouse. It is the undoing of the contract of marriage. ... If marriage is simple, divorce must be equally simple ... the mental capacity required for divorce is the same as required for entering into a marriage. ... The capacity to instruct counsel involves the ability to understand financial and legal issues. This puts it significantly higher on the competence hierarchy. ... While Mrs Calvert may have lacked the ability to instruct counsel, that did not mean she could not make the basic personal decision to separate and divorce.

Capacity to decide whether to use contraception

In *A Local Authority v Mrs A and Mr A* [2010] EWCA 1549 Fam, the court had to decide whether or not a woman had the capacity to make decisions regarding contraceptive treatment. She had a full-scale IQ of 53. Her husband had a full-scale IQ of 65. Expert evidence was given by obstetricians and gynaecologists and by a learning disability consultant. Bodey J held that the test for capacity should be so applied as to ascertain the woman's ability to understand and weigh up the immediate medical issues surrounding contraceptive treatment, including:

- The reason for contraception and what it does (which includes the likelihood of pregnancy if it is not in use during sexual intercourse);
- The types available and how each is used;
- The advantages and disadvantages of each type;
- The possible side effects of each and how they can be dealt with;
- How easily each type can be changed; and
- The generally accepted effectiveness of each.

Bodey J further held that he did not consider that questions needed to be asked as to the woman's understanding of what bringing up a child would be like in practice, how she would be likely to get on, or whether any child would be likely to be removed from her care.

Capacity to engage in sexual activity

The following factors have been identified as relevant to an individual's capacity to consent to sexual activity (British Medical Association & Law Society, 2010):

- Their understanding of the nature and character of sexual intercourse;
- Their understanding of the reasonably foreseeable consequences of sexual intercourse (including their knowledge, even if at a basic level) of the risks of pregnancy and sexually transmitted diseases;
- The kind of relationship that they have (for example, if there is a power imbalance);

- The pleasure (or otherwise) which they experience in the relationship;
- Their ability to choose or refuse intercourse; and
- Their ability to communicate their choice to their partner.

To these can be added understanding of the need to use contraception to avoid pregnancy and sexually transmitted disease. Although by its nature sexual intercourse will usually be a private activity with one other person, appropriate advice, support and assistance from others on these various matters can 'enable' capacity.

Capacity to consent to sexual activity is also an issue under the Sexual Offences Act 2003. Section 74 states that 'a person consents if he agrees by choice, and has the freedom and capacity to make that choice'. Section 30 applies to people who are 'unable to refuse because of or for a reason related to a mental disorder', where 'mental disorder' is as defined in s.1 of the MHA. The inability may involve either the inability to choose (s.30(1)(a)) or the inability to communicate the choice made (s.30(2)(b)). In such cases it is necessary to consider whether or not the person would have capacity to consent if only minor threats or inducements were made by a person seeking sexual intercourse. In other words, what level of threat or inducement would be so overbearing as to invalidate 'consent'? It may also be necessary for a psychiatric expert to assist the court as to whether or not the defendant knew, or could reasonably be expected to know, that the complainant had a mental disorder and that because of it, or for a reason related to it, was likely to be unable to refuse (s.30(1)(d)).

R v C (Respondent) (On Appeal from the Court of Appeal (Criminal Division)) [2009] UKHL 42 concerned a man who was found guilty of, but successfully appealed against, his conviction for sexual touching (oral intercourse) under s.30 of the Sexual Offences Act 2003. The complainant had a history of schizoaffective disorder, an emotionally unstable personality disorder, an IQ of less than 75 and a history of harmful alcohol use. The Crown successfully appealed to the House of Lords and in her judgment Baroness Hale held that: (1) a lack of capacity to choose can be person or situation specific and (2) an irrational fear that prevents the exercise of choice can be equated with a lack of capacity to choose. She also explained that the words 'for any other reason' in s.30:

are clearly capable of encompassing a wide range of circumstances in which a person's mental disorder may rob them of the ability to make an autonomous choice, even though they have sufficient understanding of the information relevant to making it. These could include the kind of compulsion which drives a person with schizophrenia to believe that she must do something, or the phobia (or irrational fear) which drives a person to refuse a life-saving injection (as in *Re MB*) or a blood transfusion (as in *NHS Trust v T*).

Baroness Hale held that it was not the case that to fall within s.30(2)(b) a complainant must be physically unable to communicate by reason of mental disorder. Relying on the definition of mental disorder in the MHA, she held that in the Sexual Offences Act 2003 Parliament clearly had in mind an inability to communicate that was the result of or associated with a disorder of the mind and there was no warrant at all for limiting it to a physical inability to communicate.

It is important that too high a threshold is not applied in the test for capacity to engage in sexual relations because, if it interferes with the ability of, for example, a person with an intellectual disability to develop relationships with others, this could amount to an interference with the right to respect for private life under Article 8 of the European Convention.

Capacity to litigate

Under CPR 21, people who, by reason of mental disorder within the meaning of the MHA are incapable of managing and administering their affairs, must have a 'litigation friend' to conduct proceedings on his behalf.

The most important relevant judgments in recent years are those in the case of *Masterman-Lister* but the judge at first instance in this case relied considerably on the unreported case of *White v Fell* (Rix, 1999b). This concerned a woman who was seriously injured in a road traffic accident at the age of 18 years but who sought to bring her action against the defendant more than three years later, by which time it was statute barred. There was no dispute that she had suffered significant brain damage, had suffered a fall in intellectual level from 'normal' to 'borderline subnormal' and was substantially less capable of managing her own affairs and property than she would otherwise have been. However, having regard to such evidence as how she had divorced her husband, lived on her own in sheltered accommodation, provided for her dog, arranged to visit a friend by taxi, could find her way about town, managed her benefits and took her oral contraceptive regularly, the judge decided that she had capacity to litigate. This was because: first, she had 'insight and understanding of the fact that she has a problem in respect of which she needs advice'; second, as her involvement in divorce proceedings indicated, having identified the problem, she could seek an appropriate advisor and instruct him with sufficient clarity to enable him to understand and advise appropriately; and third, she had sufficient mental capacity to understand and to make decisions based upon, or otherwise she was able to give effect to, such advice as she might receive.

In *Masterman-Lister*, the judge at first instance approved the approach of the judge in *White v Fell* and he was upheld on appeal. The Court of Appeal confirmed that, in addition to the actual medical evidence, 'that element has to be considered in conjunction with any other evidence that there may be about the manner in which the subject of the inquiry actually has conducted his everyday life and affairs' and with 'capacity at other times and in other contexts'. The Court of Appeal said that the trial judge had been right to regard the whole test as related to the individual plaintiff and her immediate problems. The Court of Appeal approved the test, now on a statutory basis in the Act, as being that the person should 'be able to absorb and retain information (including advice) relevant to the matters in question sufficiently to enable him or her to make decisions based on such information'.

It was also held by the Court of Appeal in *Masterman-Lister* that the focus should be on the capacity or ability of the individual and not the actual outcome. This is known as the 'functional' test and it is to be contrasted with a test based on 'outcomes' or a test based on 'diagnosis'. The defect of the 'diagnosis' test is that it does not follow that because someone has a condition, such as dementia or schizophrenia, they lack the capacity to make some particular decision. Outcomes are, however, relevant, as they 'can often cast a flood light on capacity'. Nevertheless, they are not determinative.

In personal injury litigation, the following matters are relevant to claimants' capacity to litigate (where appropriate, qualified by 'if necessary with suitable help from someone who knows them well'):

- knowing that potentially they have a case and being able to understand the issues in the case
- knowing who the case is against
- understanding evidence as to the nature and severity of the injuries for which compensation is sought
- the ability to seek and act on legal advice in order to investigate and bring the claim
- the ability to give instructions to solicitors
- the ability to make decisions, with appropriate advice, in the course of the proceedings:
  - to authorise proceedings to be issued
  - to approve the disclosure of witness statements and expert evidence
  - to approve an offer to settle
  - to accept a suitable offer to settle made by the defendants
  - to compromise the claim, whether on a percentage basis or in monetary terms
  - to proceed to trial
  - to withdraw the claim if there is evidence that the defendants acted lawfully
- understanding the risks involved in rejecting an offer that the claimant is reasonably advised to accept, that is:
  - withdrawal of Legal Services Commission or insurance funding for the claim
  - being awarded by the court less than an offer that was rejected
  - being ordered to pay the other side's costs from the date the offer was rejected
- understanding the advantages and disadvantages of a lump sum payment or a periodical payment.

Until 1 April 2005, compensation for injury and related financial losses, such as loss of earnings or future financial loss in buying care or assistance, was in the form of a once and only 'lump sum'. This was calculated by estimating the annual loss or expense and then multiplying that figure by the period for which the loss or expense would last, usually actuarially calculated life expectancy. Since then, there have been provisions for periodical payments. Making a choice between periodical payments and a lump sum involves a mixture of practical, financial and legal considerations.

The first advantage of periodical payments is that, as they are guaranteed for life, they more accurately meet claimants' needs by providing for them until they die, regardless of what the estimate was of their life expectancy, whereas a lump sum is based on an estimate of life expectancy, which, if it is a significant underestimate, can leave claimants with insufficient funds for their needs and possibly just when those funds are needed most. The second advantage is that the responsibility for ensuring investment sufficient to make the periodical payments is transferred from the claimant, or trustees, to the insurer. This is a not inconsiderable advantage in the present economic climate. Lump sums that are invested may perform poorly or fail to keep up with inflation. The third advantage of a periodical payment is that it is free of tax. The disadvantage of the periodical payment is that, in order to achieve the annual income, the claimant has to give up a substantial part of the lump sum so that, in effect, the defendant can buy an insurance policy to cover the claimant.

The advantages of the lump sum are that it is final, simple and offers flexibility to claimants, who can decide how to prioritise their various needs and wants (*Thompstone v Thameside and Glossop Acute Services NHS Trust* [2008] EWCA Civ 15). Claimants, or their trustees, have the power to make plans for the whole of the award at the outset. There is also the advantage, for family-minded claimants, that if they die much sooner than had been expected, their family can benefit from the residue of the compensation. Significant problems with the lump sum are that the amount of income generated will depend on the element of risk claimants are prepared to take. Also, although the lump sum itself is not taxed, income and capital gains from the investments are taxable and this may become a more important consideration if tax rates rise.

What is best for the claimant will depend on a number of factors. If the experts disagree about life expectancy, periodical payments may be particularly appropriate. Whether it is a short or long life expectancy can make a difference. If it is long, there is more time for investment of a lump sum to achieve a better than average result; if it is short, it may not be possible to do well by investing a lump sum (Braithwaite & Waldron, 2010). If there is a significant deduction for contributory negligence on the part of the claimant, a lump sum may be more appropriate (Braithwaite & Waldron, 2010). A similar consideration applies if the claim is compromised at less than 100% liability (i.e. at less than 100% of what has been claimed) because the claimant's legal advisors feel that there is a risk that if the case goes to trial the claimant might lose entirely.

177

A settlement meeting can last for several hours. There will usually be several so-called 'heads', or categories, of damage. There will be pros and cons for each. Also, for each, there will be one figure based on the claim, a second figure based on the counter schedule (the defendant's proposed settlement for the head of damage) and counsel's compromise. Each one of these has to be explained in simple enough terms for the claimant to understand. Life expectancy may be disputed. At the end of the meeting, in order to decide whether to accept or reject the offer, the claimant has to remember all of the issues, blend them together, take account of the risks on each, understand what is meant by an offer to settle and make a judgment.

This is not an exhaustive list. Sometimes instructing solicitors point out the particular decisions for which the claimant will need to have capacity. This list relates to a personal injury action. There are other proceedings where people bring or defend a case. Instructing solicitors should provide sufficient information as to the nature and extent of those proceedings for the psychiatrist to assess the person's capacity to bring or defend the case.

Lindsay v Wood is worth reading as an example of how the court approaches capacity to litigate.

Capacity to manage and administer property and affairs

The issue of capacity to manage and administer property and affairs particularly arises in personal injury cases where the claimant receives, or stands to receive, a significant amount of compensation. Experts are often instructed to deal with litigation capacity at the same time as they deal with this aspect of capacity, but in *Masterman-Lister* it was held that someone can lack the capacity to litigate but possess the capacity to manage and administer their compensation and vice versa.

In the context of a personal injury claim, capacity in relation to financial affairs and property is the central issue. In most cases the difficulty is that the amount of compensation awarded will be an amount that most people have never handled and will never handle. Although the assumption is that the person will have appropriate financial, legal and other advice, limited conclusions can be drawn from asking the person what they will do with £500,000. However, it is reasonable to explore the following areas:

- the purpose of compensation
- the distinction between general damages and damages for care, loss of earnings and so on
- an understanding of the nature and purpose of investments
- the ability to seek, understand and act on appropriate advice
- understanding of financial needs and responsibilities, including family and social responsibilities
- the degree of support the person receives or could expect to receive from others.

The claimant must understand that compensation is intended to last for life.

> **Box 37** Examples of transactions or situations to be considered under capacity to manage property and affairs
>
> - Open and close a bank account, including understanding what a bank account is and what the implications are of having a bank account
> - Pay any bills for which responsible, including making payment by standing order or direct debit
> - Work out a monthly budget to pay bills
> - Remember to pay the car insurance, get a new MOT certificate and obtain a new tax disc
> - Choose a holiday, book it, pay the deposit, organise insurance and, if necessary, save to pay the balance of the price of the holiday and spending money
> - Deal with correspondence from the Inland Revenue, Benefits Agency, insurance companies, bank and utility services
> - Appreciate the need to obtain household and buildings insurance and be able to submit a claim if anything went wrong with the property
> - Know what to do with a letter offering the opportunity to take out credit or investments
> - Be able to seek and accept advice in relation to tax, investments, savings and running a house and all that that entails

It is also necessary to explore how claimants currently manage their property and affairs and try to understand how they would do so in the future. Box 37 sets out examples of various activities and situations about which it is useful to make enquiry and Box 38 suggests an approach to exploring a claimant's current financial affairs.

Capacity to make a gift

The leading case on the capacity to make a gift is *Re Beaney (Deceased)* [1978] 2 All ER 595. The testatrix signed a deed of gift transferring her house to her older daughter a few days after being admitted to hospital suffering from advanced dementia. It was held that:

The degree or extent of understanding required in respect of any instrument is relative to the particular transaction which it is to effect. In the case of a will the degree required is always high. In the case of a contract, a deed made for consideration or a gift inter vivos, whether by deed or otherwise, the degree required varies with the circumstances of the transaction. Thus, at one extreme, if the subject matter and value of the gift are trivial in relation to the donor's other assets a low degree of understanding will suffice. But, at the other extreme, if its effect is to dispose of the donor's only asset of value and thus, for practical purposes, to pre-empt the devolution of his estate under his will or on his intestacy, then the degree of understanding is as high as that required for a will,

---

Box 38 Exploring a claimant's current financial affairs

- What is the claimant's weekly/fortnightly/monthly income?
- From what sources does the income come?
- How does the claimant access money?
- Is the claimant able to go to a cashpoint to access money and understand that this gets deducted from the bank account?
- Is the claimant able to write cheques and understand that this sum gets deducted from the bank account?
- On what does the claimant spend money?
- Does the claimant save money
- Can the claimant work out from a bank statement how much money there is left at the end of the month?
- Does the claimant understand that he or she should not spend more than his or her income?

---

and the donor must understand the claims of all potential donees and the extent of the property to be disposed of.

Thus, the assessment of capacity should include (British Medical Association & Law Society, 2010):

- understanding what a gift is – not a loan or something that the donor can ask to be returned
- whether the donor expects to receive anything in return
- when the gift is to take effect
- who the recipient is
- whether the donor has already made substantial gifts to the recipient or others
- whether it is a one-off gift or part of a larger series of transactions
- the underlying purpose of the transaction.

The assessment

The overriding principle is that people should be assessed when they are at their highest level of functioning (Ashton *et al*, 2006) and the assessing psychiatrist has a responsibility to maximise or enhance the person's mental capacity (Braithwaite & Waldron, 2010). It is important to give consideration to assessing people in their own environment, because taking all practicable steps to enable them to make a decision (s.1(3)) includes making sure that they are in an environment in which they are comfortable. Indeed, Braithwaite & Waldron (2010) suggest that it should 'probably not [be] in circumstances which might create nervousness or tension (such as hospital, surgery or office)'. 'Practicable' means the exercise of common sense, otherwise known as the combination of sound judgment with compromise (*Dedman v British Building and Engineering Appliances Ltd* [1974] 1 WLR 171, CA). Also, presentation of information in a user-friendly manner can make all the difference as to whether or not a person is determined to have capacity. Other considerations are the time of day, the assistance of a speech therapist or interpreter and any cultural, ethnic or religious factors that may influence the person's functioning.

An opinion must always take into consideration the actual assistance available, or likely to be available, as this can make a critical difference between the person having and not having capacity. Thus, it may be appropriate for part of the assessment to take place with the assistance of someone such as a family member. On the other hand, some people function better when seen without family present. Ask the person which they would prefer.

No capacity assessment should begin without knowing precisely the matter or matters about which the person is to make a decision. This should be clear either from the information provided by the instructing solicitors or by reference to the literature and case law or a combination of these. An assessment of capacity must include questions that reveal how the person responds to being asked to consider the decisions specific to the issue in question, such as those that arise in a settlement meeting. If claimants say that they will do whatever their solicitor advises, this must lead to an exploration of how, and with what information, they will evaluate and weigh in the balance what their solicitor advises.

It will usually be necessary for the expert to have some knowledge of the history of the person whose capacity is being assessed. All relevant medical records should be available. If the issue is the testamentary capacity of someone who was in hospital at the relevant time, it will be necessary to see the nursing and any other records for the day, or even the part of the day, when the instructions were given or the will executed.

As with the assessment of fitness to plead and stand trial, in most cases assessment is best approached as if the person lacked capacity (see p. 77) and conducting the examination so as to enable the person to prove, if they can, that they have capacity (Rix, 2006*b*). This means starting by providing a very limited introduction and then asking the person why they have attended. It may be obvious from the outset – and confirmed by asking about 'your case', 'solicitors' and 'court' – that the person has no idea that they have a case. Care has to be taken in the way questions are put and capabilities tested. Do not ask a personal injury claimant: 'How would you compromise your claim?' Rather, give a specific example and ask the claimant how they might proceed. If they cannot understand, use a more familiar example, such as the 'car boot sale' question: 'You want £40 for your clock and you are offered only £20. What could you do to get more?' If the person has been accompanied to the consultation, or if someone else is present if they are visited at home, find out what, if anything, they were told about the purpose of the consultation and when they were told about it. This assists in understanding the ability to understand and retain relevant information.

It may be appropriate if capacity is at issue to include in the mental state examination some tests of cognitive functioning. The Mini-Mental State Examination (Folstein *et al*, 1975) is widely used but it is for the overall grading of cognitive functioning and not very extensive. My preference is the Withers and Hinton tests of the sensorium (Withers & Hinton, 1971) because they are more extensive, although some of the items, such as those involving pre-decimal coinage, have to be updated.

As capacity is a time-specific issue, the person's mental state at the consultation is of particular importance. However, it is important to analyse carefully the documentary evidence, as this will indicate how the person functions on a day-to-day basis. Where claimants have a brain injury or other serious disability for which they have had in-patient rehabilitation, the daily records of paramedical or care staff, although time-consuming to read and sometimes voluminous, can provide a wealth of information relevant to capacity to manage property and affairs, just as nursing or care home records can provide a wealth of information relevant to the decisions to be made by elderly persons. Likewise, reliable evidence from family and friends can provide good examples of capacity or the lack of it.

Where the assessment of capacity is retrospective and entirely based on papers (medical and other records, correspondence, witness statements and so on), it is particularly important to set out the evidence in strict chronological order, so that the day, hour or even minute when the decision is taken can be seen in context. Distinguish non-contemporaneous information, such as that from witness statements, with *italic* type. Be prepared for the rival members of the family giving conflicting accounts of the mental abilities of the person whose capacity is in question. If the case goes to trial, the judge will decide on the factual evidence and unless one side's version is so obviously at odds with the contemporaneous documentary evidence, it may be necessary to give alternative opinions depending on which account is accepted.

Further reading

Ashton, G., Letts, P., Oates, L., *et al* (2006) *Mental Capacity: The New Law.* Jordans.
British Medical Association & Law Society (2010) *Assessment of Mental Capacity: A Practical Guide for Doctors and Lawyers* (3rd edn). Law Society.
Jones, R. (2007) *Mental Capacity Act Manual* (2nd edn). Sweet & Maxwell.
R v C (Respondent) (On Appeal from the Court of Appeal (Criminal Division)) [2009] UKHL 42

CHAPTER 9

Reports for tribunals, inquests and other bodies

The evidence given by expert witnesses is absolutely crucial not only to the criminal justice system but to the justice system generally (Professor Graham Zellick, Chair of the Criminal Cases Review Commission, in the Lund Lecture, delivered to the British Academy of Forensic Sciences, 22 November 2006 – see Zellick, 2010)

This chapter deals briefly with some of the tribunals and other legal settings for which expert psychiatric evidence may be admissible.

The First Tier Tribunal (Health, Education and Social Care Chamber) Mental Health

The First Tier Tribunal (Health, Education and Social Care Chamber) Mental Health used to be called the Mental Health Tribunal. It is unusual among judicial bodies in that it is inquisitorial rather than adversarial. The rules of evidence on such matters as hearsay are more relaxed. The three panel members – legal, lay and medical – have equal standing and question the patient and witnesses directly. Their main duty is to decide whether to discharge a patient who is detained under the terms of a section of the MHA.

Independent psychiatric reports are most commonly commissioned by the patient's lawyer and submitted to the Tribunal, together with other written reports, if they help the patient's case. It would be extremely rare for the author of such a report to be called to give evidence in a non-restricted Part III case or a Part II case.

Tribunals appreciate a well-written independent psychiatric report because it sometimes gives a fuller picture of the patient's condition. Often the report brings a new perspective because the author has more time available than a busy clinician.

The Tribunals Judiciary has issued a practice direction that sets out what is expected in a clinician's report to the Tribunal. Any psychiatrist instructed to prepare an independent report for the Tribunal, whether at the request of the patient's solicitor or at the request of the responsible authority or secretary of state, should have regard to this practice direction. Every psychiatrist who is responsible for detained patients should have a copy to hand, so it is not repeated here. Its content is reproduced in *Reports for Mental Health Tribunals* (Tribunals Service, 2010).

It is worth noting the emphasis in the practice direction on the detail of 'whether the patient has ever neglected or harmed himself, or has ever harmed other persons or threatened them with harm, at any time when he was mentally disordered'. Clinicians (not acting as experts) are expected to deal with this as far as it is within their knowledge. It is a fact that some clinicians do not have access to all of the relevant medical records, rely on insufficiently detailed summaries or rely on summaries that misrepresent the patient's criminal record, for example elevating actual bodily harm (ABH) to grievous bodily harm (GBH), confusing 'charge' and 'conviction' and confusing imprisonment on remand with a sentence of imprisonment. The independent expert should have the opportunity make up for these deficiencies and inaccuracies.

There is a tendency on the part of some clinicians to overlook 'the patient's strengths and any other positive factors that the Tribunal should be aware of'. The independent expert should make sure that this is covered.

The burden of proof is on the detaining authority to justify the patient's detention. Thus, the treating clinician needs to provide clear reasons for conclusions as to the nature and degree of the disorder, the need for treatment and the risks to the patient or other persons arising out of the disorder. The independent expert should pay the same regard to the reasons for their conclusions on these matters.

Independent experts are not used much in tribunals. In *MD v Nottinghamshire Health Care NHS Trust* [2010] UKUT 59 (AAC) it was said that having a psychiatrist on the panel who conducts his or her own examination of the patient and makes his or her own contribution to the expert decision-making of the tribunal panel reduces the need for patients to have their own expert evidence. In this same case the Upper Tribunal (which deals with appeals from the First Tier Tribunal) addressed the approach to disputed expert evidence. The First Tier Tribunal had directed a meeting of the experts to identify the issues on which they could and could not agree but this did not happen. It noted the procedure for experts' meetings in civil litigation and specifically the reporting on matters which inform points of disagreement. The Upper Tribunal did not make a recommendation along these lines but it did draw attention to rule 2(4) of the Tribunal Procedure (First-Tier Tribunal) (Health, Education and Social Care Chamber) Rules 2008 (SI No. 2999), which imposes a duty on parties to help the Tribunal to further the overriding objective and cooperate with the Tribunal generally. It held that these duties 'must include making their experts available to comply with any directions that are given by the tribunal'.

Some recent cases point to matters that require particular care when they are addressed. The nature and effects of the 'appropriate treatment' were some of the issues in *DL-H v Devon Partnership NHS Trust* [2010] UKUT 102 (AAC): (1) What precisely is the treatment that can be provided? (2) What discernible level of benefit may it have? (3) Is that benefit related to the patient's mental disorder or some unrelated problem? (4) Is the patient truly resistant to engagement?

The issue of 'appropriate treatment' was also central to the case of *MD v Nottinghamshire* and although the decision of the Upper Tribunal did not deal with the expert evidence in any detail, the decision is worth reading for an understanding of the Tribunal's approach to 'appropriate treatment'. It is also worth noting that on the issue of the risk of the patient violently reoffending against children, it appears that the Tribunal rejected the evidence of the patient's expert on this issue as his evidence was 'essentially statistical' and the Tribunal preferred to focus on 'the individual patient and the effect the treatment available could have on his condition' rather than 'research evidence'. Furthermore, although the Tribunal had been informed that 'there were psychiatric debates on whether personality disorder could be treated', it held that the Tribunal was not the place to resolve such debates

However familiar you regard yourself as being with the MHA, it is good practice to remind yourself of the statutory criteria for detention and of the powers to discharge detained patients. Better still, use the *Mental Health Act Manual* by Jones (2010) to do so and check his explanatory notes for the up-to-date interpretation of the law.

The UK Border Agency and the Asylum and Immigration Tribunal

Asylum seekers and those acting for them may seek psychiatric evidence where there is a history of mental disorder, or possible mental disorder, or a history, or risk, of suicide. Failed asylum seekers can appeal on mental health grounds. In such cases reports may be requested by the UK Border Agency, by the Asylum and Immigration Tribunal or by solicitors acting for the asylum seeker, and they may be sought for the Court of Appeal.

Pitman (2010) has described a framework for addressing the practical and ethical challenges in cases where experts may be uncomfortable about providing what appear to be 'life or death' decisions if the outcome is the asylum seeker's deportation to a country where he or she may be tortured or even killed. This is not work for the faint-hearted. However, this potentially vulnerable and often already greatly disadvantaged group of people should not be denied justice because psychiatrists are unwilling to report in such cases.

Where, as often happens, the request for the report is made to the treating psychiatrist there may be a grave dilemma. On the one hand, psychiatrists will want the best for their patient but on the other, if they provide a report they will have a duty to those instructing them to give an independent and impartial opinion. Furthermore, some treating psychiatrists may not feel sufficiently experienced in transcultural psychiatry or be sufficiently knowledgeable about the risks the deportee will face or about the mental health provision in different countries. If in doubt about ethics, duty or relevant expertise, the treating clinician should consider declining instructions and advising the instruction of someone more appropriately qualified by training, experience and knowledge.

Assessment in such cases may be complicated by language difficulties, which necessitate the use of an interpreter, failures to attend appointments that are beyond the asylum seeker's control and difficulties with rapport arising out of previous experiences with authority figures or their treatment by people of a different race or culture. Several assessments may be necessary in order to build up sufficient rapport.

As for any medico-legal assessment, there is a requirement for a comprehensive history and a painstaking mental state examination. Pitman (2010) calls for 'the ability to take an adequate or appropriate trauma history'. She advocates 'use of a developmental perspective [that] acknowledges past abandonments and failures of care and how these relate to an individual's experience of pre- and postmigration adversity' because it 'provides another dimension to the medico-legal opinion provided, and offers some containment where patients might doubt a Western clinician's ability to grasp the context of their situation'.

It is necessary to be alive to the possibility of malingering, exaggeration or misrepresentation of symptoms or history as a response to a real and justified fear on the part of asylum seekers that they may be deported to a country where they will suffer abuse, retribution, revenge, discrimination, torture or even death.

The particular issue that is required to be addressed is whether deportation to the country of origin would have an adverse effect on the asylum seeker's mental health. Thus, the issues to be addressed are otherwise as usual but with certain qualifications: diagnosis, but often with particular reference to post-traumatic stress disorder or complex post-traumatic stress disorder; and prognosis, (1) with or without a return to the country of origin, having regard to the impact of further detention, the impact of travel and the asylum seeker's likely treatment at the destination country, (2) with or without treatment, having regard to the availability of mental health services both in detention centres and in the country of origin where their accessibility by a failed asylum seeker may be limited, and (3) in terms of suicide risk (the expert should here point out how difficult it is to predict and how rapidly it can change). The ultimate issue may be whether or not deportation would breach the asylum seeker's human rights, in particular the right not to be deported to a country where there is a real risk of torture, or inhuman or degrading treatment, and the psychiatrist would be wise to avoid offering an opinion on this ultimate issue. However, the psychiatrist may be asked questions relating to the human rights issues.

Employment tribunals, disability discrimination and harassment

Employment tribunals deal with disputes between employers and employees. The rules of procedure are similar in Scotland, Wales and England, except that in Scotland there is no provision for written witness statements.

Psychiatric evidence may be sought where it is alleged that a person has been the subject of discrimination on the basis of a 'characteristic' that is 'protected' by the Equality Act 2010, such as sex, sexual orientation, race or disability. Expert evidence in relation to discrimination may go to the issue of the consequent psychiatric damage, as, for example, in the case of a Welshman of Somali extraction who developed clinical depression after being racially abused by his foreman when working on the construction of the Millennium Stadium in Cardiff (*Essa v Laing* [2004] IRLR 313). In a case of discrimination on the grounds of disability the expert evidence will go to the issue of the disability itself. Where the issue of discrimination arises in the context of employment, a psychiatric report may be required for an employment tribunal but other courts also deal with discrimination.

The Equality Act 2010

Under s.6(1) of the Equality Act 2010 'a person has a *disability* if (a) P has a *physical* or *mental impairment* which has a *substantial* and *long-term adverse effect* on P's ability to carry out *normal day-to-day activities*' (italic type is used here to draw attention to the essential components). As well as providing protection against discrimination in employment, the Equality Act 2010 provides protection from discrimination in the provision of goods, services and facilities and in education. For example, the issue of disability may have to be addressed by a psychiatric expert in the case of a person with psychiatric disorder who alleges discrimination in the provision of housing.

Disability

Where the issue is 'disability' it is not the role of the expert to say whether the applicant is 'disabled', as this is for the tribunal (*Abadeh v BT plc* [2001] IRLR 23), but the expert has to give an opinion as to impairment. Under the Equality Act 2010 the onus is on the claimant to prove impairment on the balance of probabilities.

The focus in all cases should be on diagnosis, condition, causation, treatment and prognosis.

Physical impairment

Where physical symptoms, sufficient to amount to an impairment, result from psychological factors, the impairment is regarded as a physical impairment. So it was held in the case of *College of Ripon and York St John v Hobbs* [2002] IRLR 185, where the applicant's case was that he had developed muscle weakness and wasting but no organic disease was identified.

Mental impairment

It is recognised that a disability can arise from mental impairments such as fluctuating or recurring depression, mental health conditions and mental illnesses, such as depression, schizophrenia, eating disorder, bipolar affective disorders, obsessive–compulsive disorders, as well as personality disorders and some self-harming behaviour.

Certain conditions were not regarded as impairments for the purposes of the now repealed Disability Discrimination Act 1995 (DDA) and they continue to be excluded under the Equality Act 2010: addiction to, or dependency on, alcohol, nicotine, or any other substance (other than in consequence of the substance being medically prescribed); tendency to set fires; tendency to steal; tendency to physical or sexual abuse of other persons; exhibitionism; voyeurism. Even where there was medical evidence to the effect that a businessman's offences of indecent exposure, committed on a business trip, were manifestations of his moderately severe depressive illness, and the employment tribunal had found that his dismissal for misconduct was discrimination on the basis of his depression, the employment appeal tribunal found that his dismissal was solely on the basis of his indecent exposures, for which he had no protection under the DDA (*Edmund Nuttall v Butterfield* [2005] IRLR 751).

Substantial

There is the matter of whether the impairment is substantial. This means more than minor or trivial. Assessment involves taking into account the time taken to carry out an activity, the way in which an activity is carried out and the cumulative effects of activities which, on their own, would reveal no more than minor or trivial impairment. It is also necessary to take into account the extent to which the person can reasonably modify their behaviour to reduce the effects because, if they can, they no longer meet the criteria.

In deciding whether the claimant's impairment amounts to a substantial, long-term effect on normal day-to-day activities, the effects of 'medical treatment' such as medication, psychological and other treatments, including counselling, have to be discounted. Disability will be decided on whether or not the claimant would be 'likely' to manifest a substantial long-term impact on normal day-to-day activities if they were not having the medication or treatment they are. Here 'likely' does not mean 'more probable than not'; it is a deliberately lower threshold and means 'may well happen' (*SCA Packaging v Boyle* [2009] IRLR 746; see also below, under 'Long-term adverse effect'). This is called the 'deduced effect' because it is necessary to deduce that there would be a substantial adverse effect on normal day-to-day activities without the medical treatment. Likewise, the expert has to disregard the successful coping strategies without which the claimant would have difficulty in carrying out normal day-to-day activities (*Vicary v BT plc* [2001] IRLR 23).

Whether or not there is a substantial impairment is for the tribunal to decide. Therefore experts should set out the evidence that will assist the tribunal and then go no further than to say that they would expect that this is evidence of substantial impairment but this is for the tribunal to decide.

Long-term adverse effect

Whether the impairment has a long-term adverse effect means that the effect has lasted, or is 'likely' to last, for at least 12 months, but this can include the cumulative effects of shorter periods than 12 months. The official guidance on the meaning of 'disability' in the DDA at one time advised that 'likely' meant 'more probable than not' but the revised guidance (SI No. 1159, 2011) published under the Equality Act 2010 (available at http://www.legislation.gov.uk/uksi/2011/1159/made) takes account of *SCA Packaging v Boyle* and now states that it means 'may well happen'. Where the person has a recurrent condition which causes fluctuating impairments they will be treated as long term if the substantial adverse effect is likely to recur over a year or more. Psychiatric evidence therefore has to deal with the prognosis of the claimant's condition.

Psychiatrists, when reaching a retrospective opinion as to prognosis, specifically the likelihood of recurrence, might reasonably be expected to take into account recurrences that have subsequently occurred. On the same basis an employment appeal tribunal had regard to the actual recurrence of a job applicant's delusional and schizoaffective disorder after her offer of employment was withdrawn and even though the psychiatrist had said at the time she applied for the post that a recurrence was unlikely. However, the Court of Appeal overturned the judgment on the basis that the tribunal must concentrate on the evidence available at the time of the alleged discriminatory act and not have regard to subsequent events because 'the statute requires a prophecy to be made' (*McDougall v Richmond Adult Community College* [2008] EWCA Civ 4). Thus the tribunal and the psychiatrist need to disregard the subsequent history.

Normal day-to-day activities

For an impairment to amount to a disability it is no longer necessary, as it was under the DDA, to show that the impairment has affected one or more of the following 'normal day to day activities': (1) mobility; (2) manual dexterity; (3) physical coordination; (4) continence; (5) ability to lift, carry or otherwise move everyday objects; (6) speech, hearing or eyesight; (7) memory or ability to concentrate, learn or understand; or (8) perceptions of the risk of physical danger. Those most obviously relevant to mental impairment are (7) and (8) and perhaps also (1), where, for example, mobility is impaired by the tiredness or fatigue that is a manifestation of a depressive illness. This could be a high hurdle to jump. It was failed by a teacher who was diagnosed as having a chronic mixed anxiety and depression as a result of which he was unable to go out and suffered intense anxiety when involved with school children; he was, though, not disabled in the terms of the DDA because there was no adverse effect on the statutory capabilities, in that he was cognitively intact and able to concentrate (*East Sussex County Council v Hancock* [2003] All ER (D) 423). It is likely that this case would now be decided differently. The Equality Act 2010 has removed the above list of 'normal day-to-day activities' but the Act provides for regulations and guidance to be issued and updated, as with Statutory Instrument 1159. Ultimately, it will be for the courts to decide what day-to-day activities are. Psychiatric experts should make sure that they are provided with any regulations or guidance and they should ask about any cases under the Equality Act 2010 that assist.

Guidance on the definition of 'disability', first issued under the DDA, was updated in 2011 in Statutory Instrument 1159. In an appendix it gives an illustrative and non-exhaustive list of factors which it would be reasonable to regard as having a substantial adverse effect on normal day-to-day activities. These include persistent general low motivation or loss of interest in everyday activities, persistently wanting to avoid people or significant difficulty taking part in normal social interaction or forming social relationships and persistent distractibility or difficulty concentrating.

Causation

In most cases causation is far from straightforward. There may be various causes. Also, importantly, employment tribunals can reduce the level of compensation awarded to an employee for psychiatric damage caused by unlawful discrimination where the psychiatric damage has resulted from a number of causes of which only one, or some, but not all are attributable to the employer's liability. They will apply a proportionate percentage reduction. In doing so, they will have regard to the psychiatric expert's causal analysis and breakdown of causal factors. For example, in *Thaine v London School of Economics* [2010] ICR 1422, the claimant alleged sex discrimination, disability discrimination and unfair dismissal. She succeeded only on the basis of sex discrimination. It was held that there was a causal link between the sex discrimination, ill-health and loss of earnings. The level of compensation, however, was reduced by 60% to reflect: (1) the tribunal's findings that a number of other 'concurrent causes' had contributed to her illness, including a history of obsessive–compulsive disorder and depressive episodes, a break-up with her boyfriend and concerns about her mother, who was suffering from cancer; and (2) the conclusion that other, non-established, accusations of sexual harassment had contributed to her ill-health. In dismissing her appeal, the employment appeal tribunal stated that:

the test for causation when more than one event causes the harm is to ask whether the conduct for which the [employer] is liable materially contributed to the harm ... the extent of its liability is another matter entirely. It is liable only to the extent of that contribution. It may be difficult to quantify the extent of the contribution, but that is the task which the Tribunal is required to undertake.

This is reassuring for experts who struggle when asked for a fractional or, worse, percentage breakdown of causation. The expert can now with greater confidence qualify an opinion by referring to the difficulty of the exercise, go no further than comparing the likely impact of the different causes in general and in the particular case, and leave the tribunal to undertake the task of quantification.

The appropriate time

The appropriate time to consider is the time of the alleged discrimination and not the time of the medical consultation.

Reasonable adjustments

If it is alleged that the employer has failed to make reasonable adjustments, it is necessary to consider both (1) what effect, if any, any specific adjustment would have made, and (2) what other adjustments (if any) would have materially mitigated the material effect of what the tribunal may find was the disability. Examples are working part time, working somewhere else in the company or business, having support, having more training, being better supervised and having scheduled meetings with supervisors or managers.

Procedure

Joint experts are preferred by employment tribunals. It is important to have access to occupational health records as well as general practitioner records.

Harassment

Under the PHA, a course of conduct amounting to harassment is both a criminal and a civil wrong. Harassment related to a protected characteristic, like sex, race or disability, is also prohibited under the Equality Act 2010. Harassment at work so severe as to result in psychiatric damage can found a civil action against the employer for negligence (*Green v DB Group Services (UK) Ltd* [2006] IRLR 764). Under both the PHA and the Equality Act 2010, compensation can be awarded for injury to feelings as well as actual psychiatric injury, but this is not possible under common law negligence. For a successful claim under the Equality Act 2010, as under the PHA, it is unnecessary to prove reasonable foreseeability (*Sheriff v Klyne Tugs*

(*Lowestoft*) *Ltd* [1999] ICR 1170), in contrast to the position at common law (see p. 148).

The Agricultural Land Tribunal

The Agricultural Land Tribunal became a court of first instance under the Agriculture Act 1958 and is roughly equivalent to a county court. It sits in public, its rules of evidence are not as strict as those of higher courts and it may admit evidence that would not be admissible elsewhere.

One of its functions is to determine the eligibility and suitability of applicants for the grant of a new tenancy. It also provides a form of dispute resolution by considering whether to uphold a landlord's notice to quit on the death of a tenant; any surviving 'close relatives' of the deceased may apply for a direction entitling them to the new tenancy of the agricultural holding on the death of the previous tenant.

The burden of proof is on applicants, who have to prove that they are both eligible and suitable. Suitability is determined by reference to s.39(8) of the Agricultural Holdings Act 1986, which provides that some of the matters to be taken into consideration are the 'age, physical health and financial standing of the applicant'. As this is not, however, an exhaustive list, it can reasonably be regarded as making provision for matters such as the mental health of the applicant to be taken into consideration. In one case before the Tribunal, an applicant's suitability to succeed was contested by the landlord, his aunt. It was the basis of her case that his drinking habits had a bearing on his physical health and therefore psychiatric evidence was admitted (Rix *et al*, 1997). This was accepted by the Tribunal, which stated that 'drinking to the level described, and [its] consequences ... had to be a relevant matter in judging suitability'.

Inquests

An inquest is the procedure used in England, Wales and Northern Ireland to investigate a sudden death for which the cause is unknown, violent or unnatural, or which has occurred in prison. The Fatal Accident Inquiry fulfils a similar function in Scotland.

In a report for a coroner, bear in mind that the coroner or coroner's court may have to decide only the identity of the deceased, and how, when and where they came by their death; or it might be a wider remit, to satisfy Article 2 of the European Convention on Human Rights ('right to life') and deal with other matters, such as in what circumstances the deceased died and in particular what care the deceased received. It is not the role of the coroner to ascertain liability or culpability or to explore issues of potential medical negligence but interested parties, such as the deceased's family, may be represented by lawyers who seek to examine the coroner's witnesses with this in mind. Whether instructed by the coroner, solicitors acting for the deceased's family or a hospital, NHS trust or prison responsible for the care of the deceased, the standard of care will be a live issue even though issues of negligence may be addressed later, in another place. However, the test for lack of care is not the same as the test for negligence. It was held in *R v HM Coroner for Coventry, ex p Chief Constable of Staffordshire Constabulary* [2000] MLC 0233 that lack of care in the context of an inquest is not necessarily sufficient to found an action for negligence, as lack of care is simply the obverse of self-neglect.

Aim to produce a sufficiently detailed account of the relevant medical history in chronological order based on the records. The report will include information that is not in the records, such as statements and sudden untoward incident reports. This should be clearly distinguishable from the information taken from the records, for example by italic type, and its source should be identified. Hearsay evidence is admissible but it must be accurate and its source identified.

As the report is likely to be read out at the inquest, it should be in a form that can be understood by the family. Essential medical and technical terms and names of drugs should therefore be explained as and when they arise, although a glossary will still assist. Explain abbreviations and initials.

Do not omit information that could be upsetting or embarrassing for family members to hear. The coroner needs to be fully briefed. A coroner may exclude delicate passages from a recital or ask you to miss out certain passages from your recital.

Avoid giving an opinion on a matter such as whether the death was through suicide. This is for the coroner or court to decide. However, it may be of assistance to draw attention to information that appears relevant, explain why, say what weight a psychiatrist would attach to it and explain how it would inform a clinical judgment as to suicidality. Acknowledge that this is only professional assistance and there is no intention to usurp the coroner's role.

Professional regulatory proceedings

Psychiatric expert evidence is often required in professional regulatory proceedings such as those of the General Medical Council, other health regulators, including the Health Professions Council, and other professional regulators, such as the General Teaching Council, the Law Society and the Bar Council.

The requirement for psychiatric evidence will usually arise from an issue as to the mental health of the professional. However, if the practitioner is not suffering from a mental disorder, the psychiatric expert needs to be aware of the limits of the assistance he or she can provide. In *Yeong v General Medical Council* [2009] LS Law Medical 582, Sales J could not fault the Fitness to

Practise Panel's approach to the evidence of a psychiatrist about the risk that the practitioner posed to his patients:

Dr Khean's evidence was to the effect that Dr Yeong did not suffer from any psychological disorder which underlay his misconduct. In light of that assessment, Dr Khean's expression as to the risk posed by Dr Yeong carried little weight attributable to any special expertise on the part of Dr Khean. The question of the possibility of a recurrence of such misconduct by Dr Yeong was a matter of the ordinary assessment of likely human behaviour, in relation to which a psychiatrist's expertise confers no special privileged insight. The assessment of risk of any particular form of future behaviour is the sort of task which courts and tribunals regularly perform without needing to refer to expert psychiatric evidence.

Sometimes in a GMC case where there is an issue of misconduct, psychiatric evidence is needed as to the boundaries or standards of normal psychiatric practice.

Although it may be *admissible* for the expert to comment on the ultimate issue of the professional's fitness to practise (Glynn & Gomez, 2005), this is a matter for the committee or panel to decide and not the expert, so it is best to avoid comment on this unless specifically invited to do so.

As the committee or panel will have to give reasons for its decision, experts need to make clear the reasons for their own opinion. This is also particularly important if there is a conflict of expert evidence and the committee or panel has to decide whose opinion to accept.

Further reading

Jones, R. (2010) *Mental Health Act Manual* (13th edn). Thomson Reuters.
Kloss, D. (2010) *Occupational Health Law* (5th edn). Wiley-Blackwell.
Pitman, A. (2010) Medicolegal reports in asylum applications: a framework for addressing the practical and ethical challenges. *Journal of the Royal Society of Medicine*, **103**, 93–97.

CHAPTER 10

Reports for the Channel Islands, the Republic of Ireland, the Isle of Man, Northern Ireland and Scotland

[A]pproved mental health professionals in Wales have one advantage over their English counterparts. While the former can section their spouses, the latter cannot. (Jones, 2009, p. v)

Overlooking the term 'section', of which I disapprove, this quotation serves to introduce the differences in statute law, common law and procedure in the nine jurisdictions of the British Isles. However, although Welsh ministers can make subordinate legislation on devolved matters, including health, and Wales has its own Code of Practice to the MHA and its own Mental Health Tribunal Rules, there do not appear to be any significant differences between England and Wales of relevance to psychiatric experts unless they are married to an approved mental health professional.

Alderney

In Alderney, the third largest of the Crown Dependencies that make up the Channel Islands, crime is rare and, if there is any, minor. Alderney has limited jurisdiction over the criminal law, as the Royal Court of Guernsey (see below) has jurisdiction for some crimes. The island has unlimited jurisdiction in civil cases.

Guernsey

Like Jersey, the law of Guernsey is rooted in Norman customary (case) law but it has been observed that 'the Jersey and Guernsey plants have frequently surfaced in different parts of the garden of jurisprudence' (*Attorney General v O'Driscoll* [2003] JLR 390). Since 1848 common law defences have developed on parallel lines to those defences in England and Wales and for the insanity defence and unfitness to plead Guernsey has adopted the law of England and Wales.

Jersey

Jersey law is a mixture of Norman customary law, statute law and English law.

Jersey's provisions for 'Persons found insane on accusation or trial' derive from art.1 of the Criminal Justice (Insane Persons) (Jersey) Law 1964 and refer to an accused being 'so insane as to be unfit to plead to the accusation or unable to understand the nature of the trial'. In *Attorney General v O'Driscoll* [2003 JLR 390] it was ruled that the test of unfitness to plead laid down in England should not be adopted and that the statutory test is satisfied if, 'as a result of unsoundness of mind or inability to communicate, he or she lacked the capacity to participate effectively in the proceedings'. This includes an inability to communicate by reason, for example, of a coma or stroke. In determining the issue the court has regard to the ability of the accused: (1) to understand the nature of the proceedings so as to instruct a lawyer and to make a proper defence; (2) to understand the substance of the evidence; (3) to give evidence on their own behalf; and (4) to make rational decisions in relation to their participation in the proceedings (including whether or not to plead guilty), which reflect true and informed choices on their part. The approach is therefore one that is based on the general principle of 'effective' participation and amounts to an 'adjudicative competence' test. The judgment adds that 'it will not be sufficient in itself to justify a finding of unfitness to plead that an accused person is someone of limited intellect or someone who, for other reasons, might find the criminal process puzzling or difficult to follow'.

In Jersey, unlike in England and Wales, where s.37(3) of the MHA provides for it, there is no mechanism or direction for fitness to plead to be determined by the lower, magistrates' court. Where the magistrates' court has doubt as to a person's fitness to enter a plea, it must immediately refer the case to the Royal Court for determination, no matter how minor the alleged offence, although it is open to the Attorney General to consider whether or not the criminal law should be engaged in the case of a relatively trivial offence (*O'Driscoll*).

Jersey's law on diminished responsibility is set out in art.3 of the Homicide (Jersey) Law 1986:

Where a person kills or is party to the killing of another, the person shall not be convicted of murder if the person was suffering from such abnormality of mind (whether arising from a condition of arrested or incomplete development of mind or any inherent causes or induced by disease or injury) as substantially impaired the person's mental responsibility for the person's acts and omissions in doing or being a party to the killing.

As this is based on the Homicide Act 1957 of England and Wales, there are many cases that assist in its interpretation. Likewise, Jersey's law on provocation follows that in the Homicide Act 1957. Article 4 of the Homicide (Jersey) Law 1986 states that:

Where on a charge of murder there is evidence on which the jury can find that the person charged was provoked (whether by things done or by things said or by both together) to lose the person's self-control, the question of whether the provocation was enough to make the reasonable person do as he or she did shall be left to be determined by the jury; and in determining that question the jury shall take into account everything both done and said according to the effect which, in their opinion, it would have on a reasonable person.

The interpretation of this statute, however, is now governed by the ruling of the Privy Council in *Holley* (see p. 99).

Insanity at the time of the commission of the offence derives from art. 2(1) of the Criminal Justice (Insane Persons) (Jersey) Law 1964:

If on the trial before the Royal Court of any person charged with any act or omission punishable with death or imprisonment, the jury is satisfied that the accused did the act or made the omission charged against him or her but that the accused was insane at the time when the act was done or omission made so as not to be responsible according to law for his or her actions, the jury shall return a special verdict to the effect that the accused did the act or made the omission charged but is not guilty on the ground that he or she was insane so as not to be responsible according to law at the time.

In *Attorney General v Prior* [2001 JLR 146] the Royal Court held that the M'Naghten Rules were not part of Jersey law and it was clear that Jersey law required a volitional test of insanity. The test adopted was that 'a person is insane … if at the time of the commission of the offence, his unsoundness of mind affected his criminal behaviour to such a substantial degree that the jury consider that he ought not to be found criminally responsible'.

The Mental Health (Jersey) Law 1969, amended in 2005, is Jersey's mental health law and art.1 should be consulted for definitions of 'addict', 'medical treatment', 'mental disorder', 'patient' and 'person requiring special care'. It includes provisions for the 'socially inefficient'. Addicts can be assessed and treated compulsorily.

Sark

Sark has its own set of laws based on Norman law but it can apply the law of Guernsey and Acts of Parliament of the United Kingdom. It does not have its own criminal law and it adopts the criminal law of Guernsey (see above).

The Isle of Man

Isle of Man lawyers are known as advocates and combine the role of solicitor and barrister. While many Manx statutes mirror their English counterparts, in some areas of law there are significant differences. Expert reports should be obtained by advocates well in advance of a trial and any directions or orders made by the court should be complied with. Any dates of non-availability should be given to the instructing advocate immediately upon request. In *R v B.E. Glover, D.P. Glover and Priestnal* 2005–06 MLR (CGGD), the Deemster (full-time High Court judge) held that 'where there is ... a failure to file non-availability ... or a failure to adduce expert evidence promptly resulting in the vacation of trial dates and wasted costs, the court may well impose adverse costs orders against advocates personally'.

Civil law

The Rules of the High Court of Justice 2009 are similar to the CPR. 'Personal injuries' include 'any disease and any impairment of a person's physical or mental condition'. Chapter 6 'Experts and Assessors' is similar to a combination of the CPR Part 35 Practice Direction combined with the *Protocol*. A 'patient' is defined as 'a person who by reason of mental disorder within the meaning of the Mental Health Act 1998 is incapable of managing and administering his property and affairs'. Expert reports have to be verified by the following statement of truth:

I confirm that insofar as the facts stated within my report are within my own knowledge, I have made clear which they are and I believe them to be true, and that the opinions I have expressed represent my true and complete professional opinion.

Under Rule 8.53(2)(c)(i), experts must make it clear when a question or issue falls outside of their expertise. In *Hawthorne v Jones* 2007 MLR 199 (CLD) the petitioner sought leave to adduce an expert report in evidence at trial. In completing the report, the expert claimed to have relied on his experience both as a general practitioner and his experience gained in accident and emergency care, his studies of relevant literature and certain disability assessment training. The expert expressed the opinion that the petitioner was suffering from post-traumatic stress disorder. The Deemster stated that he did not regard the expert opinion as admissible, because the complex and specialist area of psychiatry was outside the expert's knowledge and experience. The report was not relied on at trial.

W. J. Ward, A. M. Ward (by her next friend W. J. Ward) v Ballaughton Estate (1975) Limited 1987–89 MLR 428 (CLD) involved depressive illness in response to the illness of a close relative caused by a defendant's negligence. It was found that if the stress and mental anguish are reasonably foreseeable then the exact form of psychiatric disorder need not be foreseeable or such as a completely normal person would suffer.

Criminal law

Most criminal cases are heard in the Court of Summary Jurisdiction and more serious cases are heard in the Court of General Gaol Delivery.

The law on diminished responsibility is set out at s.22A of the Criminal Code 1872 and is much the same as the English law, whereby the offence is reduced from murder to manslaughter. The Manx courts have a discretionary power to pass a sentence of life imprisonment where the respondent would remain a potential danger to the public for such an unpredictable period of time that no assessment could be made of when their release would be appropriate. This is, however, very rare (*Attorney General's Reference in the matter of Gosling* [2005–06 MLR Note 41]).

The law on insanity is set out in the Criminal Jurisdiction Act 1993. Where it appears to a jury that a defendant did the act or made the omission charged, but was insane when doing the act or making the omission, the jury shall return a special verdict to the effect that the defendant is not guilty by reason of insanity.

In the Isle of Man, juries generally consist of 7 people, or occasionally 12 in serious matters such as murder, and their verdict must be unanimous.

Mental health law

The Isle of Man's mental health law is set out in the Mental Health Act 1998, amended in 2001 and 2006, where definitions can be found for 'mental disorder', 'severe mental impairment', 'mental impairment' and 'psychopathic disorder'. The mental health law broadly follows the English Acts.

Northern Ireland

Northern Ireland shares common law principles with England and Wales. Conduct which is criminal in England and Wales is in most instances criminal in Northern Ireland but the legislation is usually at least a year behind.

Republic of Ireland

Common law is the basis of the Irish legal system and, since the establishment of the Irish Free State, the Dáil and Seanad have made laws of binding force in the jurisdiction.

Family law

The approach to the use of expert testimony in family cases is similar to that in England and Wales.

The position of persons with a mental disorder in relation to marriage derives from the Marriage of Lunatics Act 1811 and such cases as *Turner v*

Meyers 1908 1 Hag Con 414, 161 ER 600 and *ME v AE* [1987] IR 147. In order for a marriage to be voided on the grounds of the mental disorder of one or other party, there has to be proof not only of a recognised psychiatric illness at the time of the ceremony but also that it prevented the necessary consent being given. If the marriage is not voided on this ground, the court may still grant a decree on the basis of an inability to enter into and sustain a normal marital relationship (*RSJ v JSJ* [1982] IRLM 263; *D v C* [1984] ILRM 173). In *HS v JS* [1992] 2 Fam LJ 33 it was held that immaturity would make a marriage voidable only if it was so gross or abnormal as to amount to an inability to enter into and sustain a normal marital relationship.

At present, adults and children who are incapable of looking after their property and affairs can be made subject to the wardship jurisdiction of the High Court and Circuit Court under the principle of *parens patriae*. The Child Care Act 1991 may be used where a child needs protection. The statutory language is that of the Lunacy Regulation (Ireland) Act 1871 and *In the Matter of Wards of Court and In the Matter of Francis Dolan* [2007] IESC 26 the court acknowledged the understandable umbrage of the parents of Francis Dolan when the court had to decide if he was of 'unsound mind'. This may soon change, as there is a Mental Capacity Bill 2008 under consideration. If implemented, there will be a capacity test that makes it clear that capacity is time and issue specific. A person will not be deemed to lack capacity unless all practical steps have been taken without success to help them make the decision.

Under s.71 of the Succession Act 1965 it is a requirement for testamentary capacity that the testator should be of sound disposing mind at the time of the execution of the will. The test is whether testators understand that they are giving effect to the deposition of their property after their death and that they execute it with understanding and reason.

Civil law

In the Republic of Ireland, the person who brings the case is the 'plaintiff' and the person against whom the case is brought is the 'respondent'.

The approach to the use of expert testimony in civil cases is different to that in England and Wales, in that no distinction is made between the expert and professional witness insofar as, if a patient is under the care of a particular doctor following an accident, that doctor becomes the expert witness (Casey, 2003a). There is no choice: it is a matter of obligation and a failure to comply could lead to a complaint to the Medical Council of Ireland. This does not mean that the expert is not impartial and under a duty to the court, but where a case is referred for an opinion by a solicitor it is regarded as highly advisable for that specialist to obtain a referral of the plaintiff from the claimant's general practitioner if the person is not already under the specialist's care.

The Personal Injuries Assessment Board Act 2003 has removed some cases from the courts. These include employers' liability, motor vehicle accident and public liability cases. Unlike the courts, the Board is inquisitorial rather than adversarial and it does not hold oral hearings. The Board does not deal with liability issues, so where there is an issue as to who was liable for the injuries a case is unlikely to be accepted, as it will be deemed more appropriate for the courts. There is also a specific statutory scheme for medical negligence and a scheme for claims against the Garda. Although the Board has published a *Book of Quantum* (1984), this does not refer to compensation for psychiatric injury, as such claims have to be dealt with through the courts. However, the Board does request information on mental illness in order to obtain an overall assessment of the aggregate claim.

Under s.48 of the Statute of Limitations Act 1957, in general a person of unsound mind has six years from the date on which their disability ceases to bring an action in negligence if they were under a disability at the time the tort was committed. Otherwise the limitation is two years.

In relation to employment discrimination, disability is defined in the Employment Equality Act 1998 as including: '(a) the total or partial absence of a person's bodily or mental functions ... (d) a condition or malfunction which results in a person learning differently from a person without the condition or malfunction; or (e) a condition, illness or disease which affects a person's thought processes, perception of reality, emotions or judgment or which results in disturbed behaviour'.

Criminal law

The Criminal Law (Insanity) Act 2006 governs fitness to be tried, the verdict of not guilty by reason of insanity (NGRI) and diminished responsibility. Under the Act 'mental disorder' includes 'mental illness, mental disability, dementia or any disease of the mind but does not include intoxication'.

Box 39 sets out the test for unfitness to be tried in s.4.

Box 39 Criteria for unfitness to be tried in the Republic of Ireland

Section 4(2) of the Criminal Law (Insanity) Act 2006 states:

An accused person shall be deemed unfit to be tried if he or she is unable by reason of mental disorder to understand the nature or course of the proceedings so as to –

(a) plead to the charge,
(b) instruct a legal representative,
(c) in the case of an indictable offence which may be tried summarily, elect for a trial by jury,
(d) make a proper defence,
(e) in the case of a trial by jury, challenge a juror to whom he or she might object, or
(f) understand the evidence.

Under s.5, for a successful defence of NGRI, and where the jury finds that the accused person committed the act alleged, the court has to hear evidence relating to the accused's mental condition given by a consultant psychiatrist. This evidence has to establish that:

(a) the accused person was suffering at the time from a mental disorder, and (b) the mental disorder was such that the accused person ought not to be held responsible for the act alleged by reason of the fact that he or she – (i) did not know the nature and quality of the act, or (ii) did not know that what he or she was doing was wrong, or (iii) was unable to refrain from committing the act.

A verdict of NGRI is an acquittal but the person may be committed to hospital if in need of in-patient care or treatment.

Under s.6, where a person is tried for murder and the jury or the Special Criminal Court finds that (1) the person did the act alleged, (2) the person was at the time suffering from a mental disorder and (3) the mental disorder was not such as to justify a finding of NGRI, but was such as to diminish substantially his or her responsibility for the act, the person may be found not guilty of murder but guilty of manslaughter on the ground of diminished responsibility.

Section 15(1) provides for the transfer to a designated centre of prisoners who are suffering from a mental disorder for which they cannot be afforded appropriate care or treatment within the prison in which they are detained and they voluntarily consent to transfer for this purpose. Such a transfer has to based on a certificate by a relevant officer. A similar provision under s.15(2) relates to the transfer of a prisoner who is unwilling or unable to consent voluntarily to the transfer; this requires certification by two or more relevant officers. A relevant officer is an approved medical officer, that is, a consultant psychiatrist (within the meaning of the Mental Health Act 2001) or a person on the General Register of Medical Practitioners.

Section 22 amends the Infanticide Act 1949 by substituting 'by reason of mental disorder (within the meaning of the Criminal Law (Insanity) Act 2006)' for 'by reason of the effect of lactation'. The Infanticide Act provides that in the case of a woman who by any wilful act or omission has caused the death of her child under the age of 12 months and but for this provision the act or omission would have amounted to murder, she may be tried and punished for manslaughter. The test was whether 'at the time of the act or omission the balance of her mind was disturbed by reason of her not having fully recovered from the effect of giving birth to the child or by reason of the effect of lactation consequent upon the birth of the child' (s.3(c)).

The Mental Health Act 2001 contains the provisions for the involuntary hospitalisation of persons suffering from 'mental disorder', which is defined in s.3(1) as 'mental illness, severe dementia or significant intellectual disability'. Under s.8(2)(a), involuntary hospitalisation cannot be based only on a diagnosis of personality disorder; s.8(2)(b) excludes the involuntary hospital admission of those who are only socially deviant; and s.8(2)(c) so excludes those who are only addicted to drugs or intoxicants.

'Mental illness' is defined as 'a state of mind of a person which affects the person's thinking, perceiving, emotion or judgment and which seriously impairs the mental function of the person to the extent that he or she requires care or medical treatment in his or her own interest or in the interest of other persons' (s.3(2)). 'Severe dementia' means 'a deterioration of the brain of a person which significantly impairs the intellectual function of the person thereby affecting thought, comprehension and memory and which includes severe psychiatric or behavioural symptoms such as physical aggression' (s.3(2)). 'Significant intellectual disability' means a state of arrested or incomplete development of mind of a person which includes significant impairment of intelligence and social functioning and abnormally aggressive or seriously irresponsible conduct on the part of the person (s.3(2)).

Scotland

There are important differences between Scots law and English law in the areas of criminal law, family law and the law of evidence.

Civil cases are brought by a 'pursuer' and they are defended by a 'defender'. In criminal cases those prosecuted are 'defendants'.

Evidence and procedure

Amy Whitehead's Legal Representative v Graeme John Douglas and Another (2006) CSOH 178 has made clear the differences between England and Scotland with regard to the disclosure and nature of expert evidence. In Scotland expert evidence can be admitted in the form of a written report, the terms of which have been agreed by both parties, without the need for the expert to appear and speak to the same, or it can be given orally. If given orally, it is not even necessary to prepare or lodge a written report.

There is no absolute entitlement to material upon which the expert has relied in reaching an opinion. It is up to the party to decide whether or not to lodge in court the documents on which the expert has relied and for those not lodged it is up to the other party to seek recovery under the normal rules for recovery of evidence. In particular, it does not follow that, because the expert has relied on 'precognitions' (statements), which are legally privileged documents prepared in contemplation of the litigation, the other side should have unlimited access to such documents. A party does not waive its rights of confidentiality, which are jealously guarded in Scotland, by disclosing the existence, or even some content, of documents to the expert.

Experts are often provided with little information. The precognitions are legally privileged and are not always disclosed to experts. Other documents produced in court, known as 'productions', are not routinely made available. As Chiswick (2003) has commented: 'Indeed, the information provided by the instructing agent is sometimes meagre. The general rule is "ask for what you want".'

Reports in Scotland should be addressed to the instructing party, not the court, unless the court has requested the report, as frequently happens in child custody disputes and as is the norm post-conviction in criminal cases. It should be produced with a witness statement that provides the necessary details for a witness summons to be issued and which includes a standard statement that the content of the statement is true to the best of the author's knowledge. The usual form of words is as follows ('JM' being the initials of the author of the report):

I produce a report of my findings [x] pages long as exhibit JM1, which is signed by me and dated [date of signature].

The report itself should include or end with a statement that the report is given 'on soul and conscience'. Notwithstanding that the report is not addressed to the court, the expert owes an overriding duty to the court.

Joint instructions are rare but the lawyers can submit a 'joint minute' of the evidence on which both parties agree.

Although testimony in court follows the order examination in chief, cross-examination and re-examination, after the expert has confirmed his or her qualifications and experience, counsel for the opposing party may cross-examine the expert on these and conduct a searching examination of them in order to suggest that he or she is insufficiently qualified or experienced.

Once in the witness box, the expert's evidence depends on what questions are asked. It is not for the expert to volunteer information. Chiswick (2003) advises the expert to take only minimal material into the witness box and not to refer to any document without first seeking the permission of the judge. He says that you will incur irritation if you start to thumb through case records unless they are a 'production' and have been handed to you in court. *Amy Whitehead* also established that the testing of an expert's evidence involves the analysis of the expert's oral testimony and not 'probing it with questions or using other forensic skills'. Chiswick (2003) tells experts to expect 'a searching examination of ... their opinions and the methods by which they reached those opinions'.

Experts in Scotland not only enjoy immunity from suit but for the same public policy reasons they are meant to be immune from complaint to their professional body arising from anything said in evidence unless, that is, the judge is of the opinion that the expert needs to be subjected to disciplinary action in relation to their role as an expert witness or removed from practice.

Criminal law

Criminal law relies more heavily on the common law than that of England and Wales. For insanity in bar of trial, insanity at the time of the offence and diminished responsibility it is recognised that the legal criteria do not easily translate into clinical terms. The *Mental Health (Care and*

Box 40 Information to be presented within a report to a Scottish court

The *Mental Health (Care and Treatment) (Scotland) Act 2003 Code of Practice* (Scottish Executive, 2005, ch. 6, para. 102) states that a court report should detail the following points in relation to the expert:

- Name
- Current post
- Current employer
- Qualifications
- Fully registered with the General Medical Council
- Approved under section 22 of the 2003 Act and with which health board
- A statement that the report is given on soul and conscience
- A statement as to whether the expert is related to the person
- A statement as to whether the expert has any pecuniary interest in the person's admission to hospital or placement on any community-based order
- The expert should sign the report

Treatment) (Scotland) Act 2003 Code of Practice, Volume 3: Compulsory Powers in Relation to Mentally Disordered Offenders (Scottish Executive, 2005) ('the Scottish Code of Practice') is invaluable for psychiatrists preparing reports for criminal proceedings in Scotland and, as already indicated (p. 55), some of its guidance is of more general application. Its guidance on the information expected to be presented within the report, including the expert's qualifications, goes further than the requirements in the other jurisdictions (Box 40). The Scottish Code of Practice should be read in conjunction with the Mental Health (Care and Treatment) (Scotland) Act 2003 (MH(CT)(S)A) and the Criminal Procedure (Scotland) Act 1995 (CP(S)A). *Insanity and Diminished Responsibility* (Scottish Law Commission, 2004) provides guidance on fitness to take part in a trial and what the law regards as constituting diminished responsibility.

The preparation of all criminal cases is carried out, largely, by the procurator fiscal. Serious charges are prosecuted in the name of Her Majesty's advocate. The more serious of these are prosecuted in the High Court by the Lord Advocate (and the advocates depute), while the less serious proceed in a sheriff court, being prosecuted by the procurator fiscal on behalf of the Lord Advocate. Minor charges are prosecuted in the sheriff court and run in the name of the procurator fiscal.

Reports for trial are usually requested by the Crown through the procurator fiscal, who prosecutes the case, and reports for sentencing are requested by the sentencer, who is usually a sheriff. Defence solicitors frequently seek to instruct independent experts but they find it difficult to access them because of restrictions placed on them by their health board employers. There are strict timescales, as summary cases have to come to trial within 40 days and solemn cases within 110 days.

Appropriate adults

The police should always have an appropriate adult present when they interview a person with mental disorder. 'Mental disorder' means any mental illness, personality disorder or learning disability, however caused or manifested (s.328, MH(CT)(S)A). The role of the appropriate adult is to facilitate communication between the police and the person and to provide support. It is the police who have responsibility for requesting the attendance of the appropriate adult. If a medical practitioner decides that a person with a mental disorder is fit to be interviewed, the police should be advised to contact an appropriate adult.

Vulnerable witness provisions

The Vulnerable Witnesses (Scotland) Act 2004 substitutes provisions in s.271 of the CP(S)A and defines a vulnerable witness as a child who is under the age of 16 years at the commencement of the proceedings and an adult if 'there is a significant risk that the quality of the evidence to be given by the person will be diminished by reason of (i) mental disorder within the meaning of the MH(CT)(S)A, or (ii) fear or distress in connection with giving evidence at the trial'. The quality of the evidence means its completeness, coherence and accuracy (s.271(4)). Sections 271A and B set out the special measures for child witnesses and s.271C sets out the special measures for other vulnerable witnesses. Section 271F provides for some of these measures to be applied to an accused child and a vulnerable witness who is the accused. The special measures are the taking of evidence by a commissioner appointed by the court, a live television link, a screen, a supporter, giving evidence in chief in the form of a prior statement and such other measures as may be prescribed by statutory instrument (s.271H).

Box 41 Issues expected to be addressed in a pre-conviction psychiatric report in Scotland

The Scottish Executive (2005, ch. 2, para. 23) has indicated that the following issues should be addressed in a pre-conviction psychiatric report:

- Whether the person appears to be suffering from mental disorder
- Whether an assessment or treatment order is needed
- Whether the person may be insane in bar of trial
- The risk the person poses to self or others
- Whether the person's mental condition may have a bearing on responsibility for the alleged offence
- Whether, if the person was convicted, a mental health disposal would be indicated

Pre-conviction reports and procedures

Box 12 (page 57) sets out the issues that it is expected will be addressed in a report on a person in police custody. Box 41 sets out the issues that the Scottish Executive expects to be addressed in a pre-conviction report. It is expected that, especially if limited information is available, the mental health officer (MHO) will provide useful information, and if a social circumstances report (SCR) has been prepared in accordance with s.231 of the MH(CT)(S)A, relying where available on social work records, this will be used as a source of the person's history, family or carer accounts and the circumstances leading up to the alleged offence.

Assessment and treatment orders

A recommendation for an assessment (s.52B–J, CP(S)A) or treatment (s.K–S, CP(S)A) order should be made only after the medical practitioner has discussed the case with a consultant from the unit to which the person would be admitted and only after this consultant has agreed to the admission. The expert should also seek the advice and assistance of the MHO.

Box 42 Issues to be addressed in a report recommending an assessment order in Scotland

A report recommending an assessment order under s.52(D) of the Mental Health (Care and Treatment) (Scotland) Act 2003 needs to consider the following issues:

- Does it appear that the person has a mental disorder? The category need not be specified.
- Is it likely that detention in hospital is necessary to assess whether the following conditions are met?
  - The person in respect of whom the application is made has a mental disorder.
  - Medical treatment is available which would be likely to prevent the mental disorder worsening or alleviate any of the symptoms, or effects, of the disorder.
  - If the person were not provided with such medical treatment there would be a significant risk to the health, safety or welfare of the person, or to the safety of others.
- Is it likely that there would be a significant risk to the person's health, safety or welfare or to the safety of any other person if the assessment order were not made?
- Is a suitable hospital placement available which will be able to admit the person within seven days of the order being made?
- Is there a reasonable alternative to enable the assessment to be undertaken without making an assessment order?

Box 42 sets out the matters that require specific consideration when recommending an assessment order. For the first three issues, the expert needs to be satisfied only to the extent that there are *reasonable grounds* for believing that they are the case. Discussion with the MHO is essential in order to deal with the last issue, of alternatives to an assessment order.

Insanity in bar of trial

Unfitness to plead is known formally in Scotland as insanity in bar of trial. There are two leading cases. In *HM Advocate v Wilson* (1942) JC 74 the court held that there had to be:

a mental alienation of some kind which prevents the accused giving the instruction which a sane man would give for his defence or from following the evidence as a sane man would follow it and instructing his counsel as the case goes, along any point that arises.

Similarly, in *Stewart v HM Advocate (No. 1)* (1997) JC 183, the court stated:

The question for [the trial judge] was whether the appellant, by reason of his mental handicap, would be unable to instruct his legal representatives as to his defence or to follow what went on at his trial. Without such ability he could not receive a fair trial.

The Scottish Law Commission (2004) provides guidance. It focuses on the functionality of the accused person rather than, simply, on diagnostic issues. The rationale is that a person may suffer from a mental illness or other mental disorder but that does not mean that they cannot function in relation to the role requirements of an accused person. The expert may indeed opine that the accused is disordered but, with the appropriate support and explanation which takes into account the condition, can take part in the trial.

Insanity at the time of the offence

If a person was mentally disordered at the time of the offence, this may affect their legal responsibility for their actions. The leading case is *HM Advocate v Kidd* (1960) JC 61:

in order to excuse a person from responsibility on the grounds of insanity, there must have been an alienation of reason in relation to the act committed. There must have been some mental defect … by which his reason was overpowered, and he was thereby rendered incapable of exerting his reason to control his conduct and reactions. If his reason was alienated in relation to the act committed, he was not responsible for the act, even although otherwise he may have been apparently quite rational.

It is recognised that such concepts as 'mental alienation' are difficult to translate into clinical terms but it is suggested that here this means that 'the mental disorder should be such that it played an overwhelming role in determining the occurrence of the offence. In most cases the person is suffering from a psychotic illness and there is a direct link between positive psychotic symptoms (delusions and hallucinations) and the act committed' (Scottish Code of Practice, ch. 3, para. 26).

Diminished responsibility

Reference has already been made to the 1923 case of *HM Advocate v Savage* (p. 82) and since then the legal criteria for diminished responsibility have been restated in *Galbraith v HM Advocate* (2001) SCCR 551; SLT 953:

In essence, the judge must decide whether there is evidence that, at the relevant time, the accused was suffering from an abnormality of mind which substantially impaired the ability of the accused, as compared with a normal person, to determine or control his acts.

It is recognised that, just as M'Naghten insanity is narrower in scope than diminished responsibility in England and Wales:

The conditions that come within the scope of diminished responsibility are broader than those for insanity. It would be expected that the medical practitioner or other appropriate expert would comment on the mental condition of the person at the time of the homicide and the relative contribution of any mental disorder to the occurrence of the killing. The medical practitioner or other appropriate expert should not state if the person's responsibility was diminished; this is an issue for the jury. (Scottish Code of Practice, ch. 3, para. 31)

Successful mitigation on the grounds of diminished responsibility reduces the offence from murder to culpable homicide (roughly equivalent to manslaughter).

Psychopathic personality disorder (*Carraher v HM Advocate* (1946) SLT 225; *Kennedy v HM Advocate* (1944) JC 171) and voluntary intoxication (*Brennan v HM Advocate* (1977) JC 3) cannot be the basis for a defence of diminished responsibility.

Automatism

Ross v HM Advocate (1991) SLT 564, (1991) JC 210, where the defendant had LSD and other drugs slipped into his beer and made a violent attack on others in a public house, established that intoxication can be a defence if it can be proved on evidence given that the intoxication was not self-induced and that the defendant was, as a result, incapable of forming an intention, that is, was acting in a state of non-insane automatism.

Box 43 Possible disposal recommendations in insanity cases in Scotland

- A compulsion order
- A compulsion and restriction order
- An interim compulsion order
- A guardianship order
- A supervision and treatment order
- No order

Disposal

Where it is likely that a person will be found insane in bar of trial or acquitted on the ground of insanity, the report may be required to address the most appropriate disposal.

If an accused is found insane in bar of trial, the case proceeds with an examination of the facts: if it is decided that an offence was committed, the case proceeds to determine disposal; if it is decided that an offence was not committed, that is the end of the criminal case, but if the accused suffers from a mental disorder that still needs to be addressed within the terms of the care and treatment legalisation. The disposals are very similar, but not identical. By covering both eventualities in the report, the appropriate disposal is more likely to be achieved. Recommendations for disposal will depend on the nature of the mental disorder, the person's needs and the risk they pose to others. Box 43 shows the options for disposal.

For the final disposal, where a mental health disposal is recommended, it is expected that there will be a multidisciplinary assessment (except for

---

Box 44 Possible mental health and non-mental health disposal options in Scotland for offenders with a mental disorder

If further assessment and/or treatment is required prior to final disposal:

- assessment order (s.52D)
- treatment order (s.52M)
- committal to hospital (s.200)
- interim compulsion order (s.53)

Final mental health disposals

- Hospital disposals
  - Compulsion order (s.57A)
  - Compulsion order and a restriction order (s.57A and 59)
  - Hospital direction (s.59A)
- Community disposals
  - Compulsion order (s.57A)
  - Guardianship order (s.58(1)A))
  - Treatment as a condition of probation (s.230)
  - Voluntary treatment

Non-mental health disposals

- Prison sentence
- Probation order
- Community service order
- Fine
- Deferred sentence
- Admonishment

---

probation orders with a condition of psychiatric treatment under s.230 of the CP(S)A). If psychological interventions will be a major aspect of treatment, a psychologist, or any appropriately qualified person responsible for the psychological intervention, should be consulted. Box 44 sets out all of the mental health disposals open to the court.

The criteria for special restrictions on discharge from hospital (s.59, CP(S)A) relate to: (1) the nature of the offence; (2) the antecedents of the person; and (3) the risk that as a result of the mental disorder the person would commit offences if set at large. Special restrictions, without limit of time, can be imposed for the protection of the public from serious harm. It is expected that in such a case there would be a significant link between the specified mental disorder and the offence and/or the future risk posed. Where this link is absent or small, it would be expected that the appropriate recommendation would be for a hospital direction under s.59(A) of the CP(S)A. Where such an order is considered, it is expected that an interim compulsion order would be recommended first. A report in such a case should address the role of special restrictions in facilitating future management.

For a probation order requiring treatment for a mental condition, the treatment requirement can be for the full three-year length of the order, but before making the order the court must be satisfied, on the evidence of a medical practitioner or chartered psychologist under whom the treatment will be given, that the relevant services are available and appropriate (s.230(3) CP(S)A).

Civil law

The highest civil court in Scotland is the Supreme Court of the United Kingdom. Therefore, following the doctrine of precedent, a decision of the Supreme Court in an English case will be binding in Scotland and vice versa, except where the substantive law differs, in which case the decisions of the Supreme Court would be persuasive but not binding. Decisions in other common law jurisdictions, for example Australia and New Zealand, if relevant, will be considered and may be persuasive but they are not binding.

Capacity

The Adults with Incapacity (Scotland) Act 2000 as amended by the Adult Support and Protection (Scotland) Act 2007 is the statute that governs capacity issues. Section 1(6) defines 'incapacity' as meaning that the person is incapable of (1) acting, or (2) making decisions, or (3) communicating decisions, or (4) understanding decisions or (5) retaining the memory of decisions by reason of mental disorder or of inability to communicate because of physical disability.

Under s.20(A)(3) of the Marriage (Scotland) Act 1977, a marriage is void if, at the time of the ceremony, a party to the marriage was incapable of understanding the nature of marriage or incapable of consenting to it. Such lack of capacity may arise from mental illness or mental impairment. If it is alleged that a marriage is void on such grounds, there is a very heavy burden on the person asserting this to prove it (*Long v Long* (1950) SLT (Notes) 32). Alcohol or drug intoxication can be a ground for annulment. Mary Brown's marriage was annulled on the grounds that she was so inebriated at the time of the ceremony and for the following three days that she lacked the capacity to consent (*Scott v Kelly* (1823) 25 495). Under s.20(A)(2) a marriage can be annulled on the ground that a party purported to give consent but did so only by reason of duress. Here the test of duress is a common law test and a subjective test, so personality or other psychological factors may be relevant in deciding whether or not the party was overcome by force or fear.

Personal injury cases

Delict law, which is roughly equivalent to tort law, is about putting right legal wrongs. The fundamental principle is that 'pursuers' should, as far as possible, be put into the position they would have been in had the delict not occurred. Therefore reports in personal injury cases serve a similar function to those in England and Wales.

Family cases

In Scotland, the civil courts deal with many family cases, particularly in relation to disputed residence or contact with children following the breakdown of a relationship or contact with a child where the parties were never in an established relationship. The children hearing system is concerned with children in need of protection, when such care and protection are not being appropriately provided by the family system. These children's hearings, before three members of the local children's panel, have the power to make decisions about the care of children, such as child protection orders and supervision requirements. The panels also deal with children who have committed offences, although in the case of very serious crimes or crimes committed with an adult, the child may be prosecuted in the High Court or a sheriff court. The hearings have a welfare focus but increasingly there is legal representation.

Vulnerable witnesses

Sections 11–22 of the Vulnerable Witnesses (Scotland) Act 2004 apply to civil proceedings, and make similar provisions to those that apply in criminal proceedings (see p. 206).

Further reading

Ireland

Casey, P. (2003*a*) Expert testimony in court. 1: General principles. *Advances in Psychiatric Treatment*, **9**, 177–182.

Ward, P. (2010) *Family Law in Ireland*. Kluwer Law International BV.

Jersey

Attorney General v O'Driscoll [2003 JLR 390].

Scotland

Chiswick, D. (2003) Expert testimony in court. (Invited commentary.) *Advances in Psychiatric Treatment*, **9**, 187–189.

Scottish Executive (2005) *Mental Health (Care and Treatment) (Scotland) Act 2003 Code of Practice, Volume 3: Compulsory Powers in Relation to Mentally Disordered Offenders*. Scottish Executive.

Scottish Law Commission (2004) *Insanity and Diminished Responsibility in the Criminal Law*. (Discussion Paper No. 122.) Scottish Law Commission.

Thomson, J. (2006) *Family Law in Scotland* (5th edn). Tottel.

CHAPTER 11

Going to court

The court must always be on the guard against the over-dogmatic expert, the expert whose reputation or amour proper is at stake, or the expert who has developed a scientific prejudice. (*R v Cannings* [2004] EWCA Crim 1)

Avoiding it

The best way to avoid going to court is to produce a report that enables the parties to settle the case or which is so straightforward that in a criminal case parts of it are read to the jury or it is read by the judge without your having to attend.

You can also avoid going to court by producing a report upon which those instructing you do not seek to rely and which they do not disclose. But two cases are informative here.

Dr Harry Egdell discovered that his independent mental health tribunal report was not being disclosed to the tribunal considering a patient's application for a conditional discharge. In the meantime the patient had withdrawn his application to the tribunal. Dr Egdell asked his instructing solicitors for permission to send a copy to the hospital's assistant medical director. The solicitors refused. Dr Egdell readdressed the report to the assistant medical director and sent it to him. A copy went to the Home Office and the Home Office referred the case to a tribunal under s.72(2) of the MHA. The patient brought claims against Dr Egdell and others. They were dismissed by the first-instance judge. The patient appealed unsuccessfully (*W v Egdell and Others* [1990] 4 BMLR 1990). Sir Stephen Brown P, held that:

The balance of the public interest clearly lay in the restricted disclosure of vital information to the director of the hospital and to the secretary of state who had the onerous duty of safeguarding public safety.

Bingham LJ gave a concurring judgment:

A consultant psychiatrist who becomes aware, even in the course of a confidential relationship, of information which leads him, in the exercise of what the court considered a sound professional judgment, to fear that such decisions may be made on the basis of inadequate information and with a real risk of consequent danger to the public is entitled to take such steps as are reasonable in all the circumstances to communicate the grounds of his concern to the responsible authorities.

In *R v Crozier* [1988] 8 BMLR 128, the psychiatrist who had prepared a report in a case of attempted murder, recommending a hospital order with restrictions under ss.37 and 41 of the MHA, arrived late at court to find that the defendant had been sentenced to nine years' imprisonment. His report had not been brought to the attention of defence counsel. The psychiatrist, alarmed at the sentence imposed, disclosed his report to counsel for the Crown, who then applied for a variation of sentence. The judge quashed the sentence of imprisonment and substituted the s.37/41 order. The defendant appealed against his sentence alleging, *inter alia*, that the psychiatrist had breached the duty of confidentiality between doctor and client. Referring to the case of *Egdell*, the court found that this was also a case in which there was a strong public interest in the disclosure of the psychiatrist's views, which took precedence over the confidence that he owed the appellant. They acquitted the psychiatrist of any impropriety. In a very difficult situation he had acted responsibly and reasonably.

Disclosure in the public interest is a matter about which the General Medical Council (2004) states that:

Personal information may be disclosed in the public interest, without the patient's consent, where the benefits to an individual or to society of the disclosure outweigh the public and the patient's interest in keeping the information confidential. (para. 22)

and:

Disclosure of personal information without consent may be justified in the public interest where failure to do so may expose the patient or others to risk of death or serious harm. (para. 27)

This makes it clear that if you disclose a report without the consent of the subject and/or the subject's solicitors and seek to rely on *Egdell* or *Crozier* you should do so only where there may be a risk of serious harm or death to the patient or others if the report is not disclosed.

Be prepared

If you are a party-appointed expert, you will probably be called to give evidence by the party that has instructed you, but there is 'no property in a witness'. An expert may be called by any party to the proceedings notwithstanding that the original instructions came from another party (*Harmony Shipping Co SA v Saudi Europe Line* [1979] 1 WLR 1380). This is particularly likely to happen if you have prepared a report for the CPS upon which the CPS does not want to rely. It will have been disclosed to the defence and so you may be called as a defence witness.

At present you can expect to be called to give evidence on your own. You may be called before or after the other side's expert ('back to back') so that all of the psychiatric evidence is heard at the same time. A development to be watched is 'concurrent expert evidence' or 'hot-tubbing'. Now established in Australia and undergoing a trial in the Manchester Technology and Construction Court and Mercantile Court, this involves calling all of the experts at the same time. The seating arrangements are likely to be rather ad hoc, with perhaps one side's experts in the dock and the other side's experts in the jury benches. The agenda is based on the matters not agreed at the experts' meeting, supplemented by any additional issues that have arisen in the trial thus far. In relation to each issue, the judge initiates a discussion by asking each expert for their views; the judge then has the opportunity to question the expert and so also, on the invitation of the judge, do the other experts. Then the parties' representatives are given the opportunity to ask their questions but only to test the correctness of an expert's view or clarify it. They should not cover ground already fully explored and in general a full cross-examination or re-examination is not appropriate. Finally, the judge may seek to summarise the experts' positions and ask them to confirm or correct the summary. Such an approach favours the well-prepared expert (preparations should include careful consideration of questions for the other experts), but it may require experts to learn some advocacy skills. The outcome of the trial is awaited and it may be some time before psychiatrists are involved in concurrent expert evidence.

The best preparation for going to court is to produce a quality report that enables the parties and the court to narrow down your evidence to that which needs elucidation; the report itself should deal with as much as possible of what might be put to you in cross-examination.

In many cases, there will be a conference with counsel the day before the trial starts, as well as one shortly before you give your evidence. Prepare for this as if it were the trial. Have your file properly organised and complete. 'Nothing is more annoying than the witness who fiddles about with all sorts of tatty bits of paper, in the apparently forlorn hope of finding something relevant' (Braithwaite & Waldron, 2010, p. 144). Be ready to learn from the way the barrister tests your opinion. Barristers should challenge you about your work. They want to know what you are going to say when cross-examined and your opinion is put under attack. It is in their interests to explore any potential area of uncertainty or weakness. See it as a 'dummy run'. They want to see that you are:

Confident, personable, able to explain technical issues clearly and prepared to entertain alternative points of view. Or are [you] flustered, unsure, dogmatic and possibly just outraged at the tone of your questioning...[?] (Smethurst, 2006)

Make sure that you know the questions you are likely to be asked to address by your barrister. Ask how you will be expected to give your evidence, where the barrister wants you to sit in court (usually experts sit beside the solicitor and behind the barrister) and whether you will have to hear other evidence. Be clear about the time in the proceedings at which you are expected to attend. If you are going to have to base your opinion on facts proved by the evidence of other witnesses, it is usual to be allowed to be present in court for their evidence but for this the judge will have to give permission as the court has to decide what other evidence you should be able to hear, or details of the court proceedings you should know about, before you give your own evidence. Although most court proceedings are open to the public, witnesses may be debarred until after they have given evidence.

You need to have a basic understanding of court procedures. This will help you coordinate optimally with your instructing solicitors or their counsel and engage effectively with the trial judge. If it is the first time you are going to court, it should not be. You certainly should not enter a courtroom for the first time in your life when you go to give expert evidence. Shadow another expert, sit in the public gallery in a few cases or ask your presiding judge if you can sit with a judge and benefit from some tuition. Otherwise, watch a few episodes of *Kavanagh QC* or *Judge Deed*, but not *Perry Mason*, and do not expect all judges to have such interesting private lives as Judge Deed.

On the subject of judges, at the 2010 Grange annual conference Bill Braithwaite QC recommended that you should ask *about* the judge, his or her foibles and professional background. Please note the word 'about' – although many judges joke about being the subject of a psychiatric report, they may not take too kindly to a formal psychiatric assessment before your examination in chief. Perhaps experts should contribute to a website devoted to judges' foibles. This might make as interesting reading as the files some barristers maintain on experts.

Allow sufficient time to read not only your report but also other expert reports. It is a good idea to prepare a handwritten or typed critique of the reports of the other expert or experts that identifies their strong/good and weak/bad points, as well as the points agreed and those not agreed, and why points are not agreed.

Familiarise yourself again with the factual basis for your opinions. Remind yourself of, and annotate, key evidence in medical records, witness statements or documentary exhibits. If you are allowed to take your own files into the witness box, which is almost always allowed, use coloured marker tags and highlighting to make it easy to navigate your way round the important information. Anticipate questions and have coloured tags with the subject written on it. If you know your way round the documents you will be a more confident and authoritative witness. If you have to fumble backwards and forwards through your files or retrieve scattered sheets of paper from the well of the court, your credibility may be damaged. But you need to ask counsel whether or not you can take annotated and marked files into the witness box.

If you are not going to be able to take your own files, because the court insists that you work from a 'clean copy', try to memorise some of the key points and practise reducing your opinions into a few memorable bullet points, but it is preferable to have them written down. However, giving evidence should not be a memory test or game. Be that as it may, be clear about your main points before you give evidence. Do a 'dummy run' with your secretary, some other lay person or even a teenager. Make a list of the questions that are likely to be put to you in cross-examination and what your answers would be. Some of these you will have anticipated and addressed in your report. Others should have been suggested to you by the barrister who is calling you and who should have put as many as possible of these to you in conference.

You have to appear, as you should be, the master of the facts and your opinion. If not, you will lose credibility with the judge or jury, or both. As Braithwaite & Waldron (2010, p. 145) say: 'Part of the art of being a good witness, and therefore a good expert, is to be able to communicate opinions clearly, despite provocation from opposing counsel, to someone who seems ignorant of the basics'.

Usually there will be a 'trial bundle' containing all the documents. Get this in advance and number the pages of your report to correspond to its page numbers in the trial bundle or put your copy of the report into the bundle, with corresponding numbering, so that you have everything at your fingertips. Familiarise yourself with the organisation and contents of the trial bundle and where your opinion relates to key passages in, for example, medical records, have these tagged so that you can refer to them quickly. Remember that sometimes pagination, especially of medical records, will differ from the pagination in the records as they were originally supplied and you may even have to spend time changing all the page references in your report to correspond to the numbering in the trial bundle.

Performance on the day is proportional to preparation. Never tire of rereading your report with a critical eye and cross-check carefully your references to the medical records. As a final stage in preparation remind yourself of the test which the judge will apply when evaluating your evidence (see Box 45, p. 225).

Dress, demeanour and etiquette

Dress and behaviour should convey an appropriate professional demeanour. Be punctual. Plan to arrive 30 minutes early and you will have time to get organised.

Nod or bow slightly in the direction of the judge when entering, leaving or moving about in court. If you need to speak to someone, keep your voice down. Do not speak or move about when a witness or juror is taking the oath or affirming.

Outside court

A lot of time is spent outside the courtroom. Be careful to whom you speak. You can talk to those instructing you. Do not discuss your evidence with other witnesses, especially the witnesses for the other side, without permission. Do not talk to the other side's solicitor or barrister unless specifically instructed to do so by the solicitor or barrister who is calling you. This does not mean that you cannot exchange greetings or other pleasantries. As long as the parties agree, there is usually no reason why you should not talk to your opposite number about matters unrelated to the case. Occasionally experts are asked to confer on an issue, on a 'without prejudice' basis, and report back to their respective solicitor or barrister. The court may adjourn for such a meeting to take place or continue the proceedings while it takes place. Usually you will be provided with a conference room for the purpose. Make careful notes. Such meetings can assist the parties in narrowing issues further. Remember that you will need the court's permission to refer to the contents of a 'without prejudice' meeting.

Forms of address

Etiquette requires an appropriate form of address for the judge (see Appendix 10). Ask the barrister or solicitor how to address the judge. Some courtrooms have a notice outside that gives the form of address. You may have the opportunity to hear what terms the solicitors or barristers use. If you are stuck, you may or may not want to apply the convention of calling every police 'constable' 'sergeant' and although a circuit judge will not object to being 'My Lord' instead of 'Your Honour' you will only draw attention to your ignorance if 'Your Honour' comes out as 'Your Holiness'. Fall back on 'Sir'/'Madam'. The worst is to call a judge 'Your Worship'.

Giving evidence

When you are called to give evidence, go to the witness box. The judge, jury and other side's counsel may be looking at you for the first time. Do not make extended eye contact with those instructing you, as you are there to assist the court. If you have not already been asked, whisper to the court usher and tell him or her whether you will take the oath, on an appropriate religious text, or make the affirmation.

Face the judge. If it is the oath, take the book in your right hand and hold it just below shoulder level with the elbow flexed at about 45 degrees (not with arm outstretched like a Nazi salute). Either repeat the oath after the usher or judge or read it from the card. If possible, wait for eye contact with the judge but do not wait too long! If you make eye contact at this point, you are already establishing a rapport with the judge. Alternatively, in a criminal case, look at the middle of the back row of the jury.

The judge may invite you to sit. Standing, if you are able to do so, usually makes a better impression unless you cannot see to read. The judge and jury will scrutinise your body language closely. Remember that as judges do not have to think about the next question to ask, they are well placed to observe your body language as you respond to the questions.

If there is an adjournment during your evidence, do not talk to anyone about the case. The judge should remind you of this.

Evidence in chief

Your counsel starts. You will be asked your full name, address and appointment. Give your professional address. Keep your feet facing the judge and swivel to listen to counsel ('the turning technique'). Swivel back, if there is no jury, to address your answer to the judge; if there is a jury, still address the judge but look at the furthermost juror and make sure your voice reaches that far. Addressing the judge or judge and jury is both courteous and it further assists with building rapport.

Keep your eye on the judge. Judges will often tell you to watch their pen or their fingers, as they will be usually be writing or typing a note of your evidence. If they are not, do not panic but ask yourself why not. It might be a rare situation in which there is a computer link from the court stenographer to the judge's bench. Only when the judge has finished writing or typing, turn back slowly to face counsel and signal that you are ready for the next question. Keep control.

There will probably be a microphone. This is usually to record your evidence and not to amplify your voice. If you are repeatedly reminded to speak up, or more slowly, it will adversely affect the impression you make.

You will probably be asked to look at the signature page of your report, in the trial bundle, confirm that it is your report and signature, and confirm that it continues to be your opinion, or explain if not. Correct any significant errors and indicate whether or not your opinion needs to be modified in the light of any evidence you have heard. Any other change of opinion should already have been communicated; if necessary, remind the court that you have done so. Remember, however, that in a criminal case the jury will not have seen your report, although the judge, counsel and/or solicitors will have done.

In a criminal case you may be asked for your qualifications. If you have set them out fully, in Appendix 1 to your report, you may be asked to confirm x, y and z. Counsel should have advised you how much they want to elicit. If given free reign, do not confuse the jury with letters of the alphabet in what they will see as random order. 'The basic qualification of a doctor' makes more sense than 'MB, BS', and 'MB, BChir' will have them looking for your chair. If you have an 'MD', the older ones will be telling the younger ones that you are like Dr Kildare. In a civil or family case you may be asked only to confirm that your qualifications are as set out in Appendix 1. The judge will have read the report.

If there is a jury, remember that you must be understood by the least intelligent member and remember that few lawyers and at the time of writing no judges are medically qualified. Prepare for the trial a brief summary of your opinion in simple language and rehearse delivering it to the jury. It is not enough to have a glossary of medical terms. You will have to explain medical terms so that everyone in court can understand. A few weeks after I gave evidence about hyperventilation in a rape case, I was in the same court building and responded, with two or three pathologists, to a request for any doctor in the building to make their way to the jury waiting area. On the stairs, we met the court clerk, who had been in my previous case, and he told us that there was no hurry as it was just a case of hyperventilation and the juror was recovering with the aid of a paper bag. His diagnosis and treatment were correct.

This is your evidence in chief. Questioned by your counsel, in a criminal case, you will be taken over the key points in your report. The longer this takes, the more your confidence grows. In a civil case your report stands as your evidence in chief, so do not expect much more than a request to confirm that it remains your opinion, but counsel may get you to expand on certain points or respond to questions based on evidence already given of which you are unaware or of which you were unaware when you prepared your report. Some judges, however, like to hear experts explain their relevant expertise and set out their key points.

Cross-examination

Then comes cross-examination. Remember to swivel back to face the judge and/or jury when you have heard the question. Keep calm, as a change in demeanour can give the wrong impression. Not looking at your cross-examiner helps. Console yourself in the fact that you and the other experts know more than counsel or the judge does about the subject of your evidence. Barristers are not experts in your field but they may try to give that impression. They have the advantage, however, of knowing what the next question will be; they are likely to have done extensive reading on your subject, with the help of others experts; and they may also have the advantage of being assisted by your opposite number (if there is one), who will be furiously scribbling adhesive notes that your cross-examiner will line up where you can see them in order to remind you whom they think is in control. This may seem partisan but your cross-examiner is entitled to have the assistance of an expert in order to be able to test your opinions properly.

The purpose of cross-examination is to weaken, qualify or destroy the other side's case. So, be prepared for an attack on your veracity and expertise.

Be able to explain why your qualifications and experience are relevant and why you should be regarded as at least comparable in qualifications, training and experience to the other side's expert. The bigger the case, the more likely it is that your cross-examiner will use your CV to persuade the judge that you are not qualified and use any other information, whether or not in the public domain, to discredit you. Cross-examination will include testing the validity of your opinions and bringing out evidence that supports the other side's case.

Remember a Maudsley-style case conference where several professors and other psychiatrists question your opinion. Try to bear in mind, but you should have anticipated, the stimulating, helpful and clarifying points that you would make in response to their questions.

Do not be drawn into a contest or argument. You are there to assist the court. It is the lawyers who argue:

While I am sure that both experts were trying to assist the Court, I found the evidence of Dr [X] of more assistance than that of Dr [Y]. Although Dr [X]'s measured and careful approach was more persuasive than Dr [Y]'s more argumentative and didactic approach, it was not just the manner in which they gave their evidence. It seemed to me that the content of Dr [Y]'s evidence was unconvincing: for example. ... (Simon J in *Rabone v Pennine Care NHS Trust* [2009] LS Law Med 503)

The judge wants to know your opinion, and does not want to witness, or have to referee, an argument or slanging match. The case is not about you. As soon as you start arguing, you lose your objectivity and give the impression that you are not impartial. Remember that 'anything other than a courteous, moderated and seemingly impartial response to questioning in court will damage [your] credibility' (Lewis, 2006: p. 128). If your cross-examiner does engage in fencing, the judge may not like it.

According to expert witness folklore 'crafted in the wine bars of The Strand ... [the cross examiner] has three minutes to unsettle the expert and consign the expert's opinion into the bin marked "Thank you very much for coming". If this is not achieved, it is said, the barrister's task will be that much harder' (Smethurst, 2006).

So keep calm. Do not rush into answering the question but do not delay too long. This may allow time for your counsel to object or require clarification and it allows time for your considered response.

You may be asked a very technical or medical question at an early stage and your cross-examiner will be wanting to try to unsettle you with an impression that they have an immediate and full grasp of the medical issues (Smethurst, 2006). Barristers are taught to ask only questions to which they know the answer. If you have to ask for clarification, it may be the barrister who becomes unsettled.

Even when you are asked closed ('yes'/'no') questions do not hesitate if appropriate to add some important qualifications. If you do not, you will have forgotten them later or you will not see how to introduce them. If you think that an explanation is needed, give it. If you do not say all you need to say on an issue, you have only yourself to blame if it was your only opportunity. If necessary, appeal to the judge and make it clear that the answer depends on 'x' or 'y'.

Answer the question asked. It is not in your interests to answer, however well, anything other than the question you have been asked. Wait to answer the next question, even if you know what it is, and do not be evasive. If the question takes you outside your expertise, say so and if necessary, appeal to the judge.

Do not hesitate to ask for a question to be repeated or clarified.

Do not be rushed. If it is a particularly difficult question, write it down and do not be afraid to ask for more time. The judge wants your carefully considered opinion and not the first thing that comes into your head.

Keep your answers to the point. Do not give a lecture. The longer the answer is, the more cross-examination it generates.

If your cross-examiner creates a 'pregnant pause', beware filling it. If in doubt, it is even more important to keep answers brief; otherwise this is when you are most likely to fall into hidden traps.

If you are asked several questions in one, repeat the questions you remember, write them down, answer these and then ask to be reminded of the others. There is no reason why you should not write down even a single question in order to be sure that you understand it and answer it (rather than answer another question). You will not be criticised for asking to be reminded of the questions, although counsel may be criticised for asking so many at once.

If you are interrupted, for example with 'We'll come back to this point' – perhaps because the cross-examiner does not want to hear what you have to say – politely insist on completing your answer.

If you are asked to make an assumption, do not be afraid to question it. If you do not, it might be assumed that you accept it. Even if you are not sure about its basis, it tips off your counsel, so, by the time you are re-examined, they may use your evidence to invalidate the assumption. Make it clear how your answer differs according to whether it is based on hypothesis or what appear to be the actual facts.

You may be questioned about a specific point in a document. If so, ask to be directed to the relevant part of the trial bundle. It gives you time to think, you can check exactly what is in the document, which may not be what was in the question, and you can and should read the lines before and after it so that you see it in context. If you want to draw attention to the context so that the reference is not taken in misleading isolation, address the context before you give your answer, otherwise you will be thanked for your answer and counsel may move on quickly to avoid you referring to the context.

You may be asked if the opinion of the other side's expert is within the range of reasonable opinion. If you agree, say so, but say why you think that your opinion should be preferred.

Be prepared for the fact that some of your opinions may not appear to survive cross-examination. Do not hesitate to make appropriate concessions. You will gain no respect for sticking to your opinion through thick and thin if the evidence does not justify this.

You should be able to recognise when you are being led up the garden path and the end of the path is obvious. If there do not seem to be answers that can halt your passage, do not fear. If there was no alternative but to go to the end of the path, you will be credited for having gone there. If there was another path you ought to have taken, your own counsel will probably have seen it and will take you there in re-examination.

You may be asked questions which require some memory of the evidence. However well you have prepared, there will be some evidence that you will have forgotten. Do not answer if you do not remember the evidence. Ask to be reminded. Take time, but not too long, to look through your documents.

If you are asked about a document that you have not seen previously, ask for sufficient time to read and understand it properly. Read it carefully at least twice. Do not feel that you are under pressure of time and in any case the judge may see this is an opportunity for a coffee or tea break.

Cross-examination is meant to be conducted with courtesy. Occasionally it is not. However unpleasant your cross-examiner is, remain calm and relentlessly polite. Do not lose your cool, get angry or flustered, or allow a barrister to get under your skin. Avoid being defensive or argumentative. Do not try to score points. Concentrate on the question and not how it is asked. If it appears that a question is based on a misunderstanding, answer in a way that implies counsel's misunderstanding rather than total ignorance. Appeal to the judge more in sorrow than in anger. If it seems that your cross-examiner is trying to be really offensive, appeal to the judge, but with some restraint, suggesting that you have been misunderstood. The case is not about you; unless you have failed in your duties as an expert, you should not be subjected to personal attack. When the judge or jury retires, you may have made the better impression.

Watch out for questions that tempt you to give a different answer, perhaps disguised, to that already given in evidence or in your report. Just confirm what you have already said. The more times you are asked the same question, the more desperate counsel is getting. Remain consistent and calm.

However well you think you have prepared and however good your report, you are bound to be asked something that you have not anticipated. Take your time. Remember that you are there to assist the court and it is not a contest between you and your cross-examiner. Give your answer after careful consideration. Give your opinion rather than an argument for one side or the other. Avoid being too definite. Avoid 'never' and 'always' but equally beware of 'possibly'. A degree of uncertainty on one point may make the court more likely to accept the evidence that you have given with greater certainty on another.

If you do not know the answer to a question, be up-front about it.

If questioning appears to have blown a hole in your side's case, do not try to repair the damage unless you can do so as an expert. By the time you are re-examined, your counsel will have had time to think about this and, if you missed a point, you may be led to deliver it.

If you think that you have given an incorrect answer, say so as soon as possible, even if it means interrupting another line of enquiry. It will be useless writing three weeks later to make the point.

If the cross-examiner responds with a look of disbelief or puzzlement, do not worry. Like the pregnant pause, it may be intended to encourage you to say something you might not otherwise say. Wait for the actual question. There may not be one.

Do not be taken by surprise at the suddenness of the ending of the cross-examination, but, if your cross-examiner says that she or he has only a few more points, or it will not last much longer, do not lower your guard.

Some advise that the end of cross-examination is the best time to turn to the judge, if it is appropriate, and ask to be allowed to make some further points, if you think that the thrust of your evidence has not been taken on board. But be careful. First, you should have got your message across already. Second, if permitted, it will inevitably invite further cross-examination. Third, you are about to be re-examined. Counsel should have picked up anything which needs rectifying or clarifying.

Throughout, remember that you are there to assist the court and not to support the side that has instructed you. Assisting the court depends on your ability to connect with the judge and jury. Box 45 is an example of how one judge evaluated the oral testimony of medical expert witnesses. Box 46 lists a number of 'don'ts' for experts.

Box 45 A judge's test of experts' oral testimony

Stuart Smith LJ in *Loveday v Renton and Wellcome Foundation* [1990] 1 Med LR 117–204 indicated that judges evaluate experts' oral testimony on the basis of the following:

- The internal consistency and logic of the evidence
- The care with which experts have considered the subject of the report and prepared their evidence
- Their precision and accuracy of thought as demonstrated by their answers
- How they respond to searching and informed cross-examination
- The extent to which they face up to and accept the logic of a proposition put in cross-examination or are prepared to concede points that are seen to be correct
- The extent to which they have conceived an opinion and are reluctant to re-examine it in the light of later evidence, or demonstrate a flexibility of mind which may involve changing or modifying opinions previously held
- Whether or not they are biased or lack independence
- Their demeanour in the witness box.

Box 46 'Don'ts' for the expert witness giving evidence

Babitsky *et al* (2000, p. 140) list the following 'don'ts' for experts witnesses giving evidence:

- Act in a condescending manner
- Be sharp
- Be pompous
- Be verbose
- Appear egotistical
- Change demeanour on cross-examination
- Be pedantic
- Confuse the jury
- Argue with counsel
- Patronise
- Praise yourself
- Engage in nervous habits
- Be arrogant
- Fumble for papers or documents
- Be boring
- Look or act anxious, nervous or worried
- Be cute
- Turn your back on the jury
- Be overconfident
- Overwhelm the jury.

Re-examination

After cross-examination comes re-examination. This is limited to the clarification of points made in cross-examination. It is not your opportunity to make new points or get over what you have forgotten. Only with the leave of the court can new points be introduced. This is your counsel's opportunity to regain ground lost, or repair damage sustained, during your cross-examination. As you are there to assist the court, not those instructing you, resist the temptation to join battle. Just answer the question; keep it simple. Your credibility depends upon the judge and jury seeing you as independent. Any other approach will undermine your evidence. Generally, no leading questions are allowed, lest they suggest an answer that is different to what you have given in cross-examination; so re-examination may be limited or non-existent. This is the best time to turn to the judge, if it is appropriate, and ask to be allowed to make some further points. It may be your last chance to get your points across. Just be prepared for some more cross-examination after doing so.

Remember:

The way in which you give your evidence affects the weight of credibility attached to it. Imagine that, if your evidence is clear, succinct and truthful, it will weigh down heavily on the scales of justice. ... If, however, your evidence is confusing, and you are nervous, aggressive, pompous, rambling and inflexible, it will be given little or no weight. (Bond *et al*, 2007, p. 126)

If there is no re-examination, take it as a compliment to the clarity of the evidence you have given.

Questions from the judge

Even if the judge has already asked some questions, be prepared for more and remember that your counsel and your cross-examiner may want to clarify your answers.

Afterwards

The judge will probably thank you for your attendance. Reciprocate with a simple nod and, without grovelling, express appreciation, if appropriate, for accommodating your attendance to minimise interference with your professional duties or to allow you to go on that much-deserved foreign holiday. However, if there is a jury, it is important to limit yourself to an appropriately formal response.

You may be released by the court but your counsel may want you to assist in the cross-examination of the other side's expert (if you have not already done so). To do so, you will need to sit behind counsel and pass forward handwritten notes suggesting questions. For this you need a pad of adhesive notes so that they can be attached to the back of the seat adjacent to the barrister and then you need the confidence to tug at the barrister's gown when it is necessary to draw attention to them, but also the skill to avoid distracting counsel while he or she is speaking.

Afterwards, find out about the outcome. It matters not 'which side has won'. Has your testimony assisted?

Further reading

Bond, C., Solon, M., Harper, P., *et al* (2007) *The Expert Witness: A Practical Guide* (3rd edn). Shaw & Sons.
Casey, P. (2003*b*) Expert testimony in court. 2: In the witness box. *Advances in Psychiatric Treatment*, **9**, 183–190.
Cooper, P. (2010) Cross-examination: trick or fair treatment. *Expert Witness Institute Newsletter*, autumn, 20–21.

CHAPTER 12

Maintaining and developing expertise and knowing when to stop

The more you understand about the judicial thought processes, the more valuable, I am sure, will be your contribution to the outcome of individual cases. (Wall, 2007, p. xvii)

Maintaining and developing expertise

If you want to maintain and develop your role as a psychiatric expert, you will have to keep up to date. It should go without saying that this means not just keeping up to date and fit to practise as a psychiatrist but also as a doctor, including being proficient in cardiopulmonary resuscitation. Court users in Bradford, and not least a particular judge, are likely to remember Dr Ray Travers, not for his expert psychiatric evidence in a murder trial, but for his athletic response and clinical skill, when he rendered assistance after the judge collapsed to the floor.

The following are just a few suggestions.

Maintaining clinical practice

It is important to maintain your clinical practice. Medico-legal work used to be what consultants did when they retired. Heed what Moses LJ said in *Henderson*:

The fact that an expert is in clinical practice at the time he makes his report is of significance. Clinical practice affords experts the opportunity to maintain and develop their experience. Such experts acquire experience which continues and develops. Their continuing observation, the experience of both the foreseen and unforeseen, the recognised and the unrecognised, form a powerful basis for their opinion. Clinicians learn from each case in which they are engaged. Each case makes them think and as their experience develops so does their understanding. Continuing experience gives them the opportunity to adjust previously held opinions, to alter their views. They are best placed to recognise that that which is unknown one day may be acknowledged the next. Such clinical experience ... may provide a far more reliable source of evidence than that provided by those who have ceased to practise their expertise in a continuing clinical setting and have retired from such practice. ... They have lost the opportunity, day by day to learn and develop from continuing experience.

Registration with and licensing by the General Medical Council

You should maintain your registration with the GMC. Unless your only role as an expert is to come out of retirement to give evidence as to normal psychiatric practice at the time when you were in practice, you should hold a licence to practise. If you do not, you may find that an otherwise equally well-qualified but licensed psychiatrist's evidence is preferred to your own.

Indemnity and insurance

You should have indemnity or insurance cover from an MDO or insurer for your medico-legal work. This is particularly important now that the Supreme Court in the case of *Jones v Kaney* has abolished the immunity from suit for expert witnesses, at least in respect of claims by a litigant to whom the expert owes a duty.

Section 12 approval

It is advisable to remain approved under s.12 of the MHA. This is evidence of your 'special experience in the diagnosis or treatment of mental disorder', although it is often rendered in expert reports with 'and' instead of 'or' and sometimes other variations even less accurate. In some circumstances, medical evidence is not admissible from registered and licensed medical practitioners unless they are also approved under s.12 of the Act. In such cases, one of the first questions in examination in chief is about s.12 status. I was in court when my opposite number had to admit that his approval had expired six weeks previously and this was in a case where evidence had to be given by a s.12 approved doctor.

Peer groups and personal development plans

It will help to have in your CPD peer group at least one other member who is also a psychiatric expert. You will be able to help each other formulate personal development plans (PDPs) that address your role as an expert witness.

If there is no other psychiatric expert witness in your peer group, it is even more important to have an informal peer group of psychiatric expert witnesses. Operating from the same consulting rooms or doctors' chambers can facilitate this.

A peer group is also important when professional and ethical issues arise.

Courses, training and conferences

Your PDP should include training in report writing and witness skills, seminars and lectures on developments in statute and case law and court procedure as they relate to your area of expertise, and updates on important areas of medico-legal practice as they relate to psychiatry.

At The Grange we have developed a monthly meeting at which we present cases in which we have been involved and update ourselves on areas of the law. We organise a four-day annual residential conference with mainly invited speakers from medicine and the law. The programme is generated by our peer group and the others who attend the conference. Thus, there is a close correspondence between our PDPs and the conference programme. If we identify a need for education or training on a particular subject, we usually meet that need at the next annual conference.

Books, journals, law reports and libraries

At the end of each chapter I have listed 'Further reading'. There are a number of books upon which I rely as an expert and which I consider that it would be helpful for other experts, or groups of experts, to acquire. The further reading also includes a few illustrative law reports or reports of legal cases in the medical literature.

Law reports illustrate better than any textbook what happens in court when a particular psychiatric issue is in dispute and the judge or judges have to resolve the dispute. What goes in the law report is, however, limited to what the judge considers important for the public record and as a record of the judicial decision-making. Furthermore, cases in the lower courts and cases that do not go to appeal are underrepresented in the law reports. Medical or medico-legal case reports written by one or more of the psychiatric experts in a case can be more informative on certain issues.

Aim to build up a library of the books and law reports that are relevant to your practice as an expert witness.

In addition to some of the books recommended, consider obtaining, on an annual basis, *Blackstone's Criminal Practice*. It has a companion, *Blackstone's Civil Practice*, but this is probably not as useful in civil cases as *Criminal Practice* is in criminal cases. For medical law consider purchasing *Medical Law: Text, Cases and Materials* (Jackson, 2009). A law dictionary is useful.

Many law reports are quoted in the body of the text. Look up the ones that appear especially relevant and keep copies. You can often supplement these when you go to court, as the parties often produce, for the assistance of the judge, a bundle of the relevant 'authorities' and these bundles are usually thrown away at the end of the case.

Although membership of a law library ensures access to the largest range of law reports and also law journals, many law reports are accessible online, for example from the website of the British and Irish Legal Information Institute (BAILII) at http://www.bailii.org, the website of Her Majesty's

Courts and Tribunals Service at http://www.hmcourts-service.gov.uk/, from Mental Health Law Online at http://www.mentalhealthlaw.co.uk and from http://www.familylawweek.co.uk.

Medico-legal societies and expert witness organisations

Join your local medico-legal society or the Medico-Legal Society of London and even if you do not attend the meetings in London you will get a subscription to the *Medico-Legal Journal*. The meetings of these societies are mainly academic, but many are relevant to expert witnesses and they provide the opportunity to talk with lawyers in a less formal setting.

Join an expert witness body. The two leading bodies are the Academy of Experts and the Expert Witness Institute. The Academy has an international membership, which helps when it is proposed to adopt procedures and practices from other jurisdictions. The Institute has a larger medical membership and a more national focus. Both organisations provide training for experts, publish journals or newsletters that help in keeping experts up to date and organise, like the legal training consultancy Bond Solon, annual conferences at which leading judges, as well as lawyers and experts, talk about the latest developments affecting the expert. These organisations and conferences are also valuable because there is often much to be learned from experts outside medicine.

Further education

A number of universities now offer postgraduate degrees of relevance to expert witnesses. In particular there are Master of Laws degrees in medical law, medical law and ethics and mental health law. The University of Cardiff, in association with Bond Solon, awards the Cardiff University Bond Solon Expert Witness Certificates.

Audit and case-based discussion

With fellow psychiatric experts, try to develop an audit tool for psychiatric expert witness work. In practice, the most powerful audit tool for the psychiatric expert witness is a few days in court, where three, or perhaps more, of the most incisive legal brains, assisted by a small army of experts, analyse your report and test your opinions. But something else is needed for day-to-day practice.

As case-based discussion beds down, as a part of the process of appraisals that are going to inform the process of revalidation, try to ensure that they include discussions of your expert witness cases. Through the Grange annual conferences we are in the process of developing an audit tool for expert witness case-based discussions. Our preliminary conclusions are that a case-based discussion of a medico-legal case should include assessment of areas set out in Box 47. We considered that ratings for each of these should be

---

Box 47 Areas to be assessed in case-based discussion of an expert psychiatric report

- Report is within the psychiatrist's expertise
- Evidence of consent where appropriate
- Report conforms to acceptable structure and is properly presented
- Report is 'user-friendly'
- Compliance with relevant rules
- Knowledge, understanding and correct application of legal tests
- Facts and opinions clearly separated
- Issues addressed
- Opinions supported by reasons and withstand logical analysis
- Report includes a summary of opinion/conclusions
- Evidence of independence and impartiality
- Expedition at all stages, particularly achieving all deadlines
- Probity (terms and conditions, record of time spent, detailed, itemised billing)

---

simple, should avoid the concept of 'success' or 'failure' and could perhaps involve just three categories: 'Need to develop/improve', 'Acceptable' and 'Acceptable and an example to be shared with others'. Where appropriate, a record can be made of what the psychiatrist needs to do, as part of their PDP, to remedy any deficiencies identified.

Knowing when to stop

Always be willing to learn from other experts – from their reports, when you meet them in experts' meetings or conferences and when you hear them give evidence in court. If you find that you have nothing more to learn, or have learned nothing from a book like this, it is probably time to give up being a psychiatric expert or to write your own book.

References

Academy of Medical Royal Colleges (2005) *Medical Expert Witnesses Guidance from the Academy of Medical Royal Colleges.* AMRC.

American Psychiatric Association (2000) *The Diagnostic and Statistical Manual of the American Psychiatric Association* (4th edn – text revision) (DSM-IV-TR™). APA.

Ashton, G., Letts, P., Oates, L., *et al* (2006) *Mental Capacity: The New Law.* Jordans.

Babitsky, S., Mangravati, Jr, J. J. & Todd, C. J. (2000) *The Comprehensive Forensic Services Manual: The Essential Resources For All Experts.* SEAK.

Bickle, A. (2008) The dangerous offender provisions of the Criminal Justice Act 2003 and their implications for psychiatric evidence in sentencing violent and sexual offenders. *Journal of Forensic Psychiatry and Psychology,* **19**, 603–619.

Blom-Cooper, L. (ed.) (2006) *Experts in the Civil Courts.* Oxford University Press.

Bluglass, R. (1978) Infanticide. *Bulletin of the Royal College of Psychiatrists,* August, 139–141.

Bluglass, R. (1990) Infanticide and filicide. In *Principles and Practice of Forensic Psychiatry* (eds R. Bluglass & P. Bowden), pp. 523–528. Churchill Livingstone.

Bond, C., Solon, M., Harper, P., *et al* (2007) *The Expert Witness: A Practical Guide* (3rd edn). Shaw & Sons.

Bradley, K. (2009) *People with Mental Health Problems or Learning Disabilities in the Criminal Justice System.* Home Office.

Braithwaite, B. & Waldron, W. (2010) *Brain and Spine Injuries: The Fight for Justice.* Exchange Information.

British Medical Association & Law Society (2010) *Assessment of Mental Capacity: A Practical Guide for Doctors and Lawyers* (3rd edn). Law Society.

Bryant, G. (2003) Assessing individuals for compensation. In *Handbook of Psychology in Legal Contexts* (2nd edn) (ed. D. Carson & R. Bull), pp. 89–107. Wiley.

Busby, S. (2009) *McNaughten: A Novel.* Short Books.

Casey, P. (2003*a*) Expert testimony in court. 1: General principles. *Advances in Psychiatric Treatment,* **9**, 177–182.

Casey, P. (2003*b*) Expert testimony in court. 2: In the witness box. *Advances in Psychiatric Treatment,* **9**, 183–190.

Chiswick, D. (2003) Expert testimony in court. (Invited commentary.) *Advances in Psychiatric Treatment,* **9**, 187–189.

Civil Justice Council (2005) *Protocol for the Instruction of Experts to Give Evidence in Civil Claims.* Civil Justice Council.

Cooper, P. (2010) Cross-examination: trick or fair treatment. *Expert Witness Institute Newsletter,* autumn, 20–21.

Crown Prosecution Service (2006) *Disclosure Manual – Annex K. Disclosure: Experts' Evidence and Unused Material – Guidance Booklet for Experts.* CPS.

Crown Prosecution Service (2010) *The Code for Crown Prosecutors.* CPS.

Faust, D. (1995) The detection of deception. *Neurologic Clinics,* **13**, 255–265.

Faust, D., Hart, K., Guilmette, T. J., *et al* (1988) Neuropsychologists' capacity to detect adolescent malingerers. *Professional Psychology: Research and Practice*, **19**, 508–545.

Fenwick, P. (1990) Automatism. In *Principles and Practice of Forensic Psychiatry* (ed. R. Bluglass & P. Bowden), pp. 271–285. Churchill Livingstone.

Folstein, M. F., Folstein, S. E. & McHugh, P. R. (1975) 'Mini-Mental State'. A practical method for grading the cognitive state of patients for the clinician. *Journal of Psychiatric Research*, **12**, 189–198.

General Medical Council (2004) *Confidentiality*. GMC.

General Medical Council (2006) *Good Medical Practice*. GMC.

General Medical Council (2008) *Acting as an Expert Witness*. GMC.

Gibson, B. & Cavadino, P. (2008) *The Criminal Justice System: An Introduction* (3rd edn). Waterside Press.

Glynn, J. & Gomez, D. (2005) *Fitness to Practise: Health Care Regulatory Law, Principle and Process*. Sweet & Maxwell.

Gray, N. S., O'Connor, C., Williams, T., *et al* (2001) Fitness to plead: implications from case-law arising from the Criminal Justice and Public Order Act 1994. *Journal of Forensic Psychiatry*, **12**, 52–62.

Grubin, D. H. (1996) Silence in court: psychiatry and the Criminal Justice and Public Order Act 1994. *Journal of Forensic Psychiatry*, **7**, 647–652.

Guardian (2009) Fraudulent claims reach record high, 16 April.

Gudjonsson, G. H. (2003) *The Psychology of Interrogations and Confessions: A Handbook*. Wiley.

Gunn, J. & Taylor, P. J. (eds) (1993) *Forensic Psychiatry: Clinical, Legal and Ethical Issues*. Butterworth-Heinemann.

Hale, B. (2010) *Mental Health Law* (5th edn). Sweet & Maxwell.

Handford, P. (2006) *Mullany & Handford's Tort Liability for Psychiatric Damage* (2nd edn). Lawbook Co.

Her Majesty's Courts Service (2009) *Chancery Guide* (6th edn). Ministry of Justice. Available at http://www.justice.gov.uk/guidance/courts-and-tribunals/courts/chancery-division/index.htm

Her Majesty's Courts Service (2010) *Good Practice Guidance: Commissioning, Administering and Producing Psychiatric Reports for Sentencing*. Ministry of Justice.

Hershman, D., McFarlane, A. & Ward, A. (1991) *Children, Law and Practice*. (Update 42.) Jordan Publishing.

Hickling, E. J., Blanchard, E. B., Mundy, E., *et al* (2002) Detection of malingered MVA related posttraumatic stress disorder: an investigation of the ability to detect professional actors by experienced clinicians, psychological tests, and psychophysiological assessment. *Journal of Forensic Psychology Practice*, **2**, 33–54.

Howard, R., Lovestone, S. & Levy, R. (1992) Ernest Saunders: diagnostic dilemma. *BMJ*, **304**, 1568.

Jackson, E. (2009) *Medical Law: Text, Cases, and Materials* (2nd edn). Oxford University Press.

Jones, R. (2007) *Mental Capacity Act Manual* (2nd edn). Sweet & Maxwell.

Jones, R. (2009) *Mental Health Act Manual* (12th edn). Sweet and Maxwell.

Jones, R. (2010) *Mental Health Act Manual* (13th edn). Thomson Reuters.

Judicial Studies Board (2010) *Guidelines for the Assessment of General Damages in Personal Injury Cases* (12th edn). Oxford University Press.

Kloss, D. (2010) *Occupational Health Law* (5th edn). Wiley-Blackwell.

Law Commission (2010) *Unfitness to Plead*. Consultation Paper No. 197. Law Commission.

Law Commission (2011) *Expert Evidence in Criminal Proceedings in England and Wales*. (Law Com. No. 325.) Law Commission.

Lewis, C. J. (2006) *Clinical Negligence* (6th edn). Tottel.

Livingstone, S. & Owen, T. (1999) *Prison Law* (2nd edn). Oxford University Press.

Luborsky, L. (1962) Clinicians' judgments of mental health. *Archives of General Psychiatry*, **7**, 407–417.

Mackay, R. D. (1993) The consequences of killing very young children. *Criminal Law Review*, p. 21.

Mackay, R. (1995) *Mental Condition Defences in the Criminal Law*. Oxford University Press.

Mackay, R. (2010) Mental disability at the time of the offence. In *Principles of Mental Health Law and Policy* (ed. L. Gostin, P. Bartlett, P. Fennell, *et al*), pp. 721–755. Oxford University Press.

Marks, P. (1995) Drink-driving legislation: medicine and the law. *Medico-Legal Journal*, **63**, 119–127.

Mirfield, P. (1997) *Silence, Confessions and Improperly Obtained Evidence*. Clarendon Press.

Murphy, P. (ed. in chief) (1999) *Blackstone's Criminal Practice*. Blackstone Press.

Norrie, A. (2010) The Coroners and Justice Act 2009 – partial defences to murder. (1) Loss of control. *Criminal Law Review*, p. 275.

d'Orbán, P. (1979) Women who kill their children. *British Journal of Psychiatry*, **134**, 560–571.

Ormerod, D. (2008) *Smith and Hogan Criminal Law* (12th edn). Oxford University Press.

Ormerod, D. (2011) *Smith and Hogan Criminal Law* (13th edn). Oxford University Press.

Pamplin, C. (2007) *Expert Witness Fees*. (United Kingdom Register of Expert Witnesses Little Book Series.) JS Publications.

Pamplin, C. (2010) Data protection and the expert. *Expert Witness Institute Newsletter*, autumn, 13–15.

Pamplin, C. (ed.) (for the UK Register of Expert Witnesses) (2011) *Expert Witness Year Book*. JS Publications.

Percival, T. (1803) *Medical Ethics or a Code of Institutes and Precepts Adapted to the Professional Conduct of Physicians and Surgeons*. S. Russell.

Personal Injuries Assessment Board (1984) *Book of Quantum*. Available at http://www.injuriesboard.ie/eng/Forms_and_Publications/Book_of_Quantum.pdf

Pitman, A. (2010) Medicolegal reports in asylum applications: a framework for addressing the practical and ethical challenges. *Journal of the Royal Society of Medicine*, **103**, 93–97.

Powers, M. J., Harris, N. H. & Barton, A. (2008) *Clinical Negligence* (4th edn). Tottel.

Rix, K. J. B. (1996*a*) Psychiatric reports for criminal proceedings in England and Wales. *Hospital Update*, **22**, 240–244, 282–286.

Rix, K. J. B. (1996*b*) Blood or needle phobia as a defence under the Road Traffic Act 1988. *Journal of Clinical Forensic Medicine*, **3**, 173–177.

Rix, K. J. B. (1998) Silence in interview: psychiatry and the Argent conditions. *Journal of Clinical Forensic Medicine*, **5**, 199–204.

Rix, K. J. B. (1999*a*) Expert evidence and the courts. Part 1: The history of expert evidence. *Advances in Psychiatric Treatment*, **5**, 71–77.

Rix, K. J. B. (1999*b*) Capacity to manage property and affairs: old case, new law. *Journal of Forensic Psychiatry*, **10**, 436–444.

Rix, K. J. B. (2001) 'Battered woman syndrome' and the defence of provocation: two women with something more in common. *Journal of Forensic Psychiatry*, **12**, 131–149.

Rix, K. J. B. (2006*a*) England's first expert witness? *Expert and Dispute Resolver*, **11**(2), 16–18.

Rix, K. J. B. (2006*b*) Mental capacity. *Solicitors Journal*, **150**(41), 1370–1371.

Rix, K. J. B. (2008) The psychiatrist as expert witness. Part 2: Criminal cases and Royal College of Psychiatrists' guidance. *Advances in Psychiatric Treatment*, **14**, 109–114.

Rix, K. J. B. (2011) Medico-legal work of psychiatrists: direction, not drift. Commentary on … 'You are instructed to prepare a report'. *The Psychiatrist*, **35**, 272–274.

Rix, K. J. B. & Agarwal, M. (1999) Risk of serious harm or a serious risk of harm? A trap for judges. *Journal of Forensic Psychiatry*, **10**, 187–196.

Rix, K. J. B. & Clarkson, A. (1994) Depersonalization and intent. *Journal of Forensic Psychiatry*, **5**, 409–419.

Rix, K., Thorn, S. & Neville, W. (1997) Medical evidence concerning the suitability to succeed to the tenancy of a farm: the case of 'Toad of Toad Hall'. *Journal of Clinical Forensic Medicine*, **4**, 25–32.

Rogers, R. (ed.) (2008) *Clinical Assessment of Malingering and Deception* (3rd edn). Guilford Press.

Royal College of Psychiatrists (2004) *The Impact of Extended Sentencing on the Ethical Framework of Psychiatry*. (College Report CR147.) RCPsych.

Royal College of Psychiatrists (2008a) *Supplemental Charter, Byelaws and Regulations*. (Occasional Paper OP68.) RCPsych.

Royal College of Psychiatrists (2008b) *Court Work*. RCPsych.

Royal College of Psychiatrists (2008c) *Rethinking Risk to Others in Mental Health Services*. (College Report CR150.) RCPsych.

Royal College of Psychiatrists (2009) *Good Psychiatric Practice* (3rd edn). RCPsych.

Scottish Executive (2005) *Mental Health (Care and Treatment) (Scotland) Act 2003 Code of Practice, Volume 3: Compulsory Powers in Relation to Mentally Disordered Offenders*. Scottish Executive.

Scottish Law Commission (2004) *Insanity and Diminished Responsibility in the Criminal Law*. (Discussion Paper No. 122.) Scottish Law Commission.

Shapiro, F. R. (1993) *The Oxford Dictionary of American Legal Quotations*. Oxford University Press.

Smethurst, P. D. (2006) Giving evidence – the expert view on examination. *Barrister Expert Witness*, suppl., 12–13.

Taylor, C. & Krish, J. (2010) *Advising Mentally Disordered Offenders: A Practical Guide* (2nd edn). Law Society.

Thomson, J. (2006) *Family Law in Scotland* (5th edn). Tottel.

Tribunals Service (2010) *Reports for Mental Health Tribunals*. Tribunals Service.

Ventress, M. A., Rix, K. J. B. & Kent, J. H. (2008) Keeping PACE: fitness to be interviewed by the police. *Advances in Psychiatric Treatment*, **14**, 369–381.

Wall, N. (2007) *A Handbook for Expert Witnesses in Children Act Cases*. Jordan Publishing.

Ward, P. (2010) *Family Law in Ireland*. Kluwer Law International BV.

West, D. J. & Walk, A. (1977) *Daniel McNaughton: His Trial and the Aftermath*. Royal College of Psychiatrists.

Williams, G. (1983) *Textbook of Criminal Law* (2nd edn). Stevens.

Withers, E. & Hinton, J. (1971) Three forms of the clinical tests of the sensorium and their reliability. *British Journal of Psychiatry*, **119**, 1–8.

Wood, P. J. W. & Guly, O. C. R. (1991) Unfit to plead to murder. *Medicine, Science and the Law*, **31**, 55–60.

World Health Organization (1992) *The ICD-10 Classification of Mental and Behavioural Disorders: Clinical Descriptions and Diagnostic Guidelines*. WHO.

Zellick, G. (2010) Papers presented to the Society. *Medico-Legal Journal*, **78**, 11–20.

Letter of response to request for a report

Dr John Monro, MD, FRCPsych
499 Cleckheaton Street,
London W17 5OX.
T: 020 999 1111
F: 020 999 6666
JMonro@499cleck.com
www.xxx.co.uk

Our Ref : JM/XY
Your Ref : FM/WZ

... 2011

Monteith and Company,
15 Cheapside,
London EC1 9YZ.
For the attention of ...

Dear Sirs,

Re :

Thank you for your letter dated ... 2011 (with enclosures) concerning the above case.

I believe that the work required is within my area of expertise and I have the appropriate experience. I will be pleased to provide a report in this case subject to agreement as to my Terms and Conditions.

It does not appear that acceptance of the proposed instructions will involve me in any conflict of interest but I will inform you/the lead solicitors immediately if this subsequently appears to be so.

I am familiar with the general duties of an expert.

I enclose a copy of my CV./You may wish to view my website for full details of my qualifications and experience, my CV, feedback on my reports and my oral testimony and other useful information.

I am able to offer an appointment at ... on ... at 499 Cleckheaton Street, London W17 5OX/I propose to visit your/the client at ... on ...

I am available to do the relevant work within the suggested timescale. I have noted that the trial of this case is listed for/from ... to ... at ... Court and this now appears on my commitments list. I am/am not available for the whole of this period. Please note that another case/other cases are also listed for this period./I note that the trial date has not been fixed. I need as much notice as possible to make arrangements to come to court (or to give evidence by video-link) without undue disruption to my normal professional routines. The dates and times to avoid are on my enclosed commitments list. It includes details of other cases in which I am involved in case you need to liaise with other solicitors about my availability. May I suggest that on the day that the hearing date is to be fixed you obtain an up-to-date copy from my office/consult the commitments list on my website. This is because the commitments list often changes on a daily basis.

If evidence is to be by telephone conference or video-link, I need ... days'/weeks' notice to make arrangements for a telephone conference and ... days'/weeks' notice to make arrangements for a video-link conference.

Please see my Terms and Conditions attached (2 copies enclosed). Please read, sign and return the duplicate copy. For the avoidance of doubt, these Terms and Conditions shall govern all work I undertake in this matter, including acting as an expert both before and after proceedings are issued, and shall encompass the provision of any report and attending at court should I be so instructed.

You should be aware that I will not discuss any statutory compliance obligations with clients, including money laundering or handling monies.

My hourly rate for the preparation of my evidence will be £.... The fee for the report is estimated at £..., on the basis of ... hours of reading and preparation, ... hours for the consultation and ... hours for preparing the report./The fee is estimated at £..., this being my average for similar cases./ The fee will be in the range £... to £..., this being the range for similar cases. This excludes further work on the case, such as, but not limited to, amendments, addenda and answers to questions. However, it is for you to decide whether or not such fees are proportionate because you know better than I do the value and importance of the case. It excludes travelling time and mileage (see below). These rates will go up with effect from 1 April 20....

My daily rate for attending a conference or hearing (at 2011/12 rates) is £.... This is the equivalent of 10 hours at my hourly rate for preparation of the report and it includes time spent travelling and waiting. If I am able to return to my rooms or home and engage in other fee-paid work by 2 p.m., I charge a half-day rate of £.... These rates will also go up with effect from 1 April 20....

Travel time is charged at £... per hour and ...p per mile. These rates will also go up with effect from 1 April 20.... /In this case, on the basis of ... hours travelling to and from .... and ... miles, this will be £... for travelling time and £... for mileage.

Please note that all the above charges are inclusive/exclusive of VAT at the applicable rate.

In accordance with 'The Protocol for the Instruction of Experts to Give Evidence in Civil Claims' please supply the outstanding/following information:

1 Name, address, telephone number, date of birth of the claimant/defendant/respondent, date(s) of the incident(s);

2 The purpose of requesting the advice or report, a description of the matter(s) to be investigated, the principal known issues, the identity of all parties;

3 The statement(s) of case (if any), those documents which form part of standard disclosure and the relevant witness statements;

4 Where proceedings have not been started, whether proceedings are being contemplated and, if so, whether the expert is asked only for advice;

5 Where proceedings have been started, the date(s) of any hearings (including case management conferences and/or pre-trial reviews), the name of the court, the claim number and the track to which the claim has been allocated.

I estimate that the advice or report prepared in response to my instructions will be delivered within ... working weeks of my consultation with the claimant/defendant/respondent. Please note that I will need to see the GP records at least 7 days before the consultation. If these are not available, the appointment will be postponed.

I look forward to hearing from you again.

Yours faithfully,

John Monro,
MD, FRCPsych,
Consultant Forensic Psychiatrist.
Encs.

File front sheet

CASE	Robert BRUCE	SOLICITORS	Monteith
L/A FILES	2	RING BINDERS	1

	DATE	NOTES
ENQUIRY	6.1.11	
INSTRUCTIONS	14.1.11	Downstairs room
SEEN/PAPERS RECEIVED	19.3.11	30 minutes late
Mail Out	19.3.11	Request up to date GP recs
Mail In	29.3.11	Balance of GP recs
Report	1.4.11	
Mail In	7.7.11	CPN records – 28.7.11 deadline
Amended Report	10.7.11	
Mail In	4.8.11	Report disclosed 2.8.11
Mail In	25.8.11	Questions from C's solicitors – 28 days
Mail Out	14.9.11	Answers to C's questions
Mail In	1.10.11	JS with Dr Morison
Email Out	8.10.11	Draft JS to Dr Morison
Email In	14.10.11	Draft JS back from Dr Morison
Tel. Con.	15.10.11	Discussion with Dr Morison
Email Out	16.10.11	Third draft JS to Dr Morison
Email In	17.10.11	Dr Morison – no further changes
Mail Out	18.10.11	JS to Dr M for signature and he will send to both sols
Mail In	20.10.11	File copy of JS signed by Dr M
Mail In	1.11.11	Witness summons 3.2.12 – already listed
Mail In	14.12.11	Settled

Time sheet

Time sheet (reports)

Case name: Case reference: JM.AB/
Solicitors: Their reference:
Prep/initial drafting:
Audiotapes/DVDs: Telephone con.:
Examination(s):   Travelling exp.:
Travelling time: Travelling mileage:
Parking: Pro rata: Yes/No %
Subsistence:
Report:
Setting up, summary/substance of instructions etc.
Body of report
Opinion & Summary of Conclusions
Glossary, Finalisation, Checking

Billing details

Miscellaneous: hrs mins
Reading/prep/initial drafting: hrs mins
Consultation: hrs mins
Report: hrs mins
Total: hrs mins   units @ £   = £
Travelling time: hrs mins   units @ £   = £
Travelling expenses: £
Parking: £
Subsistence etc.:   £

Grand total (exc. VAT):   £

Appointment letter

Dr John Monro, MD, FRCPsych,
499 Cleckheaton Street,
London W17 5OX.
T: 020 999 1111
F: 020 999 6666
JMonro@499cleck.com
www.xxx.co.uk

Our Ref.: JM/XY

21 April 2011

Dear Mr …,

I have arranged an appointment to see you in order to prepare a medical report. This is at the request of … Solicitors. I would be grateful if you would come and see me at … a.m./p.m. on … Please attend at the above address.

Please note that whilst I will make every effort to see you at this time, medical work is not always predictable and sometimes there are unexpected delays. Your consultation will probably last not less than an hour and some consultations can take two hours or more.

If this appointment is not convenient, please contact my secretary/assistant on the above number or by email and we will try to arrange a different appointment for you. Please also telephone, write or email to inform us if you need to be seen in a downstairs room or have any other special requirements.

Please be aware that on occasions I am asked to attend court at very short notice or have to make changes to appointments in order to respond to urgent clinical matters. Unfortunately this may mean that your appointment has to be postponed at short notice. This is why it is important to have your telephone number. I note that we have not been provided with your telephone number, so please provide this to my secretary/assistant.

It would be helpful if you could be accompanied by a partner, relative or friend who can give their views as to your condition but this is not essential.

I enclose travelling directions. I also enclose some further information that will answer frequently asked questions. You will find further information on my website.

Yours sincerely,

John Monro,
Consultant Psychiatrist
cc ... Solicitors, (reference: ...)

Information to accompany appointment letter

You have an appointment with Dr Monro –

What to expect at the consultation
- I will see you personally
- I will try to see you on time but occasionally this is not possible if, for example, another consultation takes longer than expected
- If there is a delay, we will keep you informed
- Only if you agree, a junior doctor, trainee psychiatrist or trainee psychologist may be present to observe the consultation as part of their training
- Otherwise I expect to see you on your own, unless it is appropriate for someone such as a family member, chaperone or interpreter to be present
- The consultation will probably take between one and two hours
- You will be asked to give written consent for the preparation of the report
- The consultation is likely to start with questions about your background and life story, so that I can understand you as a person; questions about your medical history; and then questions about what has happened that has led to the request for the report, for example an accident and its effects, an alleged criminal offence or an allegation of medical negligence and its effects
- There will probably not be a physical examination but if there is a chaperone will be available
- I may ask you to complete some 'pencil and paper' tests
- If we run out of time, the person after you may agree to wait, or we may have to meet again or finish by telephone

Dr Monro's role
- You have probably been asked to see me in order to prepare a report for court or similar proceedings
- I will have been asked to give an independent, unbiased opinion about your case

- This means that:
  - In a civil case, such as a road traffic accident case, I am not 'on your side' if I am instructed by your own solicitors and I am not 'against you' if I am instructed by the solicitors for the person who appears to have caused the accident
  - In a criminal case, I am not 'on your side' if instructed by your own solicitors and I am not 'against you' if I am instructed by the prosecution or the court
- My duty as an expert is to consider all of the evidence available to me at the time and reach an independent and impartial opinion, regardless of who instructs me. This means that I will give the same opinion whether I am instructed by your solicitors or the solicitors for 'the other side'.
- You need to be aware of the fact that my opinion may change if I am provided with further information or if later it appears that I have relied on information which is incorrect.

Who and what to bring
- Come by yourself if you wish
- Bring your partner, a relative or a friend if you wish
- It is best to see you on your own. Then, if you agree, I will probably see, on their own, the person who comes with you for their view of your problems
- If you need reading glasses to read my consent form, please bring these
- Some solicitors ask me to check your identity. If you have been asked to do so, bring with you means of identification such as passport, driving licence, utility bill etc., or whatever the solicitors have specified

Special needs or requirements
- Please let us know if you have any special needs or requirements
- My consulting room is up one flight of stairs. If you need to be seen in a ground floor room, we need notice to book one.
- The entrance to the consulting rooms is up four steps but we have a ramp available if wheelchair access is needed
- I cannot consult in any language other than English. If this is going to be problem, it is almost always best for us to arrange the assistance of a professional interpreter (at no cost to you) rather than a member of your family or a friend. If so, we need to know what language you speak
- You may have other needs or requirements that we have not encountered previously. Let us know in advance what they are and we will try to meet these needs or satisfy these requirements.

Refreshments, meals and other facilities
- In the reception area, we have a machine that dispenses tea, coffee and other drinks free of charge. There is also a water dispenser.
- We do not serve any meals on the premises
- We are a 10-minute walk from sandwich shops and cafés

Complaints procedure
- If there is anything with which you are not happy, it is best to say so at the time. We will try to remedy the problem and avoid giving cause for complaint
- If you want to complain, the first person to approach is me, Dr Monro, and I will try to resolve your complaint
- If you are not satisfied, there are two further levels of complaint
  - I can ask one of the other consultants at the consulting rooms to give an independent response to your complaint
  - You can complain to one of my professional bodies
- If you are considering complaining, it is probably a good idea to take advice, for example from your own solicitors, as they will help you clarify the complaint and decide how and to whom the complaint should be made.
- If you disagree with my assessment or opinion, discuss this with your solicitor

Letter requesting authorisation to use a laptop computer within a prison

Dr John Monro, MD, FRCPsych,
499 Cleckheaton Street,
London W17 5OX.
T: 020 999 1111
F: 020 999 6666
JMonro@499cleck.com
www.xxx.co.uk

My ref: JM/AB/VISITS

... 2011

The Head of Security,
HMP ...

Dear Sir/Madam

Re:

Arrangements have been made for me to visit the above named, in order to prepare a report in connection with ... [criminal/court] proceedings. The visit has been arranged for the morning/afternoon of ... 2011.

In order to record the consultation electronically, access my own files related to the prisoner and access instruments used in the process of psychiatric assessment, I wish to bring with me my laptop computer. I am aware of widely varying policies and procedures in HM Prison Service hospitals relating to laptop computers and seek by this preliminary correspondence to avoid difficulties arising on the day of the visit. On several occasions I have been advised in advance that I can bring my laptop with me but this has been refused on the day of the visit, causing delays at the gate in a number of cases and a completely wasted visit in one case.

I have been a visiting consultant psychiatrist at HMP Newgate, London, for more than 20 years and I have been familiarised with precautions necessary for security. My proof of identity on visits to prisons is my Prison Service identification card. I am aware of the risks posed to prison security by unauthorised material on laptop computers and their unauthorised use. I acknowledge that various procedures are necessary in order to avoid such and I am willing to comply with such procedures.

The following information is provided in order to assist in consideration of my application to bring my laptop into the prison. The laptop is a ..., bearing the serial number.... The general description of the laptop is: ... screen case with silver hinges. The system is password protected and the screensaver is password protected. It does/does not have an internal modem.

I agree to a competent staff member verifying the computer and software media upon entry to and exit from the prison. Some files contain confidential medical information and access to these can be permitted only to a registered medical practitioner.

So far as the files are concerned, I confirm that they will include no unauthorised correspondence, no pornography or other 'over-fleshed pictures' or so-called dubious humour. The screensaver is a view of marshland and is not 'soft core' pornography. The software does not include any that can be utilised for computer-aided designs or the production of scale drawings.

I undertake that I will not load non-Prison Service software from the laptop onto the official network or any stand-alone computers in the prison. I undertake that I will not load any Prison Service data from Prison Service systems to the laptop, such action in any event being possibly in contravention of the Data Protection Act 1998 and the IT Security Policy (POS9010). Anti-virus software is installed and kept up to date. In any event, I have no reason to connect the laptop to any computers in the prison.

The passwords will not be shared with prisoners or prison staff. The passwords will not be written down where they are accessible to unauthorised people. Indeed, I can see no reason to write down the passwords in the prison.

I undertake that the laptop will remain in my possession at all times and not be left unattended, unless locked in an office, and that the prisoner will not have access to it or to its contents.

This letter represents my disclaimer in the event that loss or damage occurs and however caused, i.e. prisoner, staff or actions of others which may include, but are not limited to, theft, damage or misuse. This will include any damage done in the searching process.

Prior to carrying out a psychiatric assessment of a prisoner, I obtain written consent to the assessment. This includes an explanation that the assessment will include information of a personal nature. It also includes, as being relevant to the electronic storage of personal information: 'The information given will be used solely for the purpose for which it was collected.'

LETTER REQUESTING USE OF LAPTOP IN PRISON

Please complete and return the copy of this letter. We will not confirm arrangements to visit the prisoner until we are satisfied that authority has been granted for me to bring the laptop into the prison.
Yours faithfully,
John Monro,
Consultant Psychiatrist.

(Please complete either section (a) or (b) and section (c).

(a) Dr Monro is hereby granted permission to bring into HMP ....
his laptop computer. In addition to the undertakings set out above, the following conditions apply (*continue on separate sheet if necessary*):
Signed:
Print name:
Grade/position:

(b) In order for Dr Monro to bring his laptop into HMP ...., further information and/or undertakings is/are required. I enclose the relevant documentation.

Signed:
Print name:
Grade/position:
Telephone number:

(c) In the event that Dr Monro has difficulties on the day of the visit, the following person or persons should be contacted by gate staff:
Name: Name:

Grade/position: Grade/position:

Telephone number: Telephone number:

Consent form

Declaration of consent to psychiatric interview, examination and report for non-treatment purposes

I understand that Dr J Monro has been instructed to prepare a report for: …

Their reference: …

I understand that this consultation is not a clinical consultation. This means that Dr Monro will not be carrying out any treatment and he will not be taking responsibility for my medical care unless it appears to him that it is urgently necessary to do so. If it is, he will advise my family doctor. He may comment upon or recommend treatment in the report and advise that my family doctor is informed of the comments and/or recommendations.

I consent to the interview, examination and preparation of the report, which will include information of a personal nature. I understand that if there are questions I do not want to answer, I am not obliged to answer them. I understand that as Dr Monro's first duty is to the court/tribunal it is an independent, expert report for the guidance of the court/tribunal. It will therefore show any weaknesses in my case as well as its strengths.

I understand that it is a confidential interview and examination but the report will be read by those who have requested it and they may disclose it to others. The information will be stored electronically. Information kept by Dr Monro and his copy of the report will not be revealed to anyone without the permission of my solicitors/my permission/the court's permission. The information given will be used solely for the purpose for which it was collected (i.e. the ongoing civil/criminal/family court/tribunal/judicial review proceedings). (If I am convicted of any offence I do/do not agree to the report being made available to the prison health service and the National Probation Service.)

If I have brought a relative or a friend and information is given by them to Dr Monro, I understand that this may be incorporated in the report.

If it is necessary for Dr Monro to see my general practice or other medical records, or copies, I agree to this and I confirm that he should have access to the complete records as he needs to assess which parts are relevant to my case. I acknowledge that my past medical history may be relevant to my claim for compensation. No legal action is being taken or is intended against the doctor and/or the hospital. Dr Monro may/may not disclose relevant extracts from the records with the report.

Signature:
Date:

Name:
D.O.B.:

General practitioner/hospital:

Covering letter for a court report

Dr John Monro, MD, FRCPsych,
499 Cleckheaton Street,
London W17 5OX.
T: 020 999 1111
F: 020 999 6666
JMonro@499cleck.com
www.xxx.co.uk

Our Reference:
Your reference:

21 April 2011

Messrs ...

Dear Sirs

Re:

I enclose my report and invoice. I respectfully refer you to my Terms and Conditions and remind you that payment is required within ... weeks/months.

Insofar as I have made recommendations as to treatment, please advise the claimant's general practitioner/private doctor or take steps to ensure that the general practitioner/private doctor is so informed. If, for whatever reason, my recommendations are not communicated to the general practitioner/private doctor you must advise me so that I can decide whether or not, having regard to my duty as a doctor, I have an overriding obligation to communicate with the general practitioner. This may be particularly likely if I have made a diagnosis of which the general practitioner is unaware, recommended treatment if the claimant is not having treatment or recommended different treatment to that which the claimant is having.

In accordance with 'The Protocol for the Instruction of Experts to Give Evidence in Civil Claims':

1   Advise me as soon as reasonably practicable whether, and if so when, the report will be disclosed to other parties; and, if so disclosed, the date of actual disclosure (14.1)

2   If my report is to be relied upon, and if I am to give oral evidence, give me the opportunity to consider and comment upon other reports within my area of expertise and which deal with relevant issues at the earliest opportunity (14.2)

3   Inform me regularly about deadlines for all matters concerning my role as an expert. This includes promptly sending me copies of all court orders and directions which concern my obligations (7.5)

4   Keep me updated with timetables (including the dates and times I am expected to attend) and the location of the court (19.21b)

5   Keep me informed of the progress of the case, including amendments to statements of case relevant to my opinion (14.3).

6   If you become aware of material changes in circumstances or that relevant information within your control was not previously provided to me, you should without delay instruct me to review and, if necessary, update the contents of my report (14.4).

If you need details of my availability for court, I suggest that on the day that the hearing date is to be fixed you obtain an up-to-date copy from my office/consult the commitments list on my website.

Yours faithfully,

John Monro,
Consultant Psychiatrist.

CPS declaration and self-certificate

Declaration

I am an expert in psychiatry and I have been requested to provide a statement. I confirm that I have read guidance contained in a booklet known as *Disclosure: Experts' Evidence and Unused Material*, which details my role and documents my responsibilities, in relation to revelation as an expert witness. I have followed the guidance and recognise the continuing nature of my responsibilities of revelation. In accordance with my duties of revelation, as documented in the guidance booklet:

- I confirm that I have complied with my duties to record, retain and reveal material in accordance with the Criminal Procedure and Investigations Act 1996, as amended.
- I have (not) compiled an Index of all material (as I have no unused material in my possession). I will ensure that the Index is updated/ prepared in the event I am provided with or generate additional material;
- In the event my opinion changes on any material issue, I will inform the investigating officer, as soon as reasonably practicable and give reasons.

Signed

Dated

Expert witnesses' self-certificate: revelation of information (Criminal Procedure and Investigations Act 1996)

Name of Expert Witness: Dr John Monro

Date of birth: 28.5.45
Business Address: 499 Cleckheaton Street, London W17 5OX.
Defendant (if known):
I have been instructed to provide expert evidence in relation to the prosecution of the above-named, or an investigation into the following criminal offence:

I confirm that I have read the booklet known as *Disclosure: Experts' Evidence and Unused Material*, that has been given to me with this form, and that I am aware of my responsibilities as an expert witness to reveal to the Prosecution Team any information that might undermine my evidence.

- Have you ever been convicted of, cautioned for, or received a penalty notice for, any criminal offence (other than minor traffic offences)? NO
- Are there any proceedings pending against you in any criminal or civil court? NO
- Are you aware of any adverse finding by a judge, magistrate or coroner about your professional competence or credibility as a witness? NO
- Have you ever been the subject of any adverse findings by a professional or regulatory body? NO
- Are there any proceedings, referrals or investigations pending against you that have been brought by a professional or regulatory body? NO
- Are you aware of any other information that you think may adversely affect your professional competence and credibility as an expert witness? NO

Should you have any queries in relation to your answers to any of the above, please contact the investigator.

Please note that the questions above apply to any proceedings, findings or other relevant information in this or any other jurisdiction.

If you have answered YES to any of the questions numbered 1–6, please give details below:
N/A

Declaration

All the information I have given in this certificate is true to the best of my knowledge and belief.

I will notify those instructing me of any change in this information.

I am aware that any false or misleading information I have given in this document, or any deliberate omission of relevant information may lead to disciplinary or criminal proceedings.

Signed:

Name (in block capitals): DR JOHN MONRO

Date:

A note on judicial titles and their abbreviations in England and Wales

Pub quiz question: When does a Knight of the Realm have the title 'Mister' and is addressed as 'My Lord'. Answer: When he is sitting as a High Court judge.

Judicial titles and their abbreviations can be confusing, not least as there is inconsistency.

The Justices of the Supreme Court, who were previously the Appellate Committee of the House of Lords, are all Peers of the Realm. They include, for example, Lord Saville of Newdigate and Baroness Hale of Richmond and this is how reference is made to them in law reports. Thus their official titles are The Rt Hon The Lord Saville of Newdigate and The Rt Hon The Baroness Hale of Richmond, although if you write to the latter you may wish to append her 'Hon FRCPsych' after her PC, DBE and FBA. Controversially, newly appointed justices of the Supreme Court are not ennobled automatically but may use the courtesy title Lord or Lady.

The judges of the Court of Appeal are appointed to the Privy Council and are knighted, so their official titles are, for example, The Rt Hon Sir Bernard Rix (no relation, as I keep being asked, and who, when addressed as 'My Lord', is not to be confused with Baron Rix of Whitehall in the City of London and of Hornsea in Yorkshire, who is also an Honorary Fellow of the College) and The Rt Hon Dame Janet Smith, DBE. They are addressed in court as 'My Lord' and 'My Lady'. In law reports they are, in the singular, Rix LJ and Smith LJ or, in the plural, Rix and Smith LJJ. However, if Rix LJ refers to a judgment of Smith LJ when she had been sitting as a High Court judge he will refer to it as 'the judgment of Smith J (as she then was)'.

The most senior judge and the head of the judiciary is at present, even more confusingly, The Rt Hon The Lord Judge. He is also addressed as 'My Lord' and in law reports he appears as Judge LCJ. Other Heads of Division include the Master of the Rolls (presently Lord Neuberger MR), the President of the Queen's Bench Division (presently Sir John Thomas P) and the President of the Family Division and Head of Family Justice (Sir Nicholas Wall P).

The High Court judges of the Queen's Bench Division, the Family Division and the Chancery Division are knighted but not appointed to the Privy Council, so their titles are 'The Hon. Sir/Dame'. The Hon. Sir Peregrine Simon sits as Mr Justice Simon, as his name will appear on the Court List, he is addressed as 'My Lord' and when his judgments are quoted he is Simon J. The Hon Dame Linda Dobbs, DBE, is Mrs Justice Dobbs on the Court List; she is addressed as 'My Lady' and she is Dobbs J when cited. If cited together they are Simon and Dobbs JJ.

Circuit judges are known as His/Her Honour and, along with recorders, who are Queen's Counsel, experienced barristers and experienced solicitors who sit from time to time as circuit judges, they are addressed in court as 'Your Honour'. In law reports, anomalously, their title goes before their name. Thus, 'in her judgment, HHJ Carr, QC, referred to...'. There are confusing exceptions. The most senior judge in a city may have the honorary title of recorder, thus 'The Hon. Recorder of Leeds, His Honour Judge P. N. Collier, QC'. He is not just a barrister 'acting up' as judge for a couple of weeks. Furthermore, he is addressed as 'My Lord' as if he were a High Court judge. In the Old Bailey (the Central Criminal Court) all of the judges, albeit that they are circuit judges, are addressed as 'My Lord/My Lady'.

The form of address otherwise goes with the court and not the person. Recently I appeared before His Honour Judge Behrens sitting as a deputy judge of the Chancery Division of the High Court and addressed him as 'My Lord' but two weeks later I appeared before him as a circuit judge sitting in the county court, where I addressed him as 'Your Honour'. You could be forgiven for thinking that he had been demoted.

I turn now to district judges. There are two sorts. First, sitting in magistrates courts, usually hearing only criminal cases, and some other courts such as the Inner London Family Proceedings Court, are legally qualified paid judges. Their full title is 'Mr District Judge Waller' or 'Miss District Judge Bradley' (only when female judges get more senior do they acquire the marital status of 'Mrs', whether they are married or not). Their abbreviated title is, for example, 'DJ(MC)' and they are addressed as 'Sir' or 'Madam'. Second, there are the district judges who sit in the county court and they are also addressed as 'Sir' or 'Madam' unless they have a 'ticket' from the President to hear contested applications and exercise the same jurisdiction as circuit judges, in which case they are addressed as 'Your Honour'.

Lay magistrates or justices of the peace are not legally qualified. They sit usually as a bench of three. They are addressed as 'Sir' or 'Madam', according to the gender of the chair, and regardless of the gender of the others, but the 'Your Worship(s)' form of address has not completely disappeared.

The bottom line is 'if in doubt, ask', or listen to how solicitors or counsel address the judge – but they sometimes get it wrong.

Specimen criminal report

This appendix aims to show how a criminal report should be set out, the sections and their content, and the prose style. The constraints of space in reproducing an A4 sheet on a smaller page while trying to preserve legibility mean that the recommendations from Box 7 (page 37) and elsewhere in this volume cannot be exactly followed.

IN THE CENTRAL CRIMINAL COURT

R v DANIEL McNAUGHTAN

Case No 20-6-1843

On the instructions of:	Monteith and Company, 15 Cheapside, London EC1
Who act on behalf of:	The Defendant
Their reference:	SM/BR
Subject matter:	Psychiatric evaluation of the Defendant
Date of report:	25 February 1843
Report reference number:	ETM/XY/1
Date of examination:	18 and 20 February 1843
Place of examination:	HMP Newgate, London
Consent:	Written

Report by
Dr. E.T. Monro,
BSc, MSc, MD, FRCPsych
Consultant Psychiatrist
499 Cleckheaton Street,
London W17 5OX

GMC No: 87654321

Tel: 020 999 1111 Fax: 020 999 6666
www.xxx.co.uk
ETMonro@499cleck.com

1

Report of: Dr. E.T. Monro
Specialism: Psychiatry
On the instructions of: Monteith and Company
Prepared for: The Central Criminal Court

CONTENTS[1]

[1] This report is based on the 'Model Form of Expert's Report' approved by the Judicial Committee for the Academy of Experts and on that of the Expert Witness Institute.

Report of Dr. E.T. Monro concerning Daniel McNaughtan, 25 February 1843   *2*
R v DANIEL MCNAUGHTAN

Report of: Dr. E.T. Monro
Specialism: Psychiatry
On the instructions of: Monteith and Company
Prepared for: The Central Criminal Court

1. INTRODUCTION

1.1. The writer

1.1.1. I am Edward Thomas Monro, a licensed and registered medical practitioner approved under section 12 of the Mental Health Act 1983 (as amended by the Mental Health Act 2007) and registered with the General Medical Council as a specialist in general psychiatry according to the provisions of Schedule 2 of the European Specialist Medical Qualifications Order 1995. Full details of my qualifications and experience entitling me to give expert opinion evidence are in **Appendix 1**.

1.2. Synopsis

1.2.1. Daniel McNaughtan ('the Defendant') is indicted that on 20 January 1843, at the parish of St. Martin's in the Fields, Middlesex, he murdered Mr Edward Drummond ('the Deceased'), the private secretary of Sir Robert Peel, the Prime Minister, against the peace of our Sovereign lady the Queen, Her Crown and Dignity, contrary to common law.

1.3. Instructions

1.3.1. I have been instructed by friends of the Defendant, through his solicitors, Monteith and Company, to visit him at Newgate and prepare a psychiatric report for his trial.

1.4. Disclosure of interests

1.4.1. The Defendant is not known to me professionally or personally. I do not know any of the parties involved. There are no conflicts of interest in respect to any of the identified parties but for the avoidance of doubt I am not a member of the Conservative Party or the Roman Catholic Church. I have no other interest which might cause a conflict based upon the nature of the case.

2. THE BACKGROUND TO THE CASE AND THE ISSUES

2.1. The relevant parties

2.1.1. Henry C. Bell	Sheriff Depute of the County of Lanark
2.1.2. Sir James Campbell	The Lord Provost of Glasgow
2.1.3. Edward Drummond	The Deceased, Private Secretary to Sir Robert Peel
2.1.4. Mrs Dutton	The Defendant's London landlady
2.1.5. William Gilchrist	Glasgow printer with whom the Defendant lodged
2.1.6. John Gordon	London acquaintance of the Defendant
2.1.7. John Hughes	Tailor and the Defendant's Glasgow landlord
2.1.8. Alexander Johnston	Member of Parliament
2.1.9. Alexander Martin	Gunmaker, Paisley
2.1.10. Daniel McNaughtan	The Defendant
2.1.11. Daniel McNaughtan (Sen)	The Defendant's father

Report of Dr. E.T. Monro concerning Daniel McNaughtan, 25 February 1843   *3*
R v DANIEL MCNAUGHTAN

Report of: Dr. E.T. Monro
Specialism: Psychiatry
On the instructions of: Monteith and Company
Prepared for: The Central Criminal Court

2.1.12. Sir Robert Peel	The Prime Minister
2.1.13. James Silver	Police Constable
2.1.14. John Tierney	Police Inspector
2.1.15. Benjamin Weston	Office Porter
2.1.16. Hugh Wilson	Commissioner of Police for Glasgow

2.2. The assumed facts and substance of all material instructions

2.2.1. The Defendant, is indicted that on 20 January 1843, at the parish of St. Martin's in the Fields, Middlesex, he murdered Mr Edward Drummond, the private secretary of Sir Robert Peel, the Prime Minister. The Deceased was on terms of intimacy and friendship with the Prime Minister and occupied apartments in the official residence of the Prime Minister. He was in the constant habit of passing from those rooms to the Prime Minister's private residence in Whitehall Gardens.

2.2.2. There is evidence that the Defendant had been seen loitering about these spots for many days and watching the persons who went in and out of the public offices and the houses in Whitehall Gardens.

2.2.3. On Friday 20 January 1843 the Deceased left his apartments in Downing Street and went to the Treasury and thence to the Admiralty, from there he visited his bank in Charing Cross and on his return, near the 'Salopian' coffee house, it is alleged that the Defendant came behind him and discharged a pistol almost close to him. After discharging it, he drew another from his breast, presented it to the Deceased and was in the act of firing it when a policeman restrained him. Although the Deceased managed to walk back to his bank, he died from his injuries on 25 January 1843.

2.2.4. It is further the case for the Crown that from the facts of the case, from the threats used by the Defendant before he committed his crime, and his declaration afterwards, it was not the life of the Deceased that he sought, it was the life of Sir Robert Peel that he desired to take, and it was his life that he believed he was destroying when he discharged the fatal pistol against the person of the Deceased.

2.2.5. The Defendant was initially arraigned at Bow Street on 21 January 1843 and he subsequently appeared before the Grand Jury on both 30 January and 2 February 1843 where he pleaded not guilty to murder.

2.2.6. I have included a brief chronology as **Appendix 3**.

2.3. The issues to be addressed

2.3.1. I have been asked:
(a) whether or not the Defendant was insane according to 'The M'Naghten Rules';
(b) whether or not the Defendant has a defence of 'diminished responsibility'; and
(c) whether or not the Defendant could have been feigning his delusions.

2.4. The assumptions adopted

2.4.1. Unless otherwise indicated, I have assumed that what the Defendant told me

Report of Dr. E.T. Monro concerning Daniel McNaughtan, 25 February 1843   **4**
R v DANIEL MCNAUGHTAN

Report of: Dr. E.T. Monro
Specialism: Psychiatry
On the instructions of: Monteith and Company
Prepared for: The Central Criminal Court

is true and that the evidence of the witnesses is true. However, the reliability of the Defendant and the witnesses is an ultimate matter for the Court to decide.

3. INVESTIGATION OF FACTS AND ASSUMED FACTS[1]

3.1. Methodology

3.1.1. Psychiatrists, as doctors, employ the time-honoured processes of history-taking and examination in order to achieve a formulation of the subject that encompasses diagnosis, aetiology (causation), treatment recommendations and prognosis. Examination may and often does include physical examination but examination of the mental state is an important psychiatric skill.

3.1.2. My approach to the process of differential diagnosis is based on normal clinical practice and a hierarchical system of psychiatric classification. By this I mean that I have considered diagnosis in the order in which mental disorders appear section by section in *The ICD-10 Classification of Mental and Behavioural Disorders* (World Health Organization, Geneva, 1992): organic, including symptomatic, mental disorders; mental and behavioural disorders due to substance misuse (including alcohol); schizophrenia and related disorders; mood disorders; neurotic, stress-related and somatoform disorders; personality and related disorders; and learning disabilities. At each level I have considered the evidence for and against the diagnosis of a mental disorder at that level and then I have proceeded to the next level. I have highlighted, if there are any, factual assumptions, deductions from factual assumptions, and any unusual, contradictory or inconsistent features of the case.

3.1.3. My approach to aetiology has been to apply to the subject's case my knowledge of the causes of psychiatric disorder in order to be able to give an opinion, if requested, as to how the psychiatric disorder came about or why it ran the course it did.

3.1.4. Where I have made recommendations for treatment, or commented on treatment already given, I have relied on approaches that have wide acceptance by psychiatrists and, if possible, given weight to treatments for which there is the strongest evidence base with regard to effectiveness and safety. However, as in medicine in general, there are many treatments which are accepted as effective but for which there have not been trials that satisfy the most stringent criteria of evidence-based medicine.

3.1.5. So far as prognosis is concerned, I have applied my knowledge of the course and outcome of psychiatric disorders to the features of this individual case. My approach to risk assessment is based on structured clinical judgment. By this I

[1] It is possible that some of the facts and assumed facts in this report are not true but this may be for the Court to decide. I have ended this report with the same declaration of truth as a witness statement made according to the provisions of the Criminal Justice Act 1967, the Magistrates' Courts Act 1980 and the Magistrates' Courts Rules 1981. Insofar as I have stated that the contents of this report are true, this must be taken to mean that it is true that the facts and assumed facts are as stated and not that each and every fact or assumed fact is in itself true.

Report of Dr. E.T. Monro concerning Daniel McNaughtan, 25 February 1843   **5**
R v DANIEL MCNAUGHTAN

mean that I have used my training, experience and skill to relate what is known about the prognoses of mental disorders in general to the specific features of the Defendant's case, endeavouring to make predictions about identified risks with which I would expect other psychiatrists to concur. It is important to realise that the value of predictions diminishes rapidly with time and this is probably because with time circumstances change so much.

3.1.6. Clinical practice, including psychiatric practice, depends in part on knowledge for which there is a sound evidence base and partly on experience-based knowledge which has stood the test of time but lacks a robust foundation in the rigorous research that now forms the basis of 'evidence-based medicine'. In relying on both categories of knowledge, I have done so in accordance with what I would regard as a responsible body of psychiatric practice.

3.2. Interview and examination

3.2.1. I have interviewed and examined the Defendant twice. On 18 February 1843 I was accompanied by Sir Alexander Morison, my colleague at Bethlem and author of the celebrated work *The Physiognomy of Mental Disease* (1840). Also present were Mr William McClure, a surgeon residing at Harley Street, and other professional gentlemen. There we met Dr A.J. Sutherland, Jnr, Physician to St Luke's Hospital, and Dr Bright, who had been instructed by the Crown. I saw the Defendant again on 20 February 1843 in the company of Dr Hutcheson and Dr Crawford. We all asked questions in turn.

3.2.2. We were able to discuss the Defendant's physical health with Dr Lavies, Physician to Newgate Gaol.

3.3. Documents

3.3.1. The documents made available or obtained are listed in **Appendix 2**.

3.3.2. There are no medical records for the Deceased. This is because he has not attended a doctor or hospital since he was a child.

3.4. Medical terms and explanations

3.4.1. I have indicated any medical or related terms in **bold type**. I have defined these terms and included them in a glossary in **Appendix 4**.

Report of Dr. E.T. Monro concerning Daniel McNaughtan, 25 February 1843   **6**
R v DANIEL MCNAUGHTAN

Report of: Dr. E.T. Monro
Specialism: Psychiatry
On the instructions of: Monteith and Company
Prepared for: The Central Criminal Court

4. THE FACTS AND ASSUMED FACTS[1]

4.1. Background history as given by the Defendant

4.1.1. The Defendant was born in Glasgow in 1813. His father was a wood turner. The Defendant was his apprentice for four and a half years, living in his father's house, and then he worked for him as a journeyman for three years but living away from home in lodgings.

4.1.2. Then the Defendant set up business on his own in 1835, as he was dissatisfied that his father would not let him have a share in his business. This was because his father wanted to provide for the Defendant's younger siblings.

4.1.3. By the time he left the business in 1840, the Defendant had saved a considerable amount of money. It had been a prosperous and thriving business. In July 1842 he responded to an advertisement in a London newspaper, *The Spectator*. It was for a partnership 'in a very genteel business in London' and with a view to succeeding to the whole business. Any gentleman having £1,000 was invited to apply. The Defendant did not have the exact amount of money specified but wrote in response to say that he had been engaged in business on his own account for a few years, was under 30 years of age and was very active and of sober habits.

4.1.4. The Defendant had first come to London in July 1841 and stayed in lodgings with a Mrs Dutton. Before doing so, he opened a deposit account with the Bank of Scotland and then shifted it to the London Joint Stock Bank.

4.1.5. In his spare time in Glasgow, the Defendant attended lectures on natural philosophy[2] at the Glasgow Mechanics' Institution. He took an active part in various alterations which were made to the rules of the Institution and also in the arrangement of the rooms and conveniences of the building. He was in the habit of getting books from the library; he was known to all the persons who frequented that institution and he attended lectures on anatomy, including attending the dissecting room every day.

4.1.6. The Defendant described himself as a person of sober habits.

4.1.7. At the time of the alleged offence, the Defendant was lodging at 7 Poplar Row, Newington, with Mrs Dutton again. He had returned to London again in July 1842.

---

[1] In order to be able to identify and distinguish different sources of information and different categories of information, this section is not set out strictly chronologically but by setting out the Defendant's background history first, the other sections should be more understandable and strict chronology is restored by taking the (alleged) offence(s) in the penultimate section and my own examination of the Defendant in the last section.
[2] In Scotland physics is known as natural philosophy.

Report of Dr. E.T. Monro concerning Daniel McNaughtan, 25 February 1843   **7**
R v DANIEL MCNAUGHTAN

Report of: Dr. E.T. Monro
Specialism: Psychiatry
On the instructions of: Monteith and Company
Prepared for: The Central Criminal Court

4.2. Personality

4.2.1. The Defendant has been described by a number of the witnesses in such terms as sullen, gloomy, reserved and unsocial and Mrs Dutton, with whom he lodged in London, said that he was not in the habit of looking people in the face. (It is not clear if these were his characteristics before he became ill [i.e. his premorbid personality] or the early signs of the illness – ETM).

4.3. Medical history as given by the Defendant[1]

4.3.1. With regard to his physical health, the Defendant responded by saying that physicians could be of no service to him. He said that if he took a ton of drugs it would be of no service to him.

4.3.2. So far as his mental health is concerned, the Defendant referred to 'the persecution' and he referred to 'grinding of the mind'.

4.3.3. He spoke of people watching him in Glasgow, pointing to him and speaking of him, saying that he was a murderer and the worst of characters. In Edinburgh, he had seen a man on horseback watching him and another had nodded to him and said: 'That's he.'

4.3.4. He was critical of Sheriff Bell for not having put an end to 'the persecution' and said that if he had had a pistol in his possession he would have shot him dead. He said that Sheriff Bell, Sheriff Alison and Sir Robert Peel could have put a stop to the system of persecution if they had wanted to do so.

4.3.5. He referred to seeing a man with a bundle of straw under his arm and he knew well enough what that meant as everything was done by signs: the straw denoted that he should lie upon straw in an asylum.

4.3.6. He had seen paragraphs in *The Times* newspaper containing allusions directed at him and he complained that there had been articles in the *Glasgow Herald* which were beastly and atrocious and insinuated things which were untrue and insufferable of him.

4.3.7. On one or two occasions pernicious things had been put in his food.

4.4. Medical history according to medical records

4.4.1. None seen.

---

[1] I have assumed that there is no truth in the allegations made by the defendant and I have assumed that he did not hear what he reported hearing said about him.

Report of Dr. E.T. Monro concerning Daniel McNaughtan, 25 February 1843   **8**
R v DANIEL MCNAUGHTAN

Report of: Dr. E.T. Monro
Specialism: Psychiatry
On the instructions of: Monteith and Company
Prepared for: The Central Criminal Court

4.5. Previous convictions

4.5.1. I understand that the Defendant has no previous convictions or cautions.

4.6. Defendant's account of the alleged offence[1]

4.6.1. We asked the Defendant more than once if he knew it was Sir Robert Peel he shot at. The Defendant hesitated and paused and at length said that he was not sure whether it was Sir Robert Peel or not.

4.6.2. The Defendant said that the person at whom he fired had given him a scowling look as he passed. He said that he was one of the crew that was destroying his health. At that moment, all the feelings of the months and years rushed into his mind and he thought that he could obtain peace only by shooting him.

4.6.3. He went on to say that he imagined that the person at whom he fired at Charing Cross was 'one of the crew – a part of the system that was destroying his health' and 'every feeling of suffering which he had endured for months and years rose up at once on his mind, and that he conceived that he should gain peace by killing him'.

4.7. Evidence of witnesses concerning the alleged offence

4.7.1. DANIEL MCNAUGHTAN, the Defendant's father, a turner residing in Glasgow, says that about two years previously the Defendant had called at his house and begged him to speak to the authorities in town to have a stop put on them. He wanted his father to speak to Mr Sheriff Alison. He said that he was being persecuted and followed day and night by spies. Although they never spoke to him, they laughed at him and shook their fists in his face and those who had sticks shook them at him. He said that one of them threw straws in his face. This he thought meant that he was to be reduced to a state of beggary. Later he wanted his father to make representations to Mr Sheriff Bell. His father never saw any of the civil authorities because he realised that he was 'labouring under some extraordinary **delusion**, and therefore considered it quite unnecessary'. He said that he did not consult any medical gentleman because he thought that the delusions would eventually pass away.

4.7.2. A Glasgow printer, WILLIAM GILCHRIST, with whom the Defendant lodged in the Gorbals, sleeping in the same bed, said that the Defendant frequently used to get up in the night and walk about the room uttering incoherent sentences and making use of ejaculations such as 'By Jove' and 'My God'. He knew him on occasions to burst out into immoderate fits of laughter without any cause whatsoever. At other times, he would moan. He said that the Defendant had told him about a visit to the House of Commons and how he was highly delighted at having heard Sir Robert Peel. This witness was asked if he had heard the Defendant speak disrespectfully of Sir Robert Peel and he said that he had not. He said that he had never heard the

[1] I have assumed that there is no truth in the allegations made by the Defendant and I have assumed that he did not hear what he reported hearing said about him.

Report of: Dr. E.T. Monro
Specialism: Psychiatry
On the instructions of: Monteith and Company
Prepared for: The Central Criminal Court

Defendant speak of Sir Robert Peel's political character nor heard him make use of any threat towards him. The last time he saw the Defendant was in July 1842. His conversation was not so connected as formerly.

4.7.3. JOHN HUGHES is a tailor and it was in his house that the Defendant and William Gilchrist had lodged. He confirmed the evidence of William Gilchrist and said that in consequence of the Defendant's strange manner he asked him to leave.

4.7.4. HENRY C. BELL, one of the sheriffs depute of the county of Lanark, said that the Defendant had been to see him and complained about being harassed to death by a system of persecution. He said that the Defendant gave a long, rambling, unintelligible statement from which it appeared that he believed that he was constantly beset by spies and considered that his life and property were in danger. It was the sheriff's conclusion that he was labouring under some extraordinary delusion.

4.7.5. Similar evidence has been given by ALEXANDER JOHNSTON, MP, whom the Defendant had consulted. The Defendant had told him that he was also being attacked through the newspapers.

4.7.6. SIR JAMES CAMPBELL, the Lord Provost of Glasgow, says that the Defendant had been to complain to him as well. He told him that he was compelled to sleep in the fields in the suburbs of the town to evade his persecutors.

4.7.7. HUGH WILSON, the Commissioner of Police for Glasgow, says that the Defendant had told him that he thought that the persecution proceeded from the priests at the Catholic chapel in Clyde Street, who were assisted by a parcel of Jesuits. Two or three days later, he returned and said that the Tories had joined the Catholics. He mentioned how, when he had fled to France, as soon as he landed at Boulogne, he had seen one of the spies peep from behind the watch-box on the Custom House Quay.

4.7.8. There is evidence from ALEXANDER MARTIN, a gunmaker of Paisley, which indicates that in July 1842 the Defendant went to the shop of a gunsmith in the neighbourhood of Glasgow where he bought the pistols used in the alleged offence along with a flask, powder and balls. The same month he travelled to London.

4.7.9. JOHN GORDON said that he had known the Defendant for six years. He had never seen anything particular about his conduct. When he met the Defendant in London in November 1842, the Defendant told him that he was in search of employment. When they walked past Sir Robert Peel's house, the Defendant said: 'Damn him, sink him'. When they passed the Treasury, he said: 'Look across the street; there is where all the treasure and worth of the world is'.

4.7.10. BENJAMIN WESTON, an office porter, witnessed the shooting and said that the Defendant had drawn his pistol 'very deliberately, but at the same time very quickly ... a very cool, deliberate act'.

4.7.11. There is evidence from JAMES SILVER, a police constable, who also witnessed the shooting and restrained the Defendant. His evidence is that on the

Report of: Dr. E.T. Monro
Specialism: Psychiatry
On the instructions of: Monteith and Company
Prepared for: The Central Criminal Court

way to the police station 'he either said "he" or "she" [he could not recollect] shall not break my peace of mind any longer'.

4.7.12. There is also evidence from a police inspector, JOHN TIERNEY, who had custody of the Defendant after his arrest. The Defendant spoke about being the object of persecution by the Tories and Inspector Tierney said to him: 'I suppose you are aware who the gentleman is you shot at?' The Defendant replied: 'It is Sir Robert Peel, is it not?' There is no evidence that he intended to shoot Sir Robert Peel save that of this police inspector.

4.8. Transcript of the Defendant's statement at Bow Street Police Court

4.8.1. When the Defendant appeared before Bow Street Police Court he made the following statement to the magistrate:
'The Tories in my native city have compelled me to do this. They follow and persecute me wherever I go, and have entirely destroyed my peace of mind. They followed me to France, into Scotland, and all over England; in fact, they follow me wherever I go. I can get no rest from them night or day. I cannot sleep at night in consequence of the course they pursue towards me. I believe they have driven me into a consumption. I am sure I shall never be the man I formerly was. I used to have good health and strength, but I have not now. They have accused me of crimes of which I am not guilty; they do everything in their power to harass and persecute me; in fact, they wish to murder me. It can be proved by evidence; that's all I have to say.'

4.9. Examination on 18 February 1843[1]

4.9.1. On examination, the Defendant presented as a young, Caucasian male, clean-shaven and of a mild and prepossessing appearance. He was tidily, if somewhat shabbily, dressed in thin overcoat, waistcoat and plain trousers. His linen was over-darned but clean. He seemed tired and his features were somewhat drawn as if from lack of sleep.

4.9.2. Eye contact was maintained only sporadically at best, the Defendant shifting his gaze at various points in the interview.

4.9.3. His manner was initially placid and contented. There was later evidence of discomfort at being interviewed, although he continued to respond thoughtfully and with unerring politeness to all the questions put to him.

4.9.4. A faint smile was observed on several occasions when giving consideration to matters of apparent and professed seriousness and import.

4.9.5. His speech was mild and not at all distracted. I noted hesitancy when discussing the character of his delusions.

[1] These are the only facts within my own knowledge.

Report of Dr. E.T. Monro concerning Daniel McNaughtan, 25 February 1843   *11*
R v DANIEL MCNAUGHTAN

Report of: Dr. E.T. Monro
Specialism: Psychiatry
On the instructions of: Monteith and Company
Prepared for: The Central Criminal Court

4.9.6. The content of his thought appeared to be dominated by a great fear that he is 'continuously dogged about' by a 'spy system' or 'crew' at Glasgow, Edinburgh, Liverpool, London and Boulogne which intended to ruin his good name. 'Go where I will, they watch over me and see me home to my lodgings and watch out for me again.' He said that he had seen in *The Times* and *The Glasgow Herald* newspapers paragraphs containing 'beastly and atrocious' allegations directed at him. On occasions he said that he had left his lodgings and remained out all night with only a fishing rod and line with which to procure food. On other occasions he has observed men pointing at him on the street and he said that he was afraid to go out at night for fear of being assassinated. He described himself as being 'like a cork tossed on the sea'.

4.9.7. His higher faculties appeared to be intact and the overall impression imparted was that of superior intelligence.

4.9.8. He expressed his beliefs with great conviction and when it was put to him that medical treatment might be of benefit, he said that a ton of drugs could not relieve him of his fears.

4.9.9. He was in apparent good physical health and this was confirmed by Dr Lavies, Physician to Newgate Gaol.

5. OPINION

5.1. This report contains conclusions based on the Defendant's account of the alleged offence. If he is pleading not guilty or if this account of the alleged offence is at variance with that given to his solicitors, it may be appropriate to delay disclosure of this report pending clarification of his instructions.

5.2. Diagnosis

5.2.1. In my opinion, the Defendant is suffering from a mental disorder within the meaning of the Mental Health Act 1983 (as amended by the Mental Health Act 2007). It is probable that it is the mental illness known as **schizophrenia** or another **psychotic** illness so like schizophrenia that it makes no difference exactly what it is called.

5.2.2. I make this diagnosis because the Defendant has a history of the following: (a) persecutory delusions, (b) **delusions of reference**, (c) what were probably auditory **hallucinations**, in that he heard people referring to him in the third person, (d) what were probably gustatory hallucinations, insofar as he thought that something had been put in his food, although this could have been a belief rather than a hallucination, (e) inappropriate **affect** and what is probably schizophrenic **thought disorder** (as evidenced by his disconnected and incoherent speech). There seems to have been a history of personality change, in particular a tendency to social withdrawal, which is consistent with this diagnosis and it is also relevant that his illness has begun in relative youth, which is when schizophrenia usually has its onset.

5.2.3. Although delusions can occur in severe depressive illness there is little or nothing to suggest this diagnosis. I cannot rule out a physical cause for his mental

Report of Dr. E.T. Monro concerning Daniel McNaughtan, 25 February 1843   *12*
R v DANIEL MCNAUGHTAN

Report of: Dr. E.T. Monro
Specialism: Psychiatry
On the instructions of: Monteith and Company
Prepared for: The Central Criminal Court

illness on the information available but if there is such a cause it must be an obscure one in view of the fact that it was not detected by Dr Lavies or any of the distinguished medical and surgical gentlemen who accompanied me. Given the evidence that the Defendant was a person of sober habits, it is unlikely that his condition is a result of the use of alcohol or other substances.

5.3. Insanity

5.3.1. According to the M'Naghten Rules, 'to establish a defence on the ground of insanity, it must be clearly proved, that at the time of the committing of the act, the party accused was labouring under such a defect of reason, from disease of the mind, as not to know the nature and quality of the act he was doing; or, if he did know it, that he did not know he was doing what was wrong'.

5.3.2. It is more probable than not that the Defendant was suffering from a disease of the mind at the material time. There is a clear history of delusions prior to the alleged offence, there has been evidence of delusions when he has been medically examined since the alleged offence and his account of the alleged offence suggests that he was deluded at the time.

5.3.3. Insofar as the Defendant came to believe that the only way that he could obtain peace from all of the suffering of the previous months and years was to shoot Mr Drummond, this makes it more probable than not that the defect of reasoning, due to his schizophrenia, which led him to believe falsely that he was subject to persecution by the Tories and the Jesuits, also led him to the false belief that he would obtain peace from the persecution by shooting Mr Drummond. In relation to this point it does not matter whether he thought that it was Sir Robert Peel or not.

5.3.4. Although it does not appear that the Defendant was questioned in depth about what he believed that he was doing, it does not appear that there is evidence which would convince a jury, on balance of probability, that he was unaware of the nature and quality of his action. Furthermore, what evidence there is suggests that he was aware of what he was doing when he shot Mr Drummond. This is also true if it is the case that he thought that he was shooting Sir Robert Peel.

5.3.5. Likewise there is nothing to indicate that the Defendant did not know that what he was doing was wrong.

5.3.6. I therefore conclude that the Defendant does not have a defence of insanity.

5.4. Diminished responsibility

5.4.1. In order to establish a defence of 'diminished responsibility' the Defendant has to satisfy the court that he was suffering from an abnormality of mental functioning such that his ability to understand his own conduct, form a rational judgment or exercise self-control was substantially impaired. Further, if the jury finds that the Defendant was suffering from an abnormality of mental functioning, they have to be satisfied that it was due to a recognised medical condition and that the abnormality of mental functioning explains the killing.

Report of Dr. E.T. Monro concerning Daniel McNaughtan, 25 February 1843   *13*
R v DANIEL MCNAUGHTAN

Report of: Dr. E.T. Monro
Specialism: Psychiatry
On the instructions of: Monteith and Company
Prepared for: The Central Criminal Court

5.4.2. I am not aware of a legal definition of 'abnormality of mental functioning' but I am aware of the legal definition of 'abnormality of mind'. Having regard to the clear evidence of serious mental illness in this case I am of the opinion that the Defendant has a basis for this defence insofar as he had, at the material time, an abnormality of mental functioning.

5.4.3. Schizophrenia, and its related disorders, are widely accepted as mental diseases or disorders and in this case I would expect that medical evidence would be unanimous to the effect that the Defendant's abnormality of mental functioning was caused by a recognised medical condition.

5.4.4. The matter of substantial impairment of ability is for the jury. However, I am mindful of the usual practice of the courts in admitting medical evidence on this issue to assist the jury.

5.4.5. My opinion is that the Defendant's ability was impaired and in my opinion that impairment was substantial. I am mindful that he was, and still is, suffering from a severe mental illness. It was not of his own making. He appears to have been in a state of steadily growing fear for his safety, albeit an irrational fear. He had no insight into the fact that he was ill, and for which reason he had not sought medical help. Thus, in his deeply distressed state he is likely to have reacted without the rational judgment which he might have applied if his mind had been functioning normally.

5.4.6. Having regard to the other aspects of his ability, it appears to me to be the evidence that he did understand his own conduct and he was capable of exercising self-control at the material time.

5.4.7. It is my opinion that the Defendant's mental illness, specifically his psychotic illness, provides an explanation for the killing of Edward Drummond.

5.4.8. Therefore, I conclude that there is a medical basis for a defence of 'diminished responsibility' on the basis that the Defendant had an abnormality of mental functioning that was caused by a recognised medical condition, as a result of which he did not form a rational judgment and his abnormality of mental functioning provides an explanation for the killing.

5.5. Feigned delusions

5.5.1. It seems improbable to me that the Defendant's delusions should be feigned. They had been present for months, indeed years, before the alleged offence, when there is no sensible reason for the Defendant feigning mental illness. The delusions he has reported are typical of those which occur in schizophrenia and related illnesses and, although, it is possible that he might have read sufficient about diseases of the mind in the library to which he had access at the Glasgow Mechanics' Institution, his account has a sophistication which I would not credit to him, having regard to his background, and again there is the question of why he should go to such lengths to present himself as mentally ill.

Report of: Dr. E.T. Monro
Specialism: Psychiatry
On the instructions of: Monteith and Company
Prepared for: The Central Criminal Court

5.5.2. In addition, and more importantly, to seemingly disinterested observers, he has displayed what are probably objective manifestations of schizophrenia and its prodromal decline, specifically social withdrawal, inappropriate affect and thought disorder.

5.5.3. I therefore conclude that on balance the Defendant is not feigning mental illness. However, I do acknowledge that ultimately the genuineness of the Defendant is a matter for the learned judge and jury.

6. Summary of conclusions

6.1. The Defendant is suffering from a mental disorder within the meaning of the Mental Health Act 1983 (as amended by the Mental Health Act 2007); it is probable that it is the mental illness known as schizophrenia.

6.2. It is more probable than not that the Defendant was suffering from a disease of the mind at the material time.

6.3. The defect of reasoning, due to his schizophrenia, which led him to believe falsely that he was subject to persecution by the Tories and the Jesuits, also led him to the false belief that he would obtain peace from the persecution by shooting Mr Drummond.

6.4. It does not appear that there is evidence which would convince a jury, on balance of probability, that he was unaware of the nature and quality of his action; what evidence there is suggests that he was aware of what he was doing when he shot Mr Drummond.

6.5. There is nothing to indicate that the Defendant did not know that what he was doing was wrong.

6.6. I therefore conclude that the Defendant does not have a defence of insanity.

6.7. The Defendant has a basis for the defence of diminished responsibility insofar as he had, at the material time, an abnormality of mental functioning.

6.8. I would expect that medical evidence would be unanimous to the effect that the Defendant's abnormality of mental functioning was caused by a recognised medical condition, namely schizophrenia.

6.9. The Defendant's ability was impaired and in my opinion that impairment was substantial because he is likely to have reacted without the rational judgment which he might have applied if his mind had been functioning normally.

6.10. He did understand his own conduct and he was capable of exercising self-control at the material time.

6.11. The Defendant's mental illness, specifically his psychotic illness, provides an explanation for the killing of Edward Drummond.

Report of Dr. E.T. Monro concerning Daniel McNaughtan, 25 February 1843   *15*
R v DANIEL MCNAUGHTAN

6.12. I conclude that the Defendant had an abnormality of mental functioning, which was caused by a recognised medical condition, as a result of which he did not form a rational judgment and his abnormality of mental functioning provides an explanation for the killing.

6.13. It seems improbable to me that the Defendant's delusions should be feigned.

6.14. In addition, and more importantly, to seemingly uninterested observers, he has displayed what are probably objective manifestations of schizophrenia and its prodromal decline.

6.15. I therefore conclude that on balance the Defendant is not feigning mental illness; however, I do acknowledge that ultimately the genuineness of the Defendant is a matter for the jury.

7. DECLARATION

I, EDWARD THOMAS MONRO, DECLARE THAT:

7.1. I understand that my duty is to help the court to achieve the overriding objective by giving assistance by way of objective, unbiased opinion on matters within my expertise, both in preparing reports and in giving oral evidence. I understand that this duty overrides any obligation to the party by whom I am engaged or the person who has paid or is liable to pay me. I confirm that I have complied with and will continue to comply with that duty.

7.2. I confirm that I have not entered into any arrangement where the amount or payment of my fees is in any way dependent on the outcome of the case.

7.3. I know of no conflict of interest of any kind, other than any which I have disclosed in this report.

7.4. I do not consider that any interest which I have disclosed affects my suitability as an expert witness on any issues about which I have expressed an opinion.

7.5. I have shown the sources of all information I have used.

7.6. I have set out in my report what I understand from those instructing me to be the questions in respect of which my opinion as an expert is required. All of the matters on which I have expressed an opinion lie within my field of expertise.

7.7. I have exercised reasonable care and skill in order to be accurate and complete in preparing this report. I have covered all relevant issues concerning the matters stated which I have been asked to address. Absence of any comment in this report does not indicate that I have no opinion on a matter. I may not have been asked to deal with it.

7.8. I have endeavoured to include in my report those matters, of which I have knowledge or of which I have been made aware, that might adversely affect the validity of my opinion. I have clearly stated any qualifications to my opinion.

Report of: Dr. E.T. Monro
Specialism: Psychiatry
On the instructions of: Monteith and Company
Prepared for: The Central Criminal Court

7.9. Where, in my view, there is a range of reasonable opinion, I have indicated the extent of that range in the report and given reasons for my own opinion.

7.10. I have not, without forming an independent view, included or excluded anything which has been suggested to me by others, including my instructing lawyers.

7.11. At the time of signing the report I consider that it is complete and accurate. I will notify those instructing me if, for any reason, I subsequently consider that the report requires any correction or qualification or if between the date of this report and the trial there is any change in circumstances which affect my declarations at 7.3 and 7.4 above.

7.12. I understand that:
(a) my report, subject to any corrections before swearing as to its correctness, will form the evidence to be given under oath;
(b) the court may at any stage direct a discussion to take place between the experts;
(c) the court may direct that, following a discussion between the experts, a statement should be prepared showing those issues which are agreed and those issues which are not agreed, together with a summary of the reasons for disagreeing;
(d) I may be required to attend court to be cross-examined on my report by a cross-examiner assisted by an expert;
(e) I am likely to be the subject of public adverse criticism by the judge if the Court concludes that I have not taken reasonable care in trying to meet the standards set out above.

7.13. This report is provided to those instructing me with the sole purpose of assisting the court in this particular case. It may not be used for any other purpose, nor may it be disclosed to any third party, other than the National Probation Service, without my express written authority or that of the Court.

7.14. I have read Part 33 of the Criminal Procedure Rules and I have complied with its requirements.

8. STATEMENT OF TRUTH

8.1. I confirm that the contents of this report are true to the best of my knowledge and belief and that I make this report knowing that, if it is tendered in evidence, I would be liable to prosecution if I have wilfully stated anything in it which I know to be false or do not believe to be true.

E.T. Monro,
BSc, MSc, MD, FRCPsych,
Consultant Psychiatrist.

Report of Dr. E.T. Monro concerning Daniel McNaughtan, 25 February 1843   *17*
R v DANIEL MCNAUGHTAN

Report of: Dr. E.T. Monro
Specialism: Psychiatry
On the instructions of: Monteith and Company
Prepared for: The Central Criminal Court

APPENDIX 1
QUALIFICATIONS AND EXPERIENCE

Qualifications
I am a medical graduate of the University of London where I obtained an intercalated **Bachelor of Science (Honours)** degree in neuropathology in 1802 and qualified **Bachelor of Medicine and Bachelor of Surgery** in 1805. I have obtained higher degrees of **Master of Science** (Manchester) and **Doctor of Medicine** (London) following study and research in psychiatry. I obtained the **Membership of the Royal College of Psychiatrists** in 1809 and was elected to the **Fellowship** in 1821. In 1825 I became a **Member of the Academy of Experts**. In 1825 I also became a **Member of the Expert Witness Institute** and in 1830 I was elected **Fellow**.

Clinical training and experience
My general professional training in psychiatry was as a **Senior House Officer** and then **Registrar in Psychiatry** in Manchester from 1806 to 1809 and I undertook higher training as **Lecturer in Psychiatry** and **Honorary Senior Registrar** at Edinburgh University between 1809 and 1813. Between 1813 and 1820 I was **Senior Lecturer and Consultant Psychiatrist** at the Royal Edinburgh Hospital and **Visiting Consultant Psychiatrist** at HMP Saughton, Edinburgh. Since 1820, I have been **Consultant Psychiatrist** at the Bethlem Hospital, an **Honorary Senior Lecturer in Psychiatry** in the University of London and a **Visiting Consultant Psychiatrist** at HMP Newgate. I am responsible for the Bow Street Police Court Mental Health Assessment and Diversion Scheme. I am a subscribing **Member of the British Academy of Forensic Sciences** and a subscribing **Member and Past President of the Medico-Legal Society of London**. I am a **Member of the Parole Board** for England and Wales.

Research and publications
I am the author of books on the classification of psychoses. My research includes studies of mentally disordered offenders in a London police court, psychiatric disorder in prison (based on my MSc dissertation), a case records study of patients in Broadmoor Hospital who had been convicted of manslaughter on the grounds of diminished responsibility and the symptomatology of schizophrenia (based on research for my MD). My published case reports include one on thyroid disease and the defence of insanity.

Report of Dr. E.T. Monro concerning Daniel McNaughtan, 25 February 1843   *18*
R v DANIEL MCNAUGHTAN

Report of: Dr. E.T. Monro
Specialism: Psychiatry
On the instructions of: Monteith and Company
Prepared for: The Central Criminal Court

APPENDIX 2
DOCUMENTS STUDIED

Indictment
Bow Street Police Court depositions
Prosecution witness statements

Report of Dr. E.T. Monro concerning Daniel McNaughtan, 25 February 1843   *19*
R v DANIEL MCNAUGHTAN

Report of: Dr. E.T. Monro
Specialism: Psychiatry
On the instructions of: Monteith and Company
Prepared for: The Central Criminal Court

APPENDIX 3
CHRONOLOGY

1813	Daniel McNaughtan born
1828	Apprenticed to father as a wood turner
1832	Completed apprenticeship and started working for father
1835	Set up his own business
1840/41	Sold his business
1841	Visited father and expressed concerns about persecution
July 1841	First visit to London
Early 1842	Expressed concerns to Commissioner of Police, Glasgow
July 1842	Purchased pistols
	Returned to London
November 1842	Walked past Sir Robert Peel's house, said 'Damn him, sink him'
20 January 1843	Shot Edward Drummond
25 January 1843	Edward Drummond died
18 February 1843	Examined in Newgate Prison
20 February 1843	Re-examined in Newgate Prison

Report of Dr. E.T. Monro concerning Daniel McNaughtan, 25 February 1843   *20*
R v DANIEL MCNAUGHTAN

Report of: Dr. E.T. Monro
Specialism: Psychiatry
On the instructions of: Monteith and Company
Prepared for: The Central Criminal Court

APPENDIX 4
GLOSSARY

affect – Synonymous with mood, the patient's emotional state. It has a subjective component which takes the form of feelings which each person can describe or recognise in himself (e.g. unhappiness) and an objective component which is the outward manifestation of the feelings (e.g. sad facial expression; dejected posture) (Rix, K.J.B. *A Handbook for Trainee Psychiatrists,* London: Baillière Tindall, 1987).

delusion – A delusion is a false belief held with total conviction and inappropriate to the patient's intelligence, social background and subcultural beliefs (Rix, K.J.B. *op. cit.*).

delusion of reference – A delusion of reference occurs when a normal perception is interpreted with delusional meaning of usually overwhelming personal significance to the patient, i.e. the normal perception refers to the patient.

hallucination – A false perception lacking an adequate basis in external stimuli (Rix, K.J.B. *op. cit.*). Hallucinations can occur in all of the sensory modalities. Auditory hallucinations commonly take the form of 'voices' but sounds of music and machinery can occur. Visual, gustatory (taste), olfactory (smell) and tactile (touch) hallucinations can also occur.

schizophrenia – Schizophrenia is a serious mental illness characterised by funda-mental distortions of thinking and perception and by inappropriate or blunted affect. Typical symptoms include: (a) disorders of the possession of thought, such as the subjective experience of thoughts being withdrawn, inserted or broadcast to others; (b) delusions, for example of being controlled, influenced or persecuted or that unconnected events or circumstances relate to the patient; (c) hallucinations, particularly in the form of voices which give a running commentary on the patient's behaviour and refer to the patient in the third person; (d) persistent grandiose delusions, including religious delusions, for example of being able to control the weather or being the Virgin Mary; (e) disorders of the form of thought (thought disorder); (f) catatonic behaviour such as excitement, mutism and stupor; (g) negative symptoms in the form of apathy, poverty of speech, blunting of emotional responses. It can occur as a single episode, as a recurrent disorder or as a chronic, progressive disorder without full recovery between episodes. When chronic there is usually a disintegration of the personality with coarsening and loss of identifying personality characteristics (*ICD-10 Classification of Mental and Behavioural Disorders: Clinical Descriptions and Diagnostic Guidelines*, World Health Organization, Geneva (1992)).

thought disorder – This is a term usually employed in relation to disturbances in the process of thinking as found in schizophrenia (q.v.). Such disorder can take a number of forms and there are a number of approaches to their classification. One of the most widely accepted identifies the following forms of thought disorder: muddling; snapping-off; fusion or literally melting of thoughts; and derailment. Careful observation and analysis of the patient's speech is necessary to classify as well as recognise these forms of thought disorder.

Report of Dr. E.T. Monro concerning Daniel McNaughtan, 25 February 1843   *21*
R v DANIEL MCNAUGHTAN

Index

Lightning Source UK Ltd.
Milton Keynes UK
UKHW022045261119
354311UK00012B/370/P